Measurement Tools
in Patient Education

2nd edition

Barbara Klug Redman, PhD, RN, FAAN, is Dean and Professor at the Wayne State University College of Nursing. She received her masters and doctoral degrees at the University of Minnesota and her BSN at South Dakota State University. She has been a Postdoctoral Fellow at The Johns Hopkins University, a fellow in Medical Ethics at Harvard Medical School, and is a Fellow of the American Academy of Nursing. Dr. Redman's career began as a staff nurse at a hospital in South Dakota. Dr. Redman has been Executive Director of the American Nurses Association, American Nurses Foundation, and American Association of Colleges of Nursing. She has also held professorships at the universities of Washington, Minnesota, Connecticut, and Johns Hopkins University. She has received honorary doctorates from Georgetown University and the University of Colorado. Dr. Redman has published numerous works in patient education including *The Practice of Patient Education*, which is now in its ninth edition and has been translated into Japanese, Finnish, Dutch, and German.

Measurement Tools in Patient Education
2nd edition

Barbara K. Redman, PhD, RN, FAAN

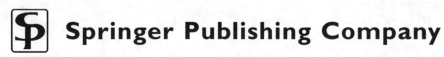

Springer Publishing Company

Springer Publishing Company, Inc.
536 Broadway
New York, NY 10012-3955

Acquisitions Editor: Ruth Chasek
Production Editor: Pamela Lankas
Cover design by Joanne E. Honigman

03 04 05 06 07 / 5 4 3 2 1

Library of Congress Cataloging-in-Publication Data

Measurement tools in patient education / [edited by] Barbara K. Redman.—2nd ed.
    p. cm.
    Includes bibliographical references and index.
    ISBN 0-8261-9859-7
    1. Patient education—Evaluation.   2. Patient education—Statistical method.
    I. Redman, Barbara Klug.
    R727.4.M4 2003
    615.5'071—dc21   2002036570
                                                                CIP

Printed in the United States of America by Sheridan Books.

Contents

Part I

Overview

1

An Introduction

Virtually all health professionals teach patients, although few think of it as a potentially full-fledged intervention with measurable outcomes. The time is long past when the field of patient education should have developed, validated, and regularly used measurement tools in both research and clinical practice. Neither practice nor research will progress without the ability to rigorously assess specific patient and group learning needs, and to hone teaching interventions to a known level of effectiveness.

The literature for patient education has always been scattered among disease-specific journals in various health disciplines and social science journals applied to health. Only one journal—*Patient Education and Counseling*—is specific to patient education, although several of the few journals in the field of health education occasionally include materials relevant to patient education. In the author's experience, formal retrieval systems have never identified more than a small portion of the relevant literature. The portion of the literature that addresses measurement tools in patient education is similarly scattered and not easily identifiable. This becomes particularly difficult when one needs to identify possible choices of tools for a particular application, or when one is trying to determine the range of measurement tools available in a field of patient education.

The first edition of this book featured 52 instruments; since it was published in 1998, the number of instruments has nearly doubled. This trend has also accelerated because evidence-based health care has quickly become the accepted norm and in all care settings there is an emphasis on documented outcomes.

The measurement instruments described in this book were collected as part of a search for patient education literature accomplished by routine searching of approximately 300 journals, indexes, and databases of nursing and medical literature. Only instruments appearing in the published literature were included; those in unpublished sources or in dissertations were not identified.

Measures of readability and health literacy are not included as they have been adequately reviewed elsewhere. Measures of quality of life are also not included as many are not oriented toward outcomes that can be expected of patient education. One journal, *Quality of Life Research,* is a good source of such instruments.

Instruments included in the first edition were updated; if they had not been further developed or used in the past 5 years, they were not included in this second edition. This time frame is important since content must be current. Authors of newly identified instruments developed and/or used in the past five years were contacted and asked for permission to include their instruments. After multiple contacts 57 responded. An effort was made to obtain a full developmental history of each instrument through references and use of the Social Science Citation Index (SSCI). Because SSCI does not index all relevant journals, including many nursing journals, authors were asked where their work had been cited.

Table 1.1 describes the focus of measurement for the 86 tools included in this volume. Twenty-nine percent measured beliefs/attitudes/behaviors; 26% were developed to measure knowledge. A number of self-efficacy (SE) scales were included because this construct

TABLE 1.1   What Is Measured

	N	Percentage
Beliefs/Attitudes/Behaviors	25	29
Decision Making	3	4
Knowledge	22	26
Learning Assessment/Instructional Design/Delivery	14	16
Self-Efficacy	16	19
Multiple/Other	6	6
TOTAL	86	100

has repeatedly been shown to be important to patient execution of behaviors and because SE beliefs are specific to a particular set of tasks. Instruments were most likely to have been published in disease-, age-, or gender-specific journals, or in nursing journals. Clearly, many disciplines are contributing to the development of these tools, and searching for them will require scholars and clinicians to look outside their fields.

There has been noticeable improvement since the first edition in the stock of measurement instruments in patient education. Although authors are still developing many new instruments whose measurement characteristics are just beginning to be understood, a significant core of instruments has been well tested. Few are oriented to the integrated concept of patient self-management, arguably the central outcome of patient education. And their availability by disease is still quite uneven, with the diabetes, cardiac, arthritis, pregnancy, childbirth, and parenting fields being the best developed. The neurological, cancer, respiratory, psychiatric, and renal fields, and the patient education program development instruments, are less frequently available.

Almost completely missing from the literature is a description of how formal measurement instruments are used in clinical practice and the outcome standards they are used to document. Also missing is a way to precisely describe the teaching intervention itself, the kinds of interactions between teacher and learner, including reinforcement and conditions to develop self-efficacy, the use and kind of teaching instruments, and the amount of time the learner spends on tasks.

Chapter 2 provides an organizing framework by which to understand measurement in patient education. It provides background information about constructs and skills measured, basic information about how one chooses and develops instruments, including their psychometric characteristics, and how the instruments might be used in clinical practice.

Next, instruments are presented, clustered by topic. The review of each instrument is organized around common sections: instrument description, including readability if available, psychometric properties, including established sensitivity to educational interventions, a summary of studies using the instrument, and a critique and summary. Particular attention was paid to the different cultures in which the instrument has been used. A summary table describing these characteristics may be found in the Appendix.

2. Measurement in Patient Education Practice and Research

Patient education is an old idea but one that has been susceptible to trends in medical practice. The old paradigm of physicians choosing what, if any, information to share with patients was first abridged with the legal and ethical doctrine of informed consent and later by the concept that psychosocial interventions are as critical to good health outcomes as are treatments based on the biomedical model.

All the trends in health care point to the need to upgrade and universalize patient education. An impressive body of research, summarized in 35 meta-analyses, shows conclusively that patient education can contribute significantly to positive health care outcomes (Redman, 2001). In some of these areas, such as diabetes education, enough research has accumulated to provide results that are robust and generalizable across gender, age, and time (Devine, 1992).

Patient education operates within each field of practice, varying widely by state of development. For example, a system of services with national accreditation standards and with certification for individual providers exists in the diabetes field and, to some extent, in the prenatal education field. Other fields of patient education practice may have model education programs that have been evaluated (asthma), or relatively available programs and educational materials (cardiac rehabilitation), or an active research community and a set of outcomes developed by consensus (arthritis), or only beginning agreement about what an educational program might look like and what it might accomplish (psychoeducation for the mentally ill). Despite this extreme variability, patient education services will face the same pressures for evidence-based practice as do all services. Yet, at this time, the field does not have a tradition of evaluation, especially not of outcome evaluation.

Purposes for the use of formal measurement tools in patient education can include the following:

1. Diagnosis or assessment of the patient's educational needs for various levels of functioning.
2. Establishment of criteria or levels of achievement known to be necessary for independent patient or family functioning.
3. Evaluation of the effectiveness of teachers and programs, including catching and correcting adverse effects of teaching.
4. Continuous improvement of care by using outcomes to improve interventions, including benchmarking.
5. In the aggregate, tracking the level of achievement of groups of patients against what is known to be necessary for effective outcomes (i.e., a "report card" on the performance of the health care system in this important area of practice).

Although little is known about how patient education is routinely practiced in this country, the author argues that its performance could be improved by routine incorporation of formal assessment and evaluation tools.

To participate in the modern practice of quality and outcomes improvement, the field will have to develop further instrumentation. For example, a wide range of age-appropriate instruments for pediatrics is needed, and few tools exist to measure the ability of patients to make informed decisions. Although approaches such as clinical paths help to assure some documentation, such approaches rarely document the quality of the measurement nor do they reveal enough about the character and length of the intervention to form a basis for improvement. In addition, we know little about whether existing tools reflect the outcomes of most importance to patients. And few instruments measure the patient's ability to competently carry out care processes and the judgments underlying them in authentic settings.

MEASUREMENT CHARACTERISTICS

Detailed technical discussions of the development and testing of measurement tools is widely available from many sources (DeVellis, 1991; Gable & Wolf, 1993). A brief conceptual review is provided here.

Validity, the central concept in measurement, is an evaluative judgment about whether an interpretation of test scores or actions based on it, are adequately supported. It involves content relevance and representativeness (content validity); generalizability including across time and raters, traditionally thought of as reliability concerns; convergent pattern of correlations between measures of the same construct (convergent validity); discriminant pattern of distinctness from measures of other constructs (discriminant validity); and lack of negative impact on individuals or groups deriving from a source of test invalidity. Population validity describes the ability to generalize results across subgroups and ecological validity the ability to generalize across settings. Validity is, therefore, an integrative summary focused on the relationship between the evidence and the inferences drawn from that evidence (Messick, 1995).

Thus, establishing validity has a judgmental element—first in examining the adequacy of operational and conceptional definitions, and second, in expert judging of the adequacy of sampling from the content universe the test is meant to represent. This occurs before the test is administered. Validity also has an empirical element, which allows examination of how the items perform when they are administered to many individuals (300 or 5 to 10 subjects per item) representative of those in the large group (Gable & Wolf, 1993). Using too few subjects means that the patterns of covariation among the items may not be stable. Items should be highly intercorrelated, with high item-scale correlations, and show relatively high item variance with means close to the center of the range of possible scores (De-Vellis, 1991).

Construct validation is an ongoing process of testing hypotheses about relationships of data from items or scales with other known instruments, with the theory on which the scale is based, and with known groups showing that a scale can differentiate members of one group from another. Factor analysis is one method used to identify or verify, within a given set of items, subsets that are clustered together by shared variation to form constructs or factors. Factor analysis may be exploratory or confirmatory to examine how the factors fit to the theory. The original pool of items is frequently three to four times larger than the final scale, with items removed as their measurement characteristics are known to improve the final scale.

Reliability has several distinct meanings—stability over time (test–retest reliability) calculated by correlating the scores from a set of subjects who take the test on two occasions, whereas internal consistency reliability is based on the average correlation among items within a test (Kline, 2000). Cronbach's alpha is the most commonly used measure of internal consistency reliability; it is an indication of the proportion of variance in the scale scores that is attributable to the true score. The Kuder Richardson formula is used to measure internal consistency for instruments with dichotomous items. A scale is internally consistent to the extent that its items are highly intercorrelated. An alpha of .65 to .70 is minimally acceptable for research, .70 to .80 is respectable, and .8 to .9 is good. Scales intended for individual diagnosis should have reliabilities in the middle .90s. More reliable scales increase statistical power for a given sample size relative to less reliable measures (DeVellis, 1991). Interrater and stability reliability measure the relationship between scores given by different raters or scores on the instrument at different periods. For knowledge tests, an overrepresentation of easy items will produce a ceiling effect, whereas overinclusion of difficult items will produce a floor effect. Generally, items with means too near the extremes of the response range will have low variances (DeVellis, 1991).

Of particular importance for interventions such as patient education is the sensitivity of a measure—evidence that it detects an important change as a result of a treatment of known efficacy. Another characteristic, sensibility, refers to characteristics of an instrument that make it usable in a clinical setting (Rowe & Oxman, 1993). Sensibility includes comprehensibility, clarity, and simplicity of questions, adequacy of instructions, ease of usage, applicability to the variety of patients with a particular problem, and acceptability to patients.

Understanding the meaning of a score is obviously important. Comparison against norms is one way to do so. Norms are any statistical data that provide a frame of reference to interpret an individual's scores relative to the scores of others. Measures based on well-developed rules including some form of norms that describe the score obtained in populations of interest are called "standardized" (Kline, 2000). The amount of score change that is clinically significant may be quite different from statistical significance. Clinical significance has been defined as a level of change recognizable by peers and patients, or by comparison with norms from fully functioning populations.

Cutoff scores are not commonly indicated for the instruments summarized in this book. Yet, for instruments with high enough reliability to influence decisions about individuals, such scores are implicitly used. A cutoff score or standard may be set using a combination of several methods, yet frequently it is finally judged by whether it is credible to the people who will be measured using it. The cutoff score (standard) is based first on the relationship between the test scores and a future criterion. It also may be based on the deliberations of several samples of judges in which they examine each item to identify the response options that a minimally competent examinee should be able to perform. The standard should differentiate masters from nonmasters in the subject matter of the test (Berk, 1986).

Before using a given instrument, it is always wise to check bibliographical sources for recent updates and revisions.

SELF-EFFICACY

Many instruments reviewed in this book measure self-efficacy (SE). Research accumulating over the past 30 years shows that with regard to many behaviors, SE is a potent predictor of important outcomes. Indeed, the total effect of SE on health behaviors is believed to exceed the effects of any other single variable (Schwarzer, 1992). Efficacy beliefs influence behavior through their effects on behavioral choice, effort expenditure, distress response to taxing conditions, and persistence in the face of difficulties. Anxiety and stress reactions are low when people cope with tasks in their perceived SE range. People tend to avoid activities they believe exceed their efficacy (Bandura, 1997).

Assessment of SE involves asking individuals to rate their ability to perform a particular behavior along some graded dimension of task difficulty such as number of repetitions or closeness to an ideal criterion. Although a general SE trait may operate in human behavior, Bandura (1997) maintains that measures of SE must be specific to the stressful event and its attendant behaviors to allow precise study of interventions designed to enhance coping in potentially aversive situations.

Routine use of these measures can help to identify individuals who, even though they are skilled, may lack the confidence to undertake behaviors critical to their treatment. Crippling anxiety that yields avoidant behaviors reflects an assessment that the individual cannot manage threatening events—a lack of SE. It is also important to know how extensive an intervention is necessary to create adequate levels of SE. For example, is a special exercise program important, or will individuals attain adequate SE simply by resumption of usual daily activities?

The elements known to develop SE can be incorporated into patient education interventions. Successfully accomplishing the behavior, positive persuasion informing the patient about his capabilities, helping the patient to accurately interpret the physical feelings that accompany performance activities, and vicarious experiences with others all provide sources of efficacy information. This information must be selected, weighed, and integrated by the individual into a judgment. Likewise, over time, repeated failure takes an increasing toll on perceived SE and beliefs about how much environmental control is possible.

There are specific concerns with measurement of SE. Even a short-term measurement of test–retest reliability may be inappropriate because it is theorized that SE is not expected to be a stable trait. Some SE measures also measure outcome expectations based on the notion that such expectations make SE more likely.

SE scales vary on three dimensions: (a) magnitude, referring to the level of difficulty of the behavior and commonly measured on scales of 0 to 10 or 0 to 100; (b) generality, referring to the number of domains of behavior in which individuals judge themselves to be efficacious over time; and (c) strength, referring to the confidence individuals have in the attainment of a specific task and usually assessed by tasks graded by level of impediment. Conceptual analysis of the domain of functioning is important to determine the competencies involved and the barriers and challenges one will have to manage. For example, perceptions of efficacy for maintaining a low-calorie diet may decrease when only fast foods are available. Conditions internal to the individual can also challenge perceptions of efficacy, for example, depression, loneliness, or intoxication. An understanding of these barriers requires interviews with members of the target population. Diagnosis is more useful when efficacy beliefs are measured for each of the competencies involved (Maibach & Murphy, 1995). A threshold of efficacy strength may be required before attempting a course of action.

Although SE is not the only psychological factor that may have an impact on outcomes, the importance of this element is underscored by the numerous studies that show its effect on health behavior. It also is alterable.

REFERENCES

Bandura, A. (1997). *Self efficacy: The exercise of control.* New York: Freeman.

Berk, R. A. (1986). A consumer's guide to setting performance standards on criterion-referenced tests. *Review of Educational Research, 56,* 137–172.

DeVellis, R. F. (1991). *Scale development: Theory and applications.* Newbury Park, NJ: Sage.

Devine, E. C. (1992). Effects of psychoeducational care with adult surgical patients: A theory-probing meta-analysis of intervention studies. In T. D. Cook, H. Cooper, D. S. Cordray, H. Hartmann, L. V. Hedges, R. J. Light, T. A. Louis, & F. Mostella (Eds.), *Meta-analysis for explanation.* New York: Russell Sage Foundation.

Gable, R. K., & Wolf, M. B. (1993). *Instrument development in the affective domain.* Boston: Kluwer Academic.

Kline, P. (2000). *Handbook of psychological testing* (2nd ed.). New York: Routledge.

Maibach, E., & Murphy, D. A. (1995). Self-efficacy in health promotion research and practice: Conceptualization and measurement. *Health Education Research, 10,* 37–50.

Messick, S. (1995). Validity of psychological assessment. *American Psychologist, 50,* 741–749.

Redman, B. K. (2001). *The practice of patient education* (9th ed.). St. Louis: Mosby.

Rowe, B. H., & Oxman, A. D. (1993). An assessment of the sensibility of a quality-of-life instrument. *American Journal of Emergency Medicine, 11,* 374–380.

Schwarzer, R. (1992). *Self-efficacy: Thought control of action.* Washington, DC: Hemisphere.

Part II

Description of Tools

Each review is organized around a common framework of (a) description, administration, and scoring guidelines; (b) psychometric properties; and (c) critique, summary, and references. The reader should keep in mind the standards for psychometric properties described in chapter 1: the variety and kinds of evidence about validity, including the number of participants used, levels of reliability needed for various kinds of uses for the instrument, and evidence of sensitivity to a patient education intervention.

Part II

Description of Tools

Section A

Basic Patient Education Needs

The instruments in this section address basic patient education needs, presumably useful across disease entities. These include assessment of learning needs, beliefs about symptoms and illness, a cluster of instruments about patient decisions, and instructional design and teaching interactions with providers.

---

3. Patient Learning Needs Scale

Developed by Susan Galloway, Natalie Bubela, Elizabeth McCay, Ann McKibbon, Eleanor Ross, and Lynn Nagle

INSTRUMENT DESCRIPTION, ADMINISTRATION, AND SCORING GUIDELINES

The Patient Learning Needs Scale (PLNS) is designed to measure patients' perceptions of learning needs to manage their health care at home at time of discharge from hospital following a medical or surgical illness. PLNS requires less than 20 minutes to complete. It yields a total score of 40 to 200, with higher scores indicating more importance placed on having information at discharge. Individual factor scores may also be calculated. Because the PLNS subscales are composed of an unequal number of questions, percentage means are calculated for subscale scores. A community version asks people who are at home how important it was to learn about each item before discharge (Galloway et al., n.d.). In nearly all of the published work on the PLNS, an earlier version was used, with 50 items scored 0 to 5 and 7 subscales, making numerical comparison of scores and items with the present scale difficult.

PSYCHOMETRIC PROPERTIES

Development and initial evaluation of the scale was based on the responses of 301 adults hospitalized with medical or surgical illnesses. Items developed from patient interviews were reviewed by nurses, doctors, patients, and healthy nonhospitalized individuals to check for item clarity, representativeness of what one needed to know to manage care at home, and ease or difficulty of completion of the items (Bubela et al., 1990). Factor analysis showed five clinically meaningful factors:

1.   Support and care in the community, defined as knowledge about negotiating the health care system, recognizing and obtaining intrapersonal support, and performing preventive skin care (items 17, 31, 13, 32, 12, 27, 22, 10, 33, 29, with a Cronbach's alpha of .91).

2.   Medications, defined as the knowledge required to understand and administer medications (items 35 to 37, 4, 25, 39, 6, 26, with a Cronbach's alpha of .90).

3.   Treatment and activities of living, defined as knowledge about treatment, and guidelines for physical activity, nutrition, and sleep (items 24, 18, 2, 28, 30, 20, 38, 23, with an alpha of .85).

4.   Complications and symptoms, defined as information needed to form expectations about the impact of the illness, and the specific information needs around recognition and management of symptoms and complications (items 8, 11, 3, 5, 21, 34, 7, 9, with an alpha of .82).

5.   Illness-related concerns, defined as how to communicate about illness and how to manage in areas such as hygiene, rest, and elimination problems (items 15, 40, 19, 1, 14, 16, with an alpha of .76). Total scale alpha is .95 (Galloway et al., n.d.).

In another study, PLNS total scale alpha was .97, with .80 to .90 for the subscales (Galloway, Bubela, McKibbon, McCay, & Ross, 1993). Convergent validity was supported by the finding that patients who perceived more uncertainty in their illness experience placed more importance on health-related information 48 hours before going home (Galloway & Graydon, 1996). It has not been possible to examine concurrent validity as there has been no parallel instrument available (Galloway et al., n.d.).

CRITIQUE AND SUMMARY

PLNS results can help health professionals focus the scope and content of educational interventions, especially because acutely ill individuals have neither the physiological stability nor the cognitive energy to learn about care at home until near the time of discharge. Length of time spent in the hospital, number of discharge medications, and patient perception of the influence of the illness on his life were positively correlated with information needs at the time of discharge. Number of medications may be an indirect indicator of the severity of problems faced by the individual and may hinder mental processing of information (Bubela & Galloway, 1990). Several studies with different populations in different countries (Bostrom, Crawford-Swent, Lazar, & Helmer, 1994; Bubela et al., 1990; Galloway, Bubela, McKibbon, McCay, & Ross, 1993) have found that medications, treatments and complications, and enhancing quality of life (symptom management) were consistently identified as most important discharge learning needs.

Although the scale will elicit the area of discharge information that is important, it does not delineate the specific content that might satisfy the learning need (Galloway et al., n.d.). For identification of gaps in existing discharge programs, subjects may be asked for each item if the information has been given and the level of satisfaction with the information.

It would be useful to study the relationship between timely identification of learning needs by PLNS, adequate meeting of these needs, and the quality of life during recovery. The PLNS has been used to study nurse- and patient-initiated call systems of follow-up after hospitalization. Mean scores for each factor on the PLNS by kind of follow-up may be found in the article by Bostrom, Caldwell, McGuide, and Everson (1996).

REFERENCES

Bostrom, J., Caldwell, J., McGuire, K., & Everson, D. (1996). Telephone follow-up after discharge from the hospital: Does it make a difference? *Applied Nursing Research, 9*, 47–52.

Bostrom, J., Crawford-Swent, C., Lazar, N., & Helmer, D. (1994). Learning needs of hospitalized and recently discharged patients. *Patient Education and Counseling, 23*, 83–89.

Bubela, N., & Galloway, S. (1990). Factors influencing patients' informational needs at time of hospital discharge. *Patient Education and Counseling, 16*, 21–28.

Bubela, N., Galloway, S., McCay, E., McKibbon, A., Nagle, L., Pringle, D., Ross, E., & Shamian, J. (1990). The Patient Learning Needs Scale: Reliability and validity. *Journal of Advanced Nursing, 15*, 1181–1187.

Galloway, S., Bubela, N., McCay, E., McKibbon, A., Ross, E., & Nagle, L. (n.d.). *Patient Learning Need Scale: Description and administration guidelines.* Unpublished manuscript.

Galloway, S. C., Bubela, N., McKibbon, A., McCay, E., & Ross, E. (1993). Perceived information needs and effect of symptoms on activities after surgery for lung cancer. *Canadian Oncology Nursing Journal, 3*, 116–119.

Galloway, S. C., & Graydon, J. E. (1996). Uncertainty, symptom distress, and information needs after surgery for cancer of the colon. *Cancer Nursing, 19*, 112–117.

PATIENT LEARNING NEEDS SCALE

Introduction for Hospital Administration

At hospital discharge, many people have some questions about how to manage once they are at home. Different people have questions about different things. The following is a list of things which some people like to know in order to care for themselves at home. For each item indicate how important it is for *you* to learn about before going home.

Introduction for Community Administration

Many people who are leaving the hospital have some questions about how to manage their care at home. Different people have questions about different things. The following is a list of things which may be important to know about to be able to care for yourself at home. Now that you are at home, please rate how important you now think each item is to learn about before hospital discharge.

Please rate how important each item is to know about before going home.

> 1 = not important
> 2 = slightly important
> 3 = moderately important
> 4 = very important
> 5 = extremely important

In order to manage my care at home it is important for me to know:

1.	What to do if I have trouble urinating.	1 2 3 4 5
2.	How to prepare the foods I am to eat.	1 2 3 4 5
3.	How to prevent a complication from occurring.	1 2 3 4 5
4.	How to take each medication.	1 2 3 4 5
5.	What symptoms I may have related to my illness.	1 2 3 4 5
6.	When to take each medication.	1 2 3 4 5
7.	How this illness will affect my life.	1 2 3 4 5
8.	How to recognize a complication.	1 2 3 4 5
9.	How this illness will affect my future.	1 2 3 4 5
10.	How to care for my feet properly.	1 2 3 4 5
11.	What complications might occur from my illness.	1 2 3 4 5
12.	How to recognize my feelings toward my illness.	1 2 3 4 5
13.	How to contact community groups for my health condition.	1 2 3 4 5
14.	When I can take a bath or a shower.	1 2 3 4 5
15.	How to talk to family/friends about my illness.	1 2 3 4 5
16.	How much rest I should be getting.	1 2 3 4 5
17.	How to get through the ''red tape'' in the health care system.	1 2 3 4 5
18.	What the possible side effects of my treatment are.	1 2 3 4 5
19.	What to do if I have trouble with my bowels.	1 2 3 4 5
20.	What to do if I cannot sleep properly.	1 2 3 4 5
21.	How to manage the symptoms I may experience.	1 2 3 4 5
22.	How I can avoid stress.	1 2 3 4 5
23.	What physical exercise I should be getting.	1 2 3 4 5
24.	What the purposes of my treatment are.	1 2 3 4 5
25.	Why I need to take each medication.	1 2 3 4 5
26.	Where I can get my medication.	1 2 3 4 5
27.	Where I can get help in handling my feelings about my illness.	1 2 3 4 5

(continued)

1 = not important
2 = slightly important
3 = moderately important
4 = very important
5 = extremely important

28. Which foods I can and cannot eat.   1   2   3   4   5

29. How to prevent my skin from getting red.   1   2   3   4   5

30. Which vitamins and supplements I should take.   1   2   3   4   5

31. How to get through the "red tape" to get services at home.   1   2   3   4   5

32. Who to talk to about my concerns about death.   1   2   3   4   5

33. How to prevent my skin from getting sore.   1   2   3   4   5

34. How to manage my pain.   1   2   3   4   5

35. When to stop taking each medication.   1   2   3   4   5

36. How each medication works.   1   2   3   4   5

37. What to do if I have a reaction to a medication.   1   2   3   4   5

38. What physical activities I cannot do such as lifting.   1   2   3   4   5

39. The possible reactions to each medication.   1   2   3   4   5

40. Where I can get help for family to deal with my illness.   1   2   3   4   5

Used with permission: Galloway, S., Bubela, N., McCay, E., McKibbon, A., Ross, E., & Nagle, L.

4.   Constructed Meaning Scale: Measuring Adaptation to Serious Illness

Developed by Betsy L. Fife

INSTRUMENT DESCRIPTION, ADMINISTRATION, AND SCORING GUIDELINES

The construction of meaning is a central aspect of adaptation to serious illness. The concept of meaning commonly refers to the relationship between individuals and their world as well as to individuals' unique perceptions of their place within that world. It encompasses the individual's perceptions of her ability to accomplish future goals, to maintain the viability of interpersonal relationships, and to sustain a sense of personal vitality, competence, and power. It is these perceptions that give a sense of coherence to life in the face of loss, change, and personal upheaval (Fife, 1994a).

Because serious illness imposes irrevocable change that totally disrupts the continuity of everyday life, individuals are forced to rapidly redefine the meanings they have assumed as fact in the routine of living. Structures of meaning are cumulative learned phenomena; in the case of an event, they are partially the outcome of an attributional search for the cause of the event and also a method of obtaining cognitive control. The Constructed Meaning Scale is based in the theoretical framework of symbolic interactionism. Because it is expected that the construction of meaning may influence future behavior, such a scale would be used to assess how the individual's perceptions of identity and social world have been affected by the illness, and would serve as a clinical marker of the quality of adaptation the individual will be able to achieve (Fife, 1994a).

The scale is scored using the values on the questionnaire, reversing the scoring of items as necessary so that the most positive response is given a value of 4 (B. L. Fife, personal communication, February 1996). The highest possible score on the scale, 32, is indicative of the most positive meaning, whereas the lowest score of 8 indicates a negative sense of the meaning.

PSYCHOMETRIC PROPERTIES

Data from which the scale was developed were gathered from interviews of 38 White persons diagnosed as having cancer. Three specific changes in self-meaning emerged: loss of personal control, threats to self-esteem or self-worth, and changes in body image (Fife, 1994a).

Studies of reliability and validity of the scale have been carried out with 422 persons diagnosed as having cancer. Nine percent were Black, and 12% were of low socioeconomic status. Items were based on and supported by data obtained from persons living with cancer and on symbolic interactionist theory, supporting content validity. Construct validity (the extent to which the scale performed in accordance with theoretical expectations) was empirically supported in several ways.

1.   Individuals newly diagnosed with nonmetastatic cancer, or those in first remission, were more likely to construct a positive meaning about their illness than those with a first recurrence or those with metastatic disease. The scale distinguished between these groups (mean scores in these groups range from 20.8 to 23.6).
2.   Prior research suggests that the construction of meaning and emotional response would be correlated. This proved to be the case with more positive meaning associated with the positive poles of the various emotional response dimensions such as composed-anxious, elated-depressed, agreeable-hostile, energetic-tired, clearheaded-confused, and confident-unsure.
3.   Social support from family, friends, and professionals was predictive of meaning, that is, the greater the support, the more positive the meaning about the implications of the illness for patients' lives.
4.   Denial and positive focusing were associated with development of a more positive meaning about the illness, whereas avoidance was strongly related to the construction of negative meaning.
5.   Formulation of meaning was associated with an attempt to develop a sense of control or mastery (Fife, 1995).
6.   In a study of 125 men and 206 women with various forms of cancer, the more positive the meaning, the more positive the adjustment (Fife, 1994b).

Item-total correlations ranged from .5 to .72, with all coefficients significant, providing support for the existence of homogeneity within the scale. Cronbach's alpha was .81. Factor analysis showed that each item in the scale contributed to the primary factor (Fife, 1995).

Fife and colleagues (2000) have recently used the Constructed Meaning Scale in a longitudinal study of the psychosocial impact of bone marrow transplantation and found that the instrument strongly correlated with measures of personal control and negatively correlated to distress—consistent with what theory would suggest. Cronbach's alpha for the scale in this study was .81.

CRITIQUE AND SUMMARY

So far, use of the tool has been limited to research and those with cancer; this work should be extended to those with other threatening or debilitating diseases. Because construction of meaning is specific to the experience with a particular disease, norms would likely be different for other diseases. Beginning work has also been done on use of the scale within the dyad of patient and partner, showing that communication within the dyad was significantly associated with the development of meaning for partners but not for patients. Extension of this work should prove helpful in understanding how to care for partners as well as for patients (Germino, Fife, & Funk, 1995).

This scale appears to have been developed and used with populations not as diverse as those with which it might be used. Further work is necessary to support validity, increase reliability, and study its sensitivity to interventions. The Constructed Meaning Scale address-es an important construct central to both the theory and practice of health care.

REFERENCES

Fife, B. L. (1994a). The conceptualization of meaning in illness. *Social Science and Medicine, 38,* 309–316.

Fife, B. L. (1994b). Gender differences and adjustment to cancer. *Research in Sociology of Health Care, 11,* 107–125.

Fife, B. L. (1995). The measurement of meaning in illness. *Social Science and Medicine, 40,* 1021–1028.

Fife, B. L., Huster, G. A., Cornetta, K. G., Kennedy, V. N., Akard, L. P., & Brown, E. R. (2000). Longitudinal study of adaptation to the stress of bone marrow transplantation. *Journal of Clinical Oncology, 18,* 1539–1549.

Germino, B. B., Fife, B. L., & Funk, S. G. (1995). Cancer and the partner relationship: What is its meaning? *Seminars in Oncology Nursing, 11,* 43–50.

CONSTRUCTED MEANING SCALE

Directions:

The items below ask how you see your life being affected by your illness. *Circle* the number that best describes how you have been feeling about your life during the *past two weeks*.

		Strongly Agree	Agree	Disagree	Strongly Disagree
1.	I feel my illness is something I will never recover from.	1	2	3	4
2.	I feel my illness is serious, but I will be able to return to life as it was before my illness.	1	2	3	4
3.	I feel my illness has changed my life permanently so it will never be as good again.	1	2	3	4
4.	I feel I have made a complete recovery from my illness.	1	2	3	4
5.	I feel that I am the same person as I was before my illness.	1	2	3	4
6.	I feel that my relationships with other people have not been negatively affected by my illness.	1	2	3	4
7.	I feel that my illness experience has made me a better or stronger person.	1	2	3	4
8.	I feel my illness has permanently interfered with my achievement of the most important goals I have set for myself.	1	2	3	4

5. Satisfaction with Decision Scale

Developed by Margaret Holmes-Rovner, Jill Kroll, Neal Schmitt, David Rovner, Lynn Breer, Marilyn L. Rothert, Georgia Padonu, and Geraldene Talarczyk

INSTRUMENT DESCRIPTION, ADMINISTRATION, AND SCORING GUIDELINES

As the passive role of patients as compliers fades, their role as decision makers moves to the fore. The Satisfaction with Decision Scale (SWD) is built on the model of an effective decision as informed, consistent with the decision-maker's values and behaviorally implemented, and measures global satisfaction with a decision incorporating these elements. The instrument was initially developed to evaluate a decision-support intervention to assist women in decision making about hormone replacement therapy (Holmes-Rovner et al., 1996) and was also used in a study of the decisions of elderly patients about influenza immunizations (O'Connor, 1994). SWD is written at an eighth-grade reading level. A higher score indicates less conflict.

PSYCHOMETRIC CHARACTERISTICS

Cronbach's alpha was .86. SWD correlated with lower levels of decisional conflict and higher confidence in the decision, and it predicted patients' levels of certainty that they would carry out the decision (Holmes-Rovner et al., 1996). In the O'Connor (1994) study SWD discriminated between those patients who were sure about what they would do and those who were less sure. Rothert and colleagues (1997) showed that SWD was sensitive to educational interventions that varied in intensity and supported menopause-related decisions. These findings support validity.

CRITIQUE AND SUMMARY

SWD is one of several instruments about patient decision making reviewed in this book. They are a welcome addition to outcome measures including informed consent, a concept that underlies all decisions.

REFERENCES

Holmes-Rovner, M., Kroll, J., Schmitt, N., Rovner, D., Breer, L., Rothert, M. L., Padonu, G., & Talarczyk, G. (1996). Patient satisfaction with health care decisions: The Satisfaction With Decision Scale. *Medical Decision-Making, 16,* 58–64.

O'Connor, A. M. (1994). Validation of a decisional conflict scale. *Medical Decision Making, 54,* 25–30.

Rothert, M. L., Holmes-Rovner, M., Rovner, D., Kroll, J., Breer, L., Talarczyk, G., Schmitt, N., Padonui, G., & Wills, C. (1997). An educational intervention as decision support for menopausal women. *Research in Nursing and Health, 20,* 377–387.

SATISFACTION WITH DECISION SCALE

You have been considering whether to consult your health care provider about hormone-replacement therapy. Answer the following questions about your decision. Please indicate to what extent each statement is true for you AT THIS TIME.

Use the following scale to answer the questions.

1 = strongly disagree
2 = disagree
3 = neither agree nor disagree
4 = agree
5 = strongly agree

1. I am satisfied that I am adequately informed about the issues important to my decision.
2. The decision I made was the best decision possible for me personally.
3. I am satisfied that my decision was consistent with my personal values.
4. I expect to successfully carry out (or continue to carry out) the decision I made.
5. I am satisfied that this was my decision to make.
6. I am satisfied with my decision.

From. Holmes-Rovner, M. et al. (1996). Patient Satisfaction with Decision Scale. *Medical Decision-Making, 16,* 58–64. Reprinted by permission of Sage Publication.

6. Decisional Conflict Scale

Developed by Annette M. O'Connor

INSTRUMENT DESCRIPTION, ADMINISTRATION, AND SCORING GUIDELINES

Informed choice rather than merely informed consent and the development of health care consumer decision aids reflect recognition of a new standard of patient autonomy. Since many decisions in health care involve high stakes and have alternatives that produce both desirable and undesirable outcomes, decisional conflict is common. It may be characterized by vacillating between choices, delayed decision making, and high levels of emotional distress. The desired outcome is an effective decision, one that is informed, consistent with values, and implemented, and one with which the patient is satisfied.

The effective-decision subscale is used only when a decision has already been made; the other two subscales can be used during deliberation or after a decision is made. The Decisional Conflict Scale (DCS) requires an eighth-grade reading level and takes five to ten minutes to complete. A simpler, low-literacy (third grade) version is now available, as are scales in French and Spanish. Responses to each statement are scored from 1 (strongly agree) to 5 (strongly disagree), with negative statements having reverse scoring so that high scores indicate higher decisional conflict (O'Connor, 1995). Patients with schizophrenia were able to respond to DCS (Bunn & O'Connor, 1996).

DCS has been evaluated with more than a thousand individuals making preventive decisions about immunization and breast screening, and persons with schizophrenia considering continuation of treatment with long-acting antipsychotic injections (Bunn & O'Connor, 1996). Items are summed and averaged. Scores range from 1 (low decisional conflict) to 5 (high decisional conflict). Scores of 2.5 or greater are associated with those who delay decisions.

PSYCHOMETRIC PROPERTIES

The uncertainty subscale has an internal consistency coefficient of .78–.92, the effective decision-making subscale, .77–.84, and the factors-contributing-to-uncertainty subscale, .58–.70, with an overall coefficient of .78–.92 (Bunn & O'Connor, 1996). Test–retest reliability was .81 for the total scale and for the uncertainty subscale. DCS discriminated significantly between those who accepted/rejected and those who were delayed/were unsure of an invitation to be immunized, with the latter showing higher decisional conflict scores. The perceived–effective–decision-making subscale was less effective in discriminating between known groups. DCS was inversely, but weakly, correlated with knowledge (O'Connor, 1995; Bunn & O'Connor, 1996). Items were developed from the construct of decisional conflict and validated by a panel of decision-making experts. The low-literacy version has an alpha of .72 and discriminated significantly between those at different stages of the decision-making process.

A study of men participating in screening for prostate cancer showed significantly lower levels of decisional conflict in those receiving information than in the control group. So, also, patients with locally advanced lung cancer showed less decisional conflict after using a decision aid (Brundage et al., 2001). These findings support DCS sensitivity to one kind of intervention (Davison et al., 1999).

CRITIQUE AND SUMMARY

Structured decision aids provide an organized approach to examining a decision problem frequently tailored to the consumer's particular clinical profile and detailing what it would be like to live with the consequences of the choice. They provide information, review alternatives and potential consequences, clarify values, and address skill deficits in implementing decisions. DCS should be useful in fine tuning the development of decision aids. For example, those who have high decisional conflict because of information deficits may need a different intervention emphasis from those who are unclear about values or anticipate having implementation problems (O'Connor, 1995).

Additional work on DCS should include checking content validity with patient experts, ability of DCS to predict a long-term commitment to a decision, and presence of regret (O'Connor, 1995). The Decisional Self-Efficacy Scale (Bunn & O'Connor, 1996) may also be of interest.

REFERENCES

Brundage, M. D., Feldman-Stewart, D., Cosby, R., Gregg, R., Dixon, P., Youssef, Y., Davies, D., & Mackillop, W. J. (2001). Phase I study of decision aid for patients with locally advanced non-small-cell lung cancer. *Journal of Clinical Oncology, 19,* 1326–1335.

Bunn, H., & O'Connor, A. L. (1996). Validation of client decision-making instruments in the context of psychiatry. *Canadian Journal of Nursing Research, 28*(3), 13–27.

Davison, B. J., Kirk, P., Degner, L. F., & Hassard, T. H. (1999). Information and patient participation in screening for prostate cancer. *Patient Education & Counseling, 37,* 255–263.

O'Connor, A. M. (1995). Validation of a decisional conflict scale. *Medical Decision Making, 15,* 25–30.

DECISIONAL CONFLICT SCALE—
"MY DIFFICULTY MAKING THIS CHOICE"

Now, thinking about the choice you just made, please look at the following comments made by some people when making decisions.

Please show how strongly you agree or disagree with these statements by circling the number from 1 (strongly agree) to 5 (strongly disagree) which best shows how you feel about the choice you just made.

1	This decision is easy for me to make	1 Strongly Agree	2 Agree	3 Neither Agree Nor Disagree	4 Disagree	5 Strongly Disagree
2	I'm sure what to do in this decision	1 Strongly Agree	2 Agree	3 Neither Agree Nor Disagree	4 Disagree	5 Strongly Disagree
3	It's clear what choice is best for me	1 Strongly Agree	2 Agree	3 Neither Agree Nor Disagree	4 Disagree	5 Strongly Disagree
4	I'm aware of the options I have in this decision	1 Strongly Agree	2 Agree	3 Neither Agree Nor Disagree	4 Disagree	5 Strongly Disagree
5	I feel I know the pros of each option	1 Strongly Agree	2 Agree	3 Neither Agree Nor Disagree	4 Disagree	5 Strongly Disagree
6	I feel I know the cons of each option	1 Strongly Agree	2 Agree	3 Neither Agree Nor Disagree	4 Disagree	5 Strongly Disagree
7	I am clear about *how important* the pros are to me in this decision	1 Strongly Agree	2 Agree	3 Neither Agree Nor Disagree	4 Disagree	5 Strongly Disagree
8	I am clear about *how important* the cons are to me in this decision	1 Strongly Agree	2 Agree	3 Neither Agree Nor Disagree	4 Disagree	5 Strongly Disagree

9	I am clear about which is *more* important to me (the pros or the cons)	1 Strongly Agree	2 Agree	3 Neither Agree Nor Disagree	4 Disagree	5 Strongly Disagree
10	I am making this choice without any pressure from others	1 Strongly Agree	2 Agree	3 Neither Agree Nor Disagree	4 Disagree	5 Strongly Disagree
11	I have the right amount of support from others in making this choice	1 Strongly Agree	2 Agree	3 Neither Agree Nor Disagree	4 Disagree	5 Strongly Disagree
12	I have enough advice about the options	1 Strongly Agree	2 Agree	3 Neither Agree Nor Disagree	4 Disagree	5 Strongly Disagree
13	I feel I have made an informed choice	1 Strongly Agree	2 Agree	3 Neither Agree Nor Disagree	4 Disagree	5 Strongly Disagree
14	My decision shows what is important to me	1 Strongly Agree	2 Agree	3 Neither Agree Nor Disagree	4 Disagree	5 Strongly Disagree
15	I expect to stick with my decision	1 Strongly Agree	2 Agree	3 Neither Agree Nor Disagree	4 Disagree	5 Strongly Disagree
16	I am satisfied with my decision	1 Strongly Agree	2 Agree	3 Neither Agree Nor Disagree	4 Disagree	5 Strongly Disagree

7.   Illness Perception Questionnaire

**Developed by John Weinman, Keith Petrie,
Rona Moss-Morris, and Rob Horne**

INSTRUMENT DESCRIPTION, ADMINISTRATION,
AND SCORING GUIDELINES

In order to make sense of and respond to problems associated with the onset of illness, patients create their own models or representations of their illnesses. The self-regulation model proposes that patients' illness representations include identity, cause, time-line, consequence, and cure/controllability of their condition. IPQ assesses these components. It is possible to replace the term "illness" with the name of a particular illness (diabetes, asthma, etc.). A significant other/carer version of the Illness Perception Questionnaire (IPQ) has also been developed (Weinman, Petrie, Moss-Morris, & Horne, 1996).

The Identity Scale is scored by summing the number of items endorsed at "occasionally" or greater with a total score of 0–12. Scores for Time-Line and Consequences and Cure/ Control Scales are obtained by summing items and dividing by the number of items. It is not appropriate to sum the cause scale as each item represents a specific causal belief (Weinman, Petrie, Moss-Morris, & Horne, 1996). Recently, a revised IPQ-R included new subscales of cyclical time-line dimension, an illness coherence scale, and an emotional representation dimension.

PSYCHOMETRIC PROPERTIES

Data from seven illness groups provide the basis for evaluating the psychometric properties of the IPQ scales. Internal consistency and 1-month test–retest reliability scores were: Identity scale .82, .84; timeline scale .73, .49; consequences scale .82, .68; and control/ cure scale .73, .68. A later study found alphas of .57–.81.

Concurrent validity is supported by the following findings. Identity scale was positively related to current reported disability and recent doctor visits, and was inversely related to self-rated health. A higher Time-Line score, indicating the belief that the illness will last a long time, was positively correlated with patients' ratings of the likelihood of a future heart attack, health distress, and recent doctor visits, and was negatively correlated with self-rated health. The Control Cure scale was significantly related to recovery SE. Scores on the Consequences scale were positively related to ratings of health distress, disability, and recent doctor visits, and were negatively related to self-rated health. Other evidence is also available.

IPQ discriminated among diabetes, rheumatoid arthritis, chronic fatigue syndrome, and chronic idiopathic pain, each of which have distinct presentations and effects on patients' lives. Predictive validity was supported (Weinman, Petrie, Moss-Morris, & Horne, 1996). Cardiac rehabilitation attendance was significantly related to a stronger belief during hospitalization that the illness could be cured or controlled, and return to work was significantly predicted by the perception that the illness would last a short time (Petrie, Weinman, Sharpe, & Buckley, 1996).

IPQ has been used in studies with a wide variety of disease entities. In a study of persons with chronic fatigue syndrome (CFS), Moss-Morris, Petrie, and Weinman (1996) found that patients who believed they had some control over CFS reported significantly more positive coping responses and significantly less behavioral disengagement—illness representations were more strongly associated with adjustment and well-being than the Coping subscales were. A study of patients with Addison's disease found that those who considered their illness to be chronic, uncontrollable, and serious reported higher levels of disability than did those who believed the opposite. Illness perceptions of patients with rheumatoid arthritis explained significant amounts of variance in the number of clinical visits and hospital admissions, pain, tiredness, and anxiety over a one-year period (predictive validity) (Schlaroo et al., 1999). Similar findings for patients with psoriasis (Scharloo, Kaptein, Weinmen, Bergmen, Vermeer, & Rooijmans, 2000) and for patients with COPD (Schlaroo, Kaptein, Weinman, Willems, & Rooijmans, 2000) provide further support. Griva, Myers, and Newman (2000) found the Perceived Control scale to be consistently related to self-reported adherence in diabetes. Fortune, Richards, Main, and Griffiths (2000) found that worry in patients with psoriasis was associated with stronger beliefs that the disease would have serious consequences and that it would be chronic or recurring. These findings are in the expected direction.

IPQ-R showed internal consistency reliability of .75–.89 and test–retest reliability ranging from .46–.88 over three weeks. Factor analysis supports the theoretically derived dimensions of patients' illness representations and further evidence of validity is forthcoming (Moss-Morris, Weinman, Petrie, Horne, Cameron, & Buick, in press).

CRITIQUE AND SUMMARY

Since patients' initial perceptions of illness are important determinants of aspects of recovery (seeking medical care, emotional reactions to symptoms, engagement in self care behaviors), these perceptions need to be identified early to optimize outcome. For example, early emergence of coherent illness perceptions after a myocardial infarction were quite consistent over time and largely unaffected by later information presented in the hospital or after discharge. Staff may not assess illness perceptions, which may be quite different from medical views, and so be unaware of the perceptions. Yet, these meanings may be more influential in determining adaption in the rehabilitation phase than are medical factors (Petrie, Weinman, Sharpe, & Buckley, 1996).

Studies of the efficacy of interventions in changing illness perceptions (encourage sense of control, alter negative illness perceptions) and thus the sensitivity of IPQ could not be located. Internal consistency relationships have been low on controllability/care and emotional attributions (Schlaroo, Kaptein, Weinman, Willems, & Rooijmans, 2000).

REFERENCES

Fortune, D. G., Richards, H. L., Main, C. J., & Griffiths, C. E. M. (2000). Pathological worrying, illness perception and disease severity in patients with psoriasis. *British Journal of Health Psychology, 5,* 71–82.

Griva, K., Myers, L. B., & Newman, S. (2000). Illness perceptions and self-efficacy beliefs in adolescents and young adults with insulin dependent diabetes mellitus. *Psychology & Health, 15,* 733–750.

Moss-Morris, R., Petrie, K. J., & Weinman, J. (1996). Functioning in chronic fatigue syndrome: Do illness perceptions play a regulatory role? *British Journal of Health Psychology, 1,* 15–25.

Moss-Morris, R., Weinman, J., Petrie, K. J., Horne, R., Cameron, L. D., & Buick, D. (in press). The revised Illness Perception Questionnaire (IPQ-R). *Psychology & Health.*

Petrie, K. J., Weinman, J., Sharpe, N., & Buckley, J. (1996). Role of patients' view of their illness in predicting return to work and functioning after myocardial infarction: Longitudinal study. *British Medical Journal, 312,* 1191–1194.

Scharloo, M., Kaptein, A. A., Weinman, J., Bergman, W., Vermeer, B. J., & Rooijmans, H. G. M. (2000). Patients' illness perceptions and coping as predictors of functional status in psoriasis: A 1-year follow-up. *British Journal of Dermatology, 142,* 899–907.

Scharloo, M., Kaptein, A. A., Weinman, J. A., Hazes, J. M. W., Breedveld, F. C., & Rooijmans, H. G. M. (1999). Predicting functional status in patients with rheumatoid arthritis. *Journal of Rheumatology, 26,* 1686–1693.

Scharloo, M., Kaptein, A. A., Weinman, J. A., Willems, L. N. A., & Rooijmans, H. G. M. (2000). Physical and psychological correlates of functioning in patients with chronic obstructive pulmonary disease. *Journal of Asthma, 37,* 17–29.

Weinman, J., Petrie, K., Moss-Morris, R., & Horne, R. (1996). The Illness Perception Questionnaire: A new method for assessing the cognitive representation of illness. *Psychology & Health, 11,* 431–445.

ILLNESS PERCEPTION QUESTIONNAIRE (IPQ-R)

Your Views About Your Illness

Listed below are a number of symptoms that you may or may not have experienced since your illness. Please indicate by circling *Yes* or *No*, whether you have experienced any of these symptoms since your illness, and whether you believe that these symptoms are related to your illness.

	I have experienced this symptom *since my illness*			This symptom is *related to my illness*	
Pain	Yes	No	_____	Yes	No
Sore Throat	Yes	No	_____	Yes	No
Nausea	Yes	No	_____	Yes	No
Breathlessness	Yes	No	_____	Yes	No
Weight Loss	Yes	No	_____	Yes	No
Fatigue	Yes	No	_____	Yes	No
Stiff Joints	Yes	No	_____	Yes	No
Sore Eyes	Yes	No	_____	Yes	No
Wheeziness	Yes	No	_____	Yes	No
Headaches	Yes	No	_____	Yes	No
Upset Stomach	Yes	No	_____	Yes	No
Sleep Difficulties	Yes	No	_____	Yes	No
Dizziness	Yes	No	_____	Yes	No
Loss of Strength	Yes	No	_____	Yes	No

We are interested in your own personal views of how you now see your current illness.

Please indicate how much you agree or disagree with the following statements about your illness by ticking the appropriate box.

(continued)

	VIEWS ABOUT YOUR ILLNESS	STRONGLY DISAGREE	DISAGREE	NEITHER AGREE NOR DISAGREE	AGREE	STRONGLY AGREE
IP1*	My illness will last a short time					
IP2	My illness is likely to be permanent rather than temporary					
IP3	My illness will last for a long time					
IP4*	This illness will pass quickly					
IP5	I expect to have this illness for the rest of my life					
IP7	My illness has major consequences on my life					
IP8*	My illness does not have much effect on my life					
IP9	My illness strongly affects the way others see me					
IP10	My illness has serious financial consequences					
IP11	My illness causes difficulties for those who are close to me					
IP12	There is a lot which I can do to control my symptoms					
IP13	What I do can determine whether my illness gets better or worse					
IP14	The course of my illness depends on me					
IP15*	Nothing I do will affect my illness					

	VIEWS ABOUT YOUR ILLNESS	STRONGLY DISAGREE	DISAGREE	NEITHER AGREE NOR DISAGREE	AGREE	STRONGLY AGREE
IP16	I have the power to influence my illness					
IP17*	My actions will have no affect on the outcome of my illness					
IP18*	My illness will improve in time					
IP19*	There is very little that can be done to improve my illness					
IP20	My treatment will be effective in curing my illness					
IP21	The negative effects of my illness can be prevented (avoided) by my treatment					
IP22	My treatment can control my illness					
IP23*	There is nothing which can help my condition					
IP24	The symptoms of my condition are puzzling to me					
IP25	My illness is a mystery to me					
IP26	I don't understand my illness					
IP27	My illness doesn't make any sense to me					
IP28*	I have a clear picture or understanding of my condition					

(continued)

	VIEWS ABOUT YOUR ILLNESS	STRONGLY DISAGREE	DISAGREE	NEITHER AGREE NOR DISAGREE	AGREE	STRONGLY AGREE
IP29	The symptoms of my illness change a great deal from day to day					
IP30	My symptoms come and go in cycles					
IP31	My illness is very unpredictable					
IP32	I go through cycles in which illness gets better and worse					
IP33	I get depressed when I think about my illness					
IP34	When I think about my illness I get upset					
IP35	My illness makes me feel angry					
IP36*	My illness does not worry me					
IP37	Having this illness makes me feel anxious					

Causes of My Illness

We are interested in what *you* consider may have been the cause of your illness. As people are very different, there is no correct answer for this question. We are most interested in your own views about the factors that caused your illness rather than what others including doctors or family may have suggested to you. Below is a list of possible causes for your illness. Please indicate how much you agree or disagree that they were causes for you by ticking the appropriate box.

	POSSIBLE CAUSES	STRONGLY DISAGREE	DISAGREE	NEITHER AGREE NOR DISAGREE	AGREE	STRONGLY AGREE
C1	Stress or worry					
C2	Hereditary—it runs in my family					
C3	A germ or virus					
C4	Diet or eating habits					
C5	Chance or bad luck					
C6	Poor medical care in my past					
C7	Pollution in the environment					
C8	My own behaviour					
C9	My mental attitude, e.g., thinking about life negatively					
C10	Family problems or worries caused my illness					
C11	Overwork					
C12	My emotional state, e.g., feeling down, lonely, anxious, empty					
C13	Ageing					
C14	Alcohol					

(continued)

	POSSIBLE CAUSES	STRONGLY DISAGREE	DISAGREE	NEITHER AGREE NOR DISAGREE	AGREE	STRONGLY AGREE
C15	Smoking					
C16	Accident or injury					
C17	My personality					
C18	Altered immunity					

In the table below, please list in rank-order the three most important factors that you now believe caused *YOUR illness*. You may use any of the items from the box above, or you may have additional ideas of your own.

The most important causes for me:

1. _____
2. _____
3. _____

Items for IPQ-R Subscales

1. Identity (sum of yes-rated symptoms in column 2 on p. 1)
2. Timeline (acute/chronic) items IP1–IP5 + IP18
3. Consequences items IP6–IP11
4. Personal control items IP12–IP17
5. Treatment control items IP19–IP23
6. Illness coherence items IP24–IP28
7. Timeline cyclical IP29–IP32
8. Emotional representations IP33–IP38
9. Causes C1–C18—do not use these as a scale. Start analysis with separate items used as grouping variables, i.e., those who do/do not believe in a specific causal factor. With a sufficient sample size ($n = 90$ or more), factor analysis can be used to identify groups of causal beliefs (e.g., lifestyle, stress, etc.), which can then be used as subscales (e.g., see Weinman et al., 2000).

SCORING—score each item for the above subscales (except Identity and Causes—*see above*) as follows—Strongly disagree = 1; disagree = 2; neither etc. = 3; agree = 4; strongly agree = 5, EXCEPT for the starred items (*) which are reverse scored (i.e., strongly disagree = 5; disagree = 4, etc.). Get total score for each subscale.

Reference

Weinman, J., Petrie, K. J., Sharpe, N., & Walker, S. (2000). Causal attributions in patients and spouses following first-time myocardial infarction and subsequent lifestyle changes. *British Journal of Health Psychology, 5,* 263–273.

8. Symptom Beliefs Questionnaire

Developed by Peter Salmon, Maria Woloshynowych, and Roland Volari

INSTRUMENT DESCRIPTION, ADMINISTRATION, AND SCORING GUIDELINES

Physical symptoms such as back or abdominal pain and respiratory complaints are common in the general population. The beliefs of individuals experiencing these symptoms and the beliefs of their families are potent factors in determining health care actions including seeking professional help and complying with the advice given. The Symptom Beliefs Questionnaire (SBQ) was designed to measure the range of symptoms at the first point of contact with the health care system, as patients describe and experience them (Salmon, Woloshynowych, & Volari, 1996). Scoring of each item and the scale to which it contributes are indicated on the questionnaire. Scale scores are the sum of scores for relevant items.

PSYCHOMETRIC PROPERTIES

To achieve content validity, SBQ was based on interviews with nearly two hundred patients described in the words they use about symptoms and what they thought caused them. Factor analysis from 406 completed questionnaires showed eight scales: stress (alpha = .87), wearing out (alpha = .81), environment (alpha – .77), internal structure (alpha = .79), internal functional (alpha = .73), life-style (alpha = .74), concern (alpha = .47), and weak constitution (alpha = .54). The last two factors should obviously be interpreted and used with caution. Gastrointestinal patients were distinguished from musculoskeletal and respiratory patients by higher scores on internal-functional and life-style beliefs. Musculoskeletal patients were higher on wearing-out and internal-structural beliefs, whereas respiratory patients had higher scores than did musculoskeletal or gastrointestinal patients on environment (known groups). The groups did not differ on stress (Salmon, Woloshynowych, & Volari, 1996).

CRITIQUE AND SUMMARY

SBQ provides a means to quantify beliefs about experienced symptoms and was able to distinguish between patients presenting with different types of questions. In clinical practice, use of SBQ could help to alert the provider to a patient's model, and in research to study the influence of beliefs on seeking help (Salmon, Woloshynowych, & Volari, 1996).

Much additional testing of SBQ remains to be done—is it sensitive to intervention, how does it perform in cultures other than the one in which it was developed (England)?

REFERENCE

Salmon, P., Woloshynowych, M., & Valori, R. (1996). The measurement of beliefs about physical symptoms in English general practice patients. *Social Science & Medicine, 42*, 1561–1567.

SBQ

Here are statements about the symptoms you have come to see your doctor about TODAY. For each set of 3 please tick the ONE statement which best applies to you. Please make sure that you answer EVERY question.

C   1.   0 ❐   I have not thought about what has caused my symptoms
             1 ❐   I have thought a little about what has caused my symptoms
             2 ❐   I have thought a lot about the cause of my symptoms

C   2.   0 ❐   I have no idea of the reason for my symptoms
             1 ❐   I have some idea of the reason for my symptoms
             2 ❐   I think I know the reason for my symptoms

C   3.   2 ❐   Whatever caused my symptoms has *probably* been going on a long while
             1 ❐   Whatever caused my symptoms *may* have been going on a long while
             0 ❐   Whatever caused my symptoms has probably *not* been going on for long

I-S   4.   2 ❐   I think there *probably* is something seriously wrong with me
             1 ❐   There *may* be something seriously wrong with me
             0 ❐   I do *not* think there is anything seriously wrong

E   5.   2 ❐   I think I *do* have an illness which others can catch from me
             1 ❐   I think I *may* have an illness which others can catch from me
             0 ❐   I do *not* think I have an illness which others can catch from me

For each of the following, show whether you think it PROBABLY WOULD HELP or PROBABLY WOULD NOT HELP to deal with the symptoms you are seeing your doctor about today. Please answer EACH item.

		PROBABLY WOULD HELP	DON'T KNOW	PROBABLY WOULD NOT HELP
		2	1	0
L	Changing my diet or lifestyle	❐	❐	❐
I-S	Seeing a specialist	❐	❐	❐
I-S	An operation	❐	❐	❐
I-S	Tests or X-rays	❐	❐	❐

For each of the following, tick whether you think it PROBABLY HAS or PROBABLY HAS NOT helped to cause the symptoms you have come to see your doctor about today.

Please answer **every** item, for **example**:

(continued)

	PROBABLY HAS HELPED TO CAUSE	DON'T KNOW	PROBABLY HAS **NOT** HELPED TO CAUSE
Working or living conditions	☐	☑	☐
Something I ate	☐	☐	☑
An allergy	☑	☐	☐

And now for **your** views:

		PROBABLY HAS HELPED TO CAUSE	DON'T KNOW	PROBABLY HAS **NOT** HELPED TO CAUSE
		2	1	0
S	Over work	☐	☐	☐
L	Not looking after myself properly	☐	☐	☐
E	Pollution	☐	☐	☐
W	A part of my body wearing out	☐	☐	☐
L	Something I ate	☐	☐	☐
W	Part of my body not working as well as it used to	☐	☐	☐
I-F	A "growth"	☐	☐	☐
WC	A "weak spot" in my body	☐	☐	☐
S	My moods/emotions	☐	☐	☐
I-S	Damage to part of my body	☐	☐	☐
S	Stress	☐	☐	☐
WC	Part of my body is inflamed	☐	☐	☐
W	Body tissues becoming harder or softer	☐	☐	☐
S	Demanding family or friends	☐	☐	☐
I-F	Poor digestion or weak stomach	☐	☐	☐
S	My personality	☐	☐	☐
E	A germ or infection	☐	☐	☐
I-F	Heart trouble	☐	☐	☐
E	Weather or changes in temperature	☐	☐	☐
W	Worn joints	☐	☐	☐
L	The food that I eat	☐	☐	☐
I-S	An accident	☐	☐	☐

		PROBABLY HAS HELPED TO CAUSE	DON'T KNOW	PROBABLY HAS **NOT** HELPED TO CAUSE
		2	1	0
W	Body tissues less firm or less supple	❐	❐	❐
S	My job/housework	❐	❐	❐
I-S	Something out of place in my body	❐	❐	❐
E	Dampness or a chill	❐	❐	❐
S	Working or living conditions	❐	❐	❐
WC	Weak constitution/low resistance	❐	❐	❐
I-S	Pressure building up somewhere in my body	❐	❐	❐
S	"Nerves"	❐	❐	❐
W	Part of my body slowing down	❐	❐	❐
S	Being run down	❐	❐	❐
1-F	Medicine or pills	❐	❐	❐
E	Something I caught from someone else	❐	❐	❐
L	Warning from my body to change the way I treat it	❐	❐	❐
I-F	Weak blood	❐	❐	❐
S	Personal, financial, or domestic problems	❐	❐	❐
L	Being over/underweight	❐	❐	❐
E	The time of year	❐	❐	❐
I-S	Part of my body is strained	❐	❐	❐
I-F	Sluggish bowels	❐	❐	❐

Notes on Scoring

Scoring of each item, and the scale to which it contributes, are indicated on the questionnaire. Scale scores are the sum of scores for relevant items.

C:	Concern
I-S:	Internal-structural
E:	Environment
S:	Stress
L:	Lifestyle
W:	Wearing out
I-F:	Internal-functional
WC:	Weak constitution

9.   Child Attitude Toward Illness Scale

Developed by Joan K. Austin

INSTRUMENT DESCRIPTION, ADMINISTRATION, AND SCORING GUIDELINES

Research has indicated that children with chronic illness are at risk for development of behavior problems, poor self-concept, and social withdrawal. The Child Attitude Toward Illness Scale (CATIS) is designed to provide systematic assessment of how favorably or unfavorably children feel about having a chronic physical condition. Initial items were generated from results of past research. To date, the tool has been used with children of middle-class background, 8 to 12 years of age, with asthma or epilepsy (Austin & Huberty, 1993).

The conceptual framework undergirding CATIS is family stress theory. Negative feelings can contribute to the stressors already placed on the family by the child's illness, and positive feelings can serve as a resource to help the family successfully adapt to the illness. Most research on adaptation to childhood chronic illness has focused on parents' perceptions and feelings about their children's illness but has failed to include perceptions from the children. Yet children who have negative feelings are more likely to engage in maladaptive coping behaviors and subsequently have a more negative adaptation to the condition than children who have positive feelings about having a chronic illness. Children's feelings are thought to be especially important when the condition has an attached stigma, such as epilepsy (Austin & Huberty, 1993).

The scale in the form for administration may be seen on the following page. The chronic condition is placed in the blank area (e.g., asthma or seizures). Ratings are on 5-point scales. Items 1, 2, 4, 5, 7, 9, 11, and 13 are reverse scored. Scores on each item are then summed and divided by 13 (Austin & Huberty, 1993). A more positive score reflects a more positive attitude toward the condition (Austin, Smith, Risinger, & McNelis, 1994). Children with epilepsy had a mean score of 3.2, whereas those with asthma had a mean score of 3.4 (Austin & Huberty, 1993). CATIS is designed to be completed independently by children as young as eight years of age and is geared toward a third-grade reading level (Heimlich, Westbrook, Austin, Cramer, & Devinsky, 2000).

PSYCHOMETRIC PROPERTIES

Initial studies showed an internal consistency reliability of .8 (coefficient alpha) or .86 (Austin, Huster, Dunn, & Risinger, 1996), with item-total correlations ranging between .27 and .59, and test–retest reliability of .8 over a two-week interval. Confirmatory factor analysis results supported one unitary construct in the scale. In a follow-up study of 136 children with epilepsy, and 133 with asthma, CATIS scores were significantly negatively correlated with school absences, anxiety, intensifying behavior problems, and depression, and significantly positively correlated with happiness, satisfaction, and self-concept scores. Attitude scores and self-concept scores were also positively correlated. These relationships lend support for construct validity of the CATIS for the measurement of children's attitudes toward having a chronic health condition (Austin & Huberty, 1993).

Subsequent studies have provided additional information about CATIS. In a study of 117 children with epilepsy, and 108 with asthma, 8–12 years of age, negative attitudes toward the condition were significantly associated with poorer academic achievement even after the effects of sex and condition severity were accounted for. This finding provides evidence that children's perceptions and feelings about having a chronic condition are important factors in possible interventions. Internal consistency reliability was .82 (Austin, Huberty, Huster, & Dunn, 1998).

Children participating in summer camps for asthma, diabetes, and spina bifida showed small but meaningful positive changes in CATIS scores. No control group was available. While this change could be seen as supportive of the sensitivity of CATIS, it is unclear what elements of the camp experience might have contributed to this change (Briery & Rabian, 1999) or how instructionally potent the intervention might be expected to be.

Heimlich and colleagues (2000) studied the validity of CATIS with 197 adolescents with epilepsy, aged 11–17 years, excluding those with other medical or psychiatric illness or inability to read at the fifth-grade level. Internal consistency reliability was .89, and test–retest reliability was .77. Adolescents with the most severe epilepsy had more negative attitudes toward their illness than did those with moderate or mild epilepsy, which is supportive of the validity of the scale.

CRITIQUE AND SUMMARY

CATIS is a short self-report scale to be used in the clinical setting to assess children's attitudes about having a chronic condition, and as a starting point for discussion of their feelings. It could also be used to evaluate whether educational programs designed to help groups of children cope with chronic conditions change these feelings (Austin & Huberty, 1993). These studies represent initial work in development of the scale. Cross-validation is needed with different samples of chronically ill children to determine if the findings are valid and reliable for these samples. CATIS was originally developed for use in research; with further development, it appears to have potential for use in the clinical setting (Austin & Huberty, 1993).

Traditionally, treatment of childhood epilepsy has emphasized neurological aspects over psychosocial factors, with seizure frequency considered to be the most important clinical outcome. Yet children with this condition have a high prevalence of behavior and learning problems not strongly correlated with seizure variables. The results of these studies indicate need for programs that prevent development of these problems for children with epilepsy (Austin, Smith, Risinger, & McNelis, 1994). Additional validation work remains, especially consideration of the sensitivity of CATIS to instructional interventions.

REFERENCES

Austin, J. K., & Huberty, T. J. (1993). Development of the Child Attitude Toward Illness Scale. *Journal of Pediatric Psychology, 18,* 467–480.

Austin, J. K., Huberty, T. J., Huster, G. A., & Dunn, D. W. (1998). Academic achievement in children with epilepsy or asthma. *Developmental Medicine and Child Neurology, 40,* 248–255.

Austin, J. K., Huster, G. A., Dunn, D. W., & Risinger, M. W. (1996). Adolescents with active or inactive epilepsy or asthma: A comparison of quality of life. *Epilepsia, 37,* 1228–1238.

Austin, J. K., Smith, M. S., Risinger, M. W., & McNelis, A. M. (1994). Childhood epilepsy and asthma: Comparison of quality of life. *Epilepsia, 35,* 608–615.

Briery, B. G., & Rabian, B. (1999). Psychosocial changes associated with participation in a pediatric summer camp. *Journal of Pediatric Psychology, 24,* 183–190.

Heimlich, T. E., Westbrook, L. E., Austin, J. K., Cramer, J. A., & Devinsky, O. (2000). Brief report: Adolescents' attitudes toward epilepsy: Further validation of the Child Attitude Toward Illness Scale (CATIS). *Journal of Pediatric Psychology, 25,* 339–345.

CHILD ATTITUDE TOWARD ILLNESS SCALE (CATIS)

Here are 13 questions that ask about you and your feelings. Read each one carefully. If there is anything that you do not understand, please ask us about it. For each question, put a check mark ✓ above the response that best describes your feelings. Answer *every* question even if some are hard to decide, but check only *one* answer. There are no right or wrong answers. Only *you* can tell us how you feel, so we hope that you will mark the way you *really* feel inside.

1. How good or bad do you feel it is that you have _____ ?

     Very Good   A Little Good   Not Sure   A Little Bad   Very Bad   _____

2. How fair is it that you have _____ ?

     Very Fair   A Little Fair   Not Sure   A Little Unfair Very Unfair   _____

3. How happy or sad is it for you to have _____ ?

     Very Sad   A Little Sad   Not Sure   A Little Happy Very Happy   _____

4. How bad or good do you feel it is to have _____ ?

     Very Good   A Little Good   Not Sure   A Little Bad   Very Bad   _____

5. How often do you feel that your _____ is your fault?

     Never   Not Often   Sometimes   Often   Very Often   _____

6. How often do you feel that your _____ keeps you from doing things you like to do?

     Very Often   Often   Sometimes   Not Often   Never   _____

7. How often do you feel that you will always be sick?

     Never   Not Often   Sometimes   Often   Very Often   _____

8. How often do you feel that your _____ keeps you from starting new things?

     Very Often   Often   Sometimes   Not Often   Never   _____

(continued)

9.   How often do you feel different from others because of your _____?

      Never   Not Often   Sometimes   Often   Very Often   _____

10. How often do you feel bad because you have _____ ?

   Very Often   Often   Sometimes   Not Often   Never   _____

11. How often do you feel sad about being sick?

      Never   Not Often   Sometimes   Often   Very Often   _____

12. How often do you feel happy even though you have _____ ?

      Never   Not Often   Sometimes   Often   Very Often   _____

13. How often do you feel just as good as other kids your age even though you have _____ ?

   Very Often   Often   Sometimes   Not Often   Never   _____

10. Bernier Instructional Design Scale

Developed by Mary Jane Bernier

INSTRUMENT DESCRIPTION, ADMINISTRATION, AND SCORING GUIDELINES

Printed educational materials (PEMs) are among the most economical and frequently used methods for educating individuals about health matters. They are portable, reusable, and permanent. Patient educators are often frustrated by the lack of quality control in the PEMs that are available (Bernier, 1993a).

The literature in patient education indicates that little evaluation of actual learning outcomes is carried out by the developers or users of PEMs. So, although congruence between desired outcomes as specified by PEM developers and the actual learning achieved by the target population represents the ultimate measure of quality in a PEM, the author seeks to develop an alternative way to evaluate them through expert consensus of important characteristics of PEMs. Criteria were selected from the literature, and a convenience sample of 11 individuals with experience in development of PEMs was used as a consensus group. The criteria include primarily content and format issues, clustered by phase of development (Bernier & Yasko, 1991).

PSYCHOMETRIC PROPERTIES

Results of the pilot study described previously established the basis for evaluating the content validity of an evaluation of a patient educational materials instrument. A pilot test of the Bernier Instructional Design Scale (BIDS) was conducted by four master's-prepared nurses who applied the BIDS to a test PEM individually and then met to discuss their ratings. Eighty-nine members of a patient education committee and graduate nursing students at a university medical center established interrater reliability for the BIDS by applying the scale to the test PEM that was used in the pilot study. The interrater agreement was only 40%, and on replication 65%, both below desirable levels. Other forms of validity were not addressed, pending achieving more adequate levels of reliability (Bernier, 1993b).

BID2, incorporating results of additional psychometric testing, was published in 1996 (Bernier, 1996). Preparation of this version included assessing content validity, interrater reliability in applying BIDS to a PEM at 86%. BIDS3 is now available and contains two subscales—comprehensibility (alpha = .92) and clarity of purpose (alpha = .89). Internal consistency reliability for the whole scale was alpha = .94 (Bernier, 2001).

CRITIQUE AND SUMMARY

The usefulness of BIDS was thought of as an empirical referent for exploring relationships between instructional design quality and achievement of patient learning outcomes (Bernier,

1993b). Evidence of this relationship would be helpful. BIDS3 reflects much work on reliability and validity.

REFERENCES

Bernier, M. J. (1993a). Developing and evaluating printed education materials: A prescriptive model for quality. *Orthopaedic Nursing, 12*(6), 39–46.

Bernier, M. J. (1993b). *Patient education in nursing: Development of a scale to evaluate the instructional design quality of printed educational materials.* Pittsburgh: University of Pittsburgh.

Bernier, M. J. (1996). Establishing the psychometric properties of a scale for evaluating quality in printed education materials. *Patient Education & Counseling, 29,* 283–299.

Bernier, M. J. (2001). Letter to author.

Bernier, M. J., & Yasko, J. (1991). Designing and evaluating printed educational materials: Model and instrument development. *Patient Education and Counseling, 18,* 253–263.

BERNIER INSTRUCTIONAL DESIGN SCALE 3 (BIDS-3) (COPYRIGHT 2000)

BIDS-3 is a checklist for rating the presence (or absence) of instructional design and learning principles contained in printed education materials (PEMs) for use with patients and families.

1. Begin the rating procedure by reading each principle on the BIDS-3.
2. Next, read the PEM to be evaluated.
3. Use the Rating Scale listed below to record the level of instructional design and learning principles contained in the PEM.
4. Re-read the PEM as many times as you need to complete the rating.

Rating Scale

0 = NOT MET
1 = PARTIALLY MET
2 = MET
NA = NOT APPLICABLE

EXAMPLE: Principle #1 states, "The font or print size can be easily read by the target group."

A PEM that is written in a print size as small as this (9-point font) would not be appropriate for a general target audience since the readers would be of many age groups and some would have difficulty reading this print size.

The appropriate rating for a PEM written in the 9-point font would be 0 = NOT MET if the PEM is intended for a general audience which would include elderly persons. You would place a check mark in the column labeled 0 for principle #1.

		Scale:		
Principles Related to Clarity of Purpose:	0	1	2	N/A
1. Titles and subtitles are clear and informative.	____	____	____	____
2. The purpose of the PEM is made clear to the target group.	____	____	____	____
3. The relevance of the educational content to the target group is clearly stated.	____	____	____	____
4. The learning objectives (either stated or implied) and the educational content of the PEM relate to one another.	____	____	____	____
5. The learning objectives (either stated or implied) relate to the intended learning outcome.	____	____	____	____
6. The content presented is accurate.	____	____	____	____

(continued)

	Scale:			
Principles Related to Clarity of Purpose:	0	1	2	N/A
7. The content is current.	___	___	___	___
8. The content is presented in concrete terms rather than as abstract concepts.	___	___	___	___
9. The content is presented in a style that is patient-centered so that the needs of the patients are foremost.	___	___	___	___
10. The content focuses upon what the target group should *do* as well as *know*.	___	___	___	___
11. The main ideas of the PEM are divided into meaningful content units.	___	___	___	___
12. The content of the PEM builds from the familiar to the unfamiliar.	___	___	___	___
13. Specific, precise instructions are given if the target group is expected to carry out some self-care activity.	___	___	___	___
14. The ideas in the PEM are logically related and present a coherent structure for the information being conveyed.	___	___	___	___

	Scale:			
Principles Related to Comprehensibility:	0	1	2	N/A
15. The font or print size can be easily read by the target group.	___	___	___	___

This is a 14-point font recommended for the elderly; this is a 12-point font recommended for general audiences; and this is a 10-point font.

16. Drawings and illustrations represent racial and ethnic groups.	___	___	___	___
17. The vocabulary of the PEM reflects words commonly used by the target group.	___	___	___	___
18. Necessary health terms are defined.	___	___	___	___
19. Only the most important information is presented using not more than 3–4 main points.	___	___	___	___

	Scale:			
Principles Related to Comprehensibility:	0	1	2	N/A
20. The content is presented in a way that relates and integrates new information to what is already known and understood by the target group.	____	____	____	____
21. Examples are used to bridge the gap between what the target group knows and the content to be taught.	____	____	____	____
22. The content is presented in a manner that is respectful of the customs and traditions of the target group.	____	____	____	____
23. The information load of the material is appropriate to the target group. Information load = amount + obscurity or novelty of information. Content that is unfamiliar represents a larger information load than content that is familiar to the target group.	____	____	____	____
24. Important ideas and points of content are repeated as reinforcement throughout the PEM.	____	____	____	____
25. Sentences are kept in logical order.	____	____	____	____
26. Accurate, coherent summaries and synopses of the message being delivered are included throughout the PEM.	____	____	____	____
27. The PEM is written at a reading level that is appropriate to the target group. Material intended for the general public should be written at the 6th to 8th grade level.	____	____	____	____

Bernier, M. J. Used with permission.

11. Perceived Efficacy in Patient–Physician Interactions Questionnaire

Developed by Rose C. Maly, Janet C. Frank, Grant N. Marshall, M. Robin DiMatteo, and David B. Reuben

INSTRUMENT DESCRIPTION, ADMINISTRATION, AND SCORING GUIDELINES

Effective patient–physician communication has been shown to be associated with a broad range of improved outcomes of care including health and functional status, physiologic outcomes, patient satisfaction, and patient adherence to medical care recommendations. Sociocultural factors specific to older persons may affect their actions with physicians adversely including their being less effective than younger persons in getting their physicians to attend to their health concerns and thus obtaining potentially poorer medical outcomes (Maly, Frank, Marshall, DiMatteo, & Reuben, 1998).

The full ten-item (and a five-item short form) Perceived Efficacy in Patient–Physician Interactions (PEPPI) were developed to measure patients' confidence in their ability to elicit and understand information from, and communicate information to, their physicians as well as confidence in their ability to get their physicians to address and act on their medical concerns.

Total score is obtained by summing item scores, ranging from 10–50, with 50 representing highest patient perceived SE, and for the five-item PEPPI, 5–25 (Maly et al., 1998).

PSYCHOMETRIC PROPERTIES

Items were based on issues older patients raised about their interactions with physicians. The five-item version uses those items demonstrating the most variability. Internal reliability coefficient for the ten-item PEPPI was .91, and for the five-item short form, .83. Factor analysis of the full questionnaire confirmed the presence of one distinct domain. PEPPI correlated negatively with avoidant coping style, and positively with active coping style. It appeared to have no association with health-related self-mastery but did correlate significantly with a general SE measure. PEPPI-5 demonstrated essentially the same relationships (Maly et al., 1998). These findings support construct validity.

CRITIQUE AND SUMMARY

The authors believe that the PEPPI may be useful in measuring the impact of empowerment interventions to increase older patients' personal sense of effectiveness in obtaining needed health care. Since female gender was associated negatively with SE in patient-physician interactions, further studies of women, including investigation of PEPPI's sensitivity to interventions, seems warranted. PEPPI's relationship with two measures of self-efficacy/self-mastery was not consistent (Maly et al., 1998) and needs additional research. Studies with populations other than ambulatory Caucasian and female are needed, as is a noncross-sectional design.

PEPPI-10 approaches the alpha reliability needed for clinical applications with individuals.

REFERENCE

Maly, R. C., Frank, J. C., Marshall, G. N., DiMatteo, M. R., & Reuben, D. B. (1998). Perceived efficacy in patient–physician interactions (PEPPI): Validation of an instrument in older persons. *Journal of the American Geriatric Society, 46,* 889–894.

PERCEIVED EFFICACY IN PHYSICIAN–
PATIENT INTERACTIONS ("PEPPI")

"The following questions are about how you interact with doctors as a patient. Please tell us how CONFIDENT you feel in your ability to do each of the following things.

Rate your confidence level with a number from one to five, with five being most confident, and one not feeling confident at all." INTERVIEWER CIRCLE GIVEN NUMBER FOR EACH ITEM:

HOW CONFIDENT ARE YOU IN YOUR ABILITY:

1.   To get doctors to pay attention to what you have to say:

CONFIDENCE   LEVEL

1............................ 2 .... 3 .... 4............................. 5
Not at all   Very
Confident   Confident

2.   To know what questions to ask doctors:

CONFIDENCE   LEVEL

1............................ 2 .... 3 .... 4............................. 5
Not at all   Very
Confident   Confident

3.   To get doctors to answer all of your questions:

CONFIDENCE   LEVEL

1............................ 2 .... 3 .... 4............................. 5
Not at all   Very
Confident   Confident

4.   To ask your doctors questions about your chief health concern:

CONFIDENCE   LEVEL

1............................ 2 .... 3 .... 4............................. 5
Not at all   Very
Confident   Confident

5.   To make the most of your visits with your doctors:

CONFIDENCE   LEVEL

1............................ 2 .... 3 .... 4............................. 5
Not at all   Very
Confident   Confident

6.   To get your doctors to take your chief health concern seriously:

C O N F I D E N C E   L E V E L

1............................ 2 .... 3 .... 4 5
Not at all   Very
Confident   Confident

7.   To understand what doctors tell you:

C O N F I D E N C E   L E V E L

1............................ 2 .... 3 .... 4 5
Not at all   Very
Confident   Confident

8.   To get doctors to do something about your chief health concern:

C O N F I D E N C E   L E V E L

1............................ 2 .... 3 .... 4 5
Not at all   Very
Confident   Confident

9.   To explain your chief health concern to doctors:

C O N F I D E N C E   L E V E L

1............................ 2 .... 3 .... 4 5
Not at all   Very
Confident   Confident

10.   To ask doctors for more information if you don't understand what he or she said:

C O N F I D E N C E   L E V E L

1............................ 2 .... 3 .... 4 5
Not at all   Very
Confident   Confident

PEPPI 5-Item Version
Perceived Efficacy in Patient–Physician Interactions

Interviewer:

"The following 5 questions are about how you interact with doctors as a patient. Please tell me how CONFIDENT you feel in your ability to do each of the following things. Remember, these questions are about your ability to do these things *in general* and not about any particular doctor."

Rate your confidence on a scale of 0 to 10, with 10 meaning extremely confident and 0 meaning not confident at all.

How *confident* are you in your *ability*:
1. To know what questions to ask a doctor:

   CONFIDENCE LEVEL, 0–10 _____ [0 = not confident at all, 10 = extremely
   confident]

How *confident* are you in your *ability*:
2. To get a doctor to answer all of your questions:

   CONFIDENCE LEVEL, 0–10 _____ [0 = not confident at all, 10 = extremely
   confident]

How *confident* are you in your *ability*:
3. To make the most of your visits with your doctors:

   CONFIDENCE LEVEL, 0–10 _____ [0 = not confident at all, 10 = extremely
   confident]

How *confident* are you in your *ability*:
4. To get a doctor to take your chief health concern seriously:

   CONFIDENCE LEVEL, 0–10 _____ [0 = not confident at all, 10 = extremely
   confident]

How *confident* are you in your *ability*:
5. To get a doctor to do something about your chief health concern:

   CONFIDENCE LEVEL, 0–10 _____ [0 = not confident at all, 10 = extremely
   confident]

12. The Purdue Pharmacist Directive Guidance Scale

Developed by Gireesh V. Gupchup, Alan P. Wolfgang, and Joseph Thomas III

INSTRUMENT DESCRIPTION, ADMINISTRATION, AND SCORING GUIDELINES

As pharmacists become more accountable for patient outcomes, measurement of the type and quality of their services is increasingly important. Pharmacists are to take an active role in helping each patient effectively use medications. Examples of activities that can be considered directive guidance are: providing information about proper use of medications, how to manage adverse effects, and encouragement to take medications appropriately. The Purdue Pharmacist Directive Guidance Scale (PPDG) was developed to measure patients' perceptions of the directive guidance they received from pharmacists. Total PPDG scale and subscale scores are calculated by summing responses (Gupchup, Wolfgang, & Thomas, 1996).

PSYCHOMETRIC PROPERTIES

In an effort to support content validity, items for the PPDG were developed to capture activities outlined from the directive guidance dimensions of the Inventory of Socially Supportive Behaviors. The instrument was tested with three hundred persons, eighteen years or older, who reported taking prescription medications in the past three months for asthma, hypertension, or diabetes, or a combination. It was expected that individuals with these disorders would interact with pharmacists to obtain their maintenance medications.

Factor analysis showed two components: 1) instruction (alpha = .84), feedback, and goal setting (alpha = .71), with alpha = .86 for the total PPDG. The total and subscale scores were significantly and positively related to a measure of family and friend support, offering some evidence of convergent validity. The total number of prescription medications taken in the past three months was positive and significantly related to total and subscale scores, perhaps an indicator of therapeutic complexity, in which case more directive guidance would be expected (Gupchup, Wolfgang, & Thomas, 1996).

A separate study of persons with hypertension (Sen & Thomas, 2000) showed alpha reliabilities of .83 (total scale), .78 (instruction subscale), and .68 (feedback and goal-setting subscale), with factor analysis results similar to those in the prior study, that is, scores from 0 to 39 with a mean of 13.6. This study found limited support for convergent validity with no significant correlation between PPDG scores and pharmacists' perceptions of the level of pharmaceutical care provided or with patient reports of medication adherence but a positive correlation with perceived support from family and friends.

CRITIQUE AND SUMMARY

Divergent validity studies would be helpful, as would evidence of sensitivity of the scales to instruction and to change in pharmacists' skills and work environment including incentives to deliver this kind of care. In the population of pharmacists studied, the level of directive guidance behaviors was low.

REFERENCES

Gupchup, G. V., Wolfgang, A. P., & Thomas, J. (1996). Development of a scale to measure directive guidance by pharmacists. *Annals of Pharmacotherapy, 30,* 1369–1375.
Sen, S. S., & Thomas, J. (2000). Assessment of a patient-based pharmaceutical care scale. *American Journal of Health-System Pharmacists, 57,* 1592–1598.

PURDUE PHARMACIST DIRECTIVE GUIDANCE SCALE

The statements in this section describe the services that may be performed by your pharmacist. After reading each statement, please indicate *how often* during the *past three months* the pharmacist that you usually meet has performed these services.

Item	Never	Rarely	Sometimes	Often	Very often
1) Your pharmacist gave you some information on how to take your medication.	0	1	2	3	4
2) Your pharmacist gave you feedback on how you were doing without saying it was good or bad.	0	1	2	3	4
3) Your pharmacist made it clear what is expected of you with regard to your medication.	0	1	2	3	4
4) Your pharmacist gave you some information to help you understand your disease better.	0	1	2	3	4
5) Your pharmacist checked back with you to see if you followed the advice you were given.	0	1	2	3	4
6) Your pharmacist taught you how to take your medication.	0	1	2	3	4
7) Your pharmacist told you who you should contact in case you need assistance with your medication.	0	1	2	3	4
8) Your pharmacist told you what to expect from your medication.	0	1	2	3	4
9) Your pharmacist said things that made it easier to understand how to take your medication.	0	1	2	3	4
10) Your pharmacist assisted you in setting goal for yourself with respect to taking your medication correctly.	0	1	2	3	4

SCORING:
1) Entire scale score obtained by adding all 10 items; possible range = 0–40.
2) Instruction subscale score: Add first 6 items; possible range = 0–24.
3) Feedback and goal setting subscale score: Add items 7–10; possible range = 0–16.

Section B

Diabetes

Diabetes is the disease entity with the longest established record in patient education, and several strong research centers have excelled in instrument development. Besides the commonly available knowledge and self-efficacy instruments, the field of diabetes management has instruments that purport to measure diabetes-related distress, beliefs, cognitive representations of the disease, and management independence in children and adults. Many of these instruments are psychological in focus and those that measure self-management skill levels use self-report. Thus, further work to develop solid outcome measures for self-management preparation remains.

---

13. MDRTC Diabetes Knowledge Test

Developed by James. T. Fitzgerald, Martha M. Funnell, George E. Hess, Patricia A. Barr, Robert M. Anderson, Roland G. Hiss, and Wayne K. Davis

INSTRUMENT DESCRIPTION, ADMINISTRATION, AND SCORING GUIDELINES

The Michigan Diabetes Research and Training Center began in the mid-1980s to develop a series of valid and reliable knowledge tests that could be used by diabetes educators and researchers throughout the country. The general test segment of this diabetes knowledge test has 14 items and is appropriate for adults with Type 1 and Type 2 diabetes. An additional nine items constitute the insulin-use subscale appropriate for these same kinds of patients. Completion time is about 15 minutes; reading level is sixth grade, and the instrument can generally be self-administered. Item scores are summed (Fitzgerald et al., 1998).

PSYCHOMETRIC PROPERTIES

A national group of expert professionals identified content areas and judged items. Patients with Type 1 diabetes scored better than did those with Type 2, hypothesized because Type

2 is more severe and its treatment more complex. Scores increased as the years of formal education increased, and those who had received diabetes education scored higher than did those who had not. All of these comparisons support validity of this instrument. Cronbach's alpha for the general test and the insulin use test with two different Michigan populations were in the low to mid .70s (Fitzgerald et al., 1998).

CRITIQUE AND SUMMARY

This is a general test of diabetes knowledge and may not contain enough detail to comprehensively assess specific components of knowledge or self-care. Its usefulness as an outcome measure for educational interventions remains to be determined (Fitzgerald et al., 1998).

REFERENCE

Fitzgerald, J. T., Funnell, M. M., Hess, G. E., Barr, P. A., Anderson, R. M., Hiss, R. G., & Davis, W. K. (1998). The reliability and validity of a brief diabetes knowledge test. *Diabetes Care, 21,* 706–710.

MDRTC DIABETES KNOWLEDGE TEST

1. The diabetes diet is:
   a. the way most American people eat
   b. a healthy diet for most people*
   c. too high in carbohydrate for most people
   d. too high in protein for most people

2. Which of the following is highest in carbohydrate?
   a. Baked chicken
   b. Swiss cheese
   c. Baked potato*
   d. Peanut butter

3. Which of the following is highest in fat?
   a. Low fat milk*
   b. Orange juice
   c. Corn
   d. Honey

4. Which of the following is a "free food"?
   a. Any unsweetened food
   b. Any dietetic food
   c. Any food that says "sugar free" on the label
   d. Any food that has less than 20 calories per serving*

5. Glycosylated hemoglobin (hemoglobin A1) is a test that is a measure of your average blood glucose level for the past:

   a. day
   b. week
   c. 6–10 weeks*
   d. 6 months

6. Which is the best method for testing blood glucose?
   a. Urine testing
   b. Blood testing*
   c. Both are equally good

7. What effect does unsweetened fruit juice have on blood glucose?
   a. Lowers it
   b. Raises it*
   c. Has no effect

8. Which should not be used to treat low blood glucose?
   a. 3 hard candies
   b. 1/2 cup orange juice
   c. 1 cup diet soft drink*
   d. 1 cup skim milk

9. For a person in good control, what effect does exercise have on blood glucose?
   a. Lowers it*
   b. Raises it
   c. Has no effect

10. Infection is likely to cause:
    a. an increase in blood glucose*
    b. a decrease in blood glucose
    c. no change in blood glucose

11. The best way to take care of your feet is to:
    a. look at and wash them each day*
    b. massage them with alcohol each day
    c. soak them for one hour each day
    d. buy shoes a size larger than usual

12. Eating foods lower in fat decreases your risk for:
    a. nerve disease
    b. kidney disease
    c. heart disease*
    d. eye disease

13. Numbness and tingling may be symptoms of:
    a. kidney disease
    b. nerve disease*
    c. eye disease
    d. liver disease

14. Which of the following is usually not associated with diabetes:
    a. vision problems
    b. kidney problems
    c. nerve problems
    d. lung problems*

15. Signs of ketoacidosis include:
    a. shakiness
    b. sweating
    c. vomiting*
    d. low blood glucose

16. If you are sick with the flu, which of the following changes should you make?
    a. Take less insulin
    b. Drink less liquids

c. Eat more proteins

d. Test for glucose and ketones more often*

17. If you have taken intermediate-acting insulin (NPH or Lente), you are most likely to have an insulin reaction in:
    a. 1–3 h
    b. 6–12 h*
    c. 12–15 h
    d. more than 15 h

18. You realize just before lunch time that you forgot to take your insulin before breakfast. What should you do now?
    a. Skip lunch to lower your blood glucose
    b. Take the insulin that you usually take at breakfast
    c. Take twice as much insulin as you usually take at breakfast

d. Check your blood glucose level to decide how much insulin to take*

19. If you are beginning to have an insulin reaction, you should:
    a. exercise
    b. lie down and rest
    c. drink some juice*
    d. take regular insulin

20. Low blood glucose may be caused by:
    a. too much insulin*
    b. too little insulin
    c. too much food
    d. too little exercise

21. If you take your morning insulin but skip breakfast your blood glucose level will usually:
    a. increase
    b. decrease*
    c. remain the same

22. High blood glucose may be caused by:
    a. not enough insulin*
    b. skipping meals
    c. delaying your snack
    d. large ketones in your urine

23. Which one of the following will most likely cause an insulin reaction:
    a. heavy exercise*
    b. infection
    c. overeating
    d. not taking your insulin

*Correct answer

Fitzgerald, J. T. et al. (1998). The reliability and validity of a brief diabetes knowledge test. *Diabetes Care, 21,* 706–710. Used with permission.

14.   Diabetes Attitudes Scale

Developed by Robert M. Anderson, Michael B. Donnelly, and Robert F. Dedrick

INSTRUMENT DESCRIPTION, ADMINISTRATION, AND SCORING GUIDELINES

Some of the major theories of health behavior, such as the health belief model and the theory of reasoned action, emphasize that attitudes and beliefs are a major component of health behavior. The theory of reasoned action also posits the importance of how other people whom the patient views as important feel about the action. The Diabetes Attitudes Scale (DAS) is not intended to be, or to replace, a diabetes attitude scale focusing exclusively on the concerns of persons with diabetes. Rather, its special purpose as expressed by its authors is to allow identification of differences in opinion that could interfere with the quality of the patient–health care provider relationship and ultimately affect the management and treatment of the disease.

The DAS was originally designed to measure the attitudes of health care professionals and was revised for use with patients to make items less technical. The rewording lowered the reading level from 12th to 10th grade. Items are scored with 5 for strongly agree; 4, agree; 3, neither agree nor disagree; 2, disagree; and 1, strongly disagree. Scores for each scale are averaged by the number of items. Positive attitudes are defined as those over 3 and negative as those less than 3.

Findings from the comparison suggest that a significant number of young and well-educated patients do not wish to be told what they should do to care for their diabetes; health care professionals tend to underestimate the perceived negative impact diabetes has on the lives of patients who are required to take insulin; a significant number of older patients do not desire an independent self-care role, although nurses and dietitians place strong value on patient autonomy (Anderson, Donnelly, & Dedrick, 1990; Anderson, Fitzgerald, Gorenflo, & Oh, 1993).

DAS can also be used to assess the impact of diabetes education programs on the attitudes of patients and to explore the relationship between attitudes and behavior (Anderson et al., 1998). Mean scores for each item and each scale may be found in Anderson and colleagues (1998).

PSYCHOMETRIC PROPERTIES

For DAS-2 most respondents believed that health care professionals need special training to care for persons with diabetes, good blood glucose control reduces the likelihood that complications will develop, diabetes has a significant negative impact on the patient's life, and a team approach is essential to diabetes care. Although the respondents generally agreed that noninsulin dependent diabetes mellitus (NIDDM) is a serious disease and were supportive of patients being in charge of their diabetes management, these issues generated the widest differences of opinion (Anderson et al., 1990).

A study of self-reported adherence to 10 diabetes self-care behaviors showed that patients in the high-adherence group had more positive attitudes on the DAS than did patients in the low-adherence group. This finding is believed to provide evidence of construct validity for the DAS (Anderson, Fitzgerald, & Oh, 1993). Differences in the DAS by gender have been investigated. Similarities across gender were common, although men were more passive than women in their diabetes care (Fitzgerald, Anderson, & Davis, 1995)

Using selected subscales for the DAS, Via and Salyer (1999) found a .45 correlation with psychosocial self-efficacy, and no significant correlation with glycosylated hemoglobin.

Recently, a third version of DAS, congruent with current scientific knowledge about diabetes, has been developed (Anderson et al., 1998). It has 33 items, some new and some old, and the following subscales: (1) need for special training to provide diabetes care; (2) seriousness of Type 2 diabetes; (3) value of tight control; (4) psychosocial impact of diabetes; and (5) attitude toward patient autonomy.

Items for DAS-3 were written by professional and patient experts to reflect content validity. It was then administered to 1,814 persons with diabetes, physicians, nurses, and dietitians. Reliabilities of the subscales ranged from .65 to .80. Findings with use of DAS-3 are similar to those with DAS-2—patients using insulin report more psychosocial impact than patients who do not take insulin, and health care professionals who spend more time treating diabetes are likely to have a more favorable attitude toward the disease than those who spend less time.

CRITIQUE AND SUMMARY

The reading level is high for a number of persons with diabetes. Race and socioeconomic class of patients was not reported.

Additional validity studies would be useful. Although the authors report that content validity was assured through the use of a Delphi process for item construction and selection, this process involved only health professionals and not patients. Thus, it is unknown whether the comparisons that can be obtained with the DAS are with attitudes and beliefs held primarily by health professionals. Construct validity support cited previously depends on self-reported adherence to the self-care components as well as the assumption that compliance with self-care is directly related to each subscale.

It is expected that differences in attitudes among patients with diabetes will affect how they receive and act on the content from educational sessions and that it is useful to compare the attitudes of patients and health professionals (Anderson et al., 1990). Further evidence exploring these two expectations would be useful.

REFERENCES

Anderson, R. M., Donnelly, M. B., & Dedrick, R. F. (1990). Measuring the attitudes of patients toward diabetes and its treatment. *Patient Education and Counseling, 16,* 231–245.

Anderson, R. M., Fitzgerald, J. T., Funnell, M. M., & Gruppen, L. D. (1998). The third version of the Diabetes Attitude Scale. *Diabetes Care, 21,* 1403–1407.

Anderson, R. M., Fitzgerald, J. T., Gorenflo, D. W., & Oh, M. S. (1993). A comparison of the diabetes-related attitudes of health care professionals and patients. *Patient Education and Counseling, 21,* 41–50.

Anderson, R. M., Fitzgerald, J. T., & Oh, M. S. (1993). The relationship between diabetes-related attitudes and patients' self-reported adherence. *Diabetes Educator, 19,* 287–292.

Fitzgerald, J. T., Anderson, R. M., & Davis, W. K. (1995). Gender differences in diabetes attitudes and adherence. *Diabetes Educator, 21,* 523–529.

Via, P. S., & Salyer, J. (1999). Psychosocial self-efficacy and personal characteristics of veterans attending a diabetes education program. *Diabetes Educator, 25,* 727–737.

DIABETES ATTITUDES SCALE

Below are some statements about diabetes. Each numbered statement finishes the sentence "In general, I believe that . . . " You may believe that a statement is true for one person but not for another person, or may be true one time but not be true another time. Mark the answer that you believe is true most of the time or is true for most people. Place a check mark in the box below the word or phrase that is closest to your opinion about each statement. It is important that you answer *every* statement.

Note: The term "health care professionals" in this survey refers to doctors, nurses, and dietitians.

In general, I believe that:	Strongly Agree	Agree	Neutral	Disagree	Strongly Disagree
1. . . . health care professionals who treat people with diabetes should be trained to communicate well with their patients.	❐	❐	❐	❐	❐
2. . . . people who do *not* need to take insulin to treat their diabetes have a pretty mild disease.	❐	❐	❐	❐	❐
3. . . . there is not much use in trying to have good blood sugar control because the complications of diabetes will happen anyway.	❐	❐	❐	❐	❐
4. . . . diabetes affects almost every part of a diabetic person's life.	❐	❐	❐	❐	❐
5. . . . the important decisions regarding daily diabetes care should be made by the person with diabetes.	❐	❐	❐	❐	❐
6. . . . health care professionals should be taught how daily diabetes care affects patients' lives.	❐	❐	❐	❐	❐
7. . . . older people with Type 2* diabetes do not usually get complications.	❐	❐	❐	❐	❐

(continued)

In general, I believe that:	Strongly Agree	Agree	Neutral	Disagree	Strongly Disagree
8. . . . keeping the blood sugar close to normal can help to prevent the complications of diabetes.	❑	❑	❑	❑	❑
9. . . . health care professionals should help patients make informed choices about their care plans.	❑	❑	❑	❑	❑
10. . . . it is important for the nurses and dietitians who teach people with diabetes to learn counseling skills.	❑	❑	❑	❑	❑
11. . . . people whose diabetes is treated by just a diet do not have to worry about getting many long-term complications.	❑	❑	❑	❑	❑
12. . . . a lmost everyone with diabetes should do whatever it takes to keep their blood sugar close to normal.	❑	❑	❑	❑	❑
13. . . . the emotional effects of diabetes are pretty small.	❑	❑	❑	❑	❑
14. . : . people with diabetes should have the final say in setting their blood glucose goals.	❑	❑	❑	❑	❑
15. . . . blood sugar testing is not needed for people with Type 2* diabetes.	❑	❑	❑	❑	❑
16. . . . low blood sugar reactions make tight control too risky for most people.	❑	❑	❑	❑	❑
17. . . . health care professionals should learn how to set goals with patients, not just tell them what to do.	❑	❑	❑	❑	❑

In general, I believe that:	Strongly Agree	Agree	Neutral	Disagree	Strongly Disagree
18. . . . diabetes is hard because you never get a break from it.	❐	❐	❐	❐	❐
19. . . . the person with diabetes is the most important member of the diabetes care team.	❐	❐	❐	❐	❐
20. . . . to do a good job, diabetes educators should learn a lot about being teachers.	❐	❐	❐	❐	❐
21. . . . Type 2* diabetes is a very serious disease.	❐	❐	❐	❐	❐
22. . . . having diabetes changes a person's outlook on life.	❐	❐	❐	❐	❐
23. . . . people who have Type 2* diabetes will probably not get much payoff from tight control of their blood sugar.	❐	❐	❐	❐	❐
24. . . . people with diabetes should learn a lot about the disease so that they can be in charge of their own diabetes care.	❐	❐	❐	❐	❐
25. . . . Type 2* is as serious as Type 1[†] diabetes.	❐	❐	❐	❐	❐
26. . . . tight control is too much work.	❐	❐	❐	❐	❐
27. . . . what the patient does has more effect on the outcome of diabetes care than anything a health professional does.	❐	❐	❐	❐	❐
28. . . . tight control of blood sugar makes sense only for people with Type 1[†] diabetes.	❐	❐	❐	❐	❐

(continued)

In general, I believe that:	Strongly Agree	Agree	Neutral	Disagree	Strongly Disagree
29. ... it is frustrating for people with diabetes to take care of their disease.	❐	❐	❐	❐	❐
30. ... people with diabetes have a right to decide how hard they will work to control their blood sugar.	❐	❐	❐	❐	❐
31. ... people who take diabetes pills should be as concerned about their blood sugar as people who take insulin.	❐	❐	❐	❐	❐
32. ... people with diabetes have the right *not* to take good care of their diabetes.	❐	❐	❐	❐	❐
33. ... support from family and friends is important in dealing with diabetes.	❐	❐	❐	❐	❐

*Type 2 diabetes usually begins after age 40. Many patients are overweight and weight loss is often an important part of the treatment. Insulin and/or diabetes pills are sometimes used in the treatment. Type 2 diabetes is also called noninsulin-dependent diabetes mellitus or NIDDM; formerly it was called "adult diabetes."

†Type 1 diabetes usually begins before age 40 and always requires insulin as part of the treatment. Patients are usually not overweight. Type 1 diabetes is also called insulin-dependent diabetes mellitus or IDDM; formerly it was called "juvenile diabetes."

Diabetes Attitude Scale - 3 Formulae*

Scale Name	Scale Equation	Special Instructions
Need for Special Training	Σ (Q1, Q6, Q10, Q17, Q20)/Number of nonmissing items	
Seriousness of NIDDM	Σ (Q2, Q7, Q11, Q15, Q21, Q25, Q31)/ Number of nonmissing items	Reverse scores for Q2, Q7, Q11, and Q15.
Value of Tight Control	Σ (Q3, Q8, Q12, Q16, Q23, Q26, Q28)/ Number of nonmissing items	Reverse scores for Q3, Q16, Q23, Q26, and Q28.
Psychosocial Impact of DM	Σ (Q4, Q13, Q18, Q22, Q29, Q33)/Number of nonmissing items	Reverse scores for Q13.
Patient Autonomy	Σ (Q5, Q9, Q14, Q19, Q24, Q27, Q30, Q32)/ Number of nonmissing items	

Note: Strongly Agree = 5, Agree = 4, Neutral = 3, Disagree = 2, and Strongly Disagree = 1.
Note: If 50% of the items of a scale are missing, the scale should be considered as missing.

15. Problem Areas in Diabetes Survey

Developed by William H. Polonsky, Barbara J. Anderson, Patricia A. Lohrer, Garry Welch, Alan M. Jacobson, Jennifer E. Aponte, and Carolyn E. Schwartz

INSTRUMENT DESCRIPTION, ADMINISTRATION, AND SCORING GUIDELINES

For those living with diabetes, illness-related emotional distress stemming from the self-care demands and worry about long-term complications and frustrations of the regimen and illness may not be uncommon. In the complex adjustment to life with diabetes, patients may feel defeated, and become unmotivated to adhere to the diabetes regimen. Anger, guilt, frustration, denial, fear of hypoglycemia, and loneliness have also been observed. Recent evidence suggests that emotional distress as represented by the presence of affective disorders or poor coping skills may be linked to poor adherence to the self-care regimen, especially among adolescents with insulin-dependent diabetes mellitus. The primary aims of the Problem Areas in Diabetes Survey (PAID) are to serve as a screening measure for clinical and research purposes, and to help clinicians identify patients experiencing high levels of diabetes related distress, so that treatment interventions may be developed around specific problem areas (Polonsky et al., 1995).

Each item represents an aspect of emotional distress in the psychosocial adjustment to diabetes. Summing the item responses creates a total score hypothesized to reflect the overall level of distress, which can range from 0 to 100 (transformed scores) with higher scores indicating greater emotional distress.

PSYCHOMETRIC PROPERTIES

Items for the tool were solicited from 10 health care providers at the Joslin Clinic and patient comments that focused on the range of difficulties encountered by persons living with diabetes. Early drafts of the items were piloted, and then the tool was tested on 451 female patients, all of whom required insulin and had diabetes for at least 1 year. Approximately 60% of the sample reported at least one serious diabetes-related concern, most frequently worrying about the future and the possibility of serious complications (42%) (Polonsky et al., 1995).

There is no absolute criterion or gold standard for emotional adjustment to diabetes. PAID scores were positively associated with measures of general emotional distress, fear of hypoglycemia, and disordered eating attitudes and behaviors; and negatively associated with adherence to recommendations for blood glucose testing, insulin usage, meal planning, reported self-care behaviors, and diabetes-specific coping skills. Greater distress was associated with poorer glycemic control and more frequent short- and long-term complications of diabetes. Patterns of correlations between PAID and other tests measuring theoretically related constructs including self-efficacy, further support concurrent validity (Polonsky et al., 1995; Welch, Jacobson, & Polonsky, 1997). Recent work on construct validity found that patients with IDDM (and therefore a more complicated regimen and greater demands associated with earlier illness onset) reported higher scores than did those with NIDDM. This finding provides evidence of discriminant validity. The most recent study (Nichols, Hillier, Javor, & Brown, 2000) showed that increased emotional distress as measured by PAID was a significant predictor of worse glycemic control in adults with Type 2 diabetes, which would be expected.

Cronbach's alpha (measure of internal consistency) was .95. Factor analysis showed the presence of a large general factor representing diabetes emotional functioning, and it supports summation of the items into a total score. Correlations of PAID with measures of glycemic control were not statistically significant (Welch, Jacobson, & Polonsky, 1997). Snoek, Pouwer, Welch, and Polonsky (2000) found PAID to be psychometrically equivalent in Dutch and U.S. patients. Weininger and Jacobson (2001) found in an observational study without a control group of patients undergoing intensive diabetes treatment/education to improve glycemic control, that change in PAID scores was associated with change in glycemic control. The authors suggest that the emotional distress surrounding diabetes may become a barrier to the implementation of self-care behaviors, and thus interferes with efforts to improve glycemic control.

CRITIQUE AND SUMMARY

Since the first edition of this book, initial development work on the PAID has been considerably extended. The populations on which the instrument has been developed were White and well-educated volunteers from the Joslin Clinic, now extended to Dutch patients. Although explicit domains of emotional adjustment were apparently not established, the inclusion of patient comments as a source of items is helpful. Further testing will be necessary to see if scores are sensitive to clinically important changes in patient status and in response to appropriate additional forms and amounts of education or psychosocial interventions known to promote significant decrease in diabetes-related emotional distress. Further evidence of PAID's ability to predict glycemic control in the future will be important, as will establishing a score indicative of a pathological level of distress.

PAID may serve as a useful clinical tool to identify high levels of diabetes-related distress and as an outcome measure in clinical trials. PAID total scores have been used as an overall measure of the emotional burden of diabetes. Individual PAID items should be considered only as a rough initial screen for the identification of emotional problems in management but should be examined to identify specific sources of diabetes distress. The data presented are consistent with the hypothesis that diabetes-related emotional distress is an independent major contributor to poor adherence, separate from the contribution of general emotional distress (Polonsky et al., 1995).

REFERENCES

Nichols, G. A., Hillier, T. A., Javor, K., & Brown, J. B. (2000). Predictors of glycemic control in insulin-using adults with Type 2 diabetes. *Diabetes Care, 23,* 273–277.

Polonsky, W. H., Anderson, B. J., Lohrer, P. A., Welch, G., Jacobson, A. M., Aponte, J. E., & Schwartz, C. E. (1995). Assessment of diabetes-related distress. *Diabetes Care, 18,* 754–760.

Polonsky, W. H., & Welch, G. M. (1996). Listening to our patients' concerns; understanding and addressing diabetes-specific emotional distress. *Diabetes Spectrum, 9*(1), 8–11.

Snoek, F. J., Pouwer, F., Welch, G. W., & Polonsky, W. H. (2000). Diabetes-related emotional distress in Dutch and U.S. diabetic patients. *Diabetes Care, 23,* 1305–1309.

Weinger, K., & Jacobson, A. M. (2001). Psychosocial and quality of life correlates of glycemic control during intensive treatment of Type 1 diabetes. *Patient Education & Counseling, 42,* 1213–131.

Welch, G. W., Jacobson, A. M., & Polonsky, W. H. (1997). The Problem Areas in Diabetes Scale; An evaluation of its clinical utility. *Diabetes Care, 20,* 760–766.

PROBLEM AREAS IN DIABETES (PAID) QUESTIONNAIRE

INSTRUCTIONS: Which of the following diabetes issues are currently a problem for you? Circle the number that gives the best answer for you. Please provide an answer for each question.

	Not a problem	Minor problem	Moderate problem	Somewhat serious problem	Serious problem
1. Not having clear and concrete goals for your diabetes care?	0	1	2	3	4
2. Feeling discouraged with your diabetes treatment plan?	0	1	2	3	4
3. Feeling scared when you think about living with diabetes?	0	1	2	3	4
4. Uncomfortable social situations related to your diabetes care (e.g., people telling you what to eat)?	0	1	2	3	4
5. Feelings of deprivation regarding food and meals?	0	1	2	3	4
6. Feeling depressed when you think about living with diabetes?	0	1	2	3	4
7. Not knowing if your mood or feelings are related to your diabetes?	0	1	2	3	4
8. Feeling overwhelmed by your diabetes?	0	1	2	3	4
9. Worrying about low blood sugar reactions?	0	1	2	3	4
10. Feeling angry when you think about living with diabetes?	0	1	2	3	4
11. Feeling constantly concerned about food and eating?	0	1	2	3	4

(continued)

	Not a problem	Minor problem	Moderate problem	Somewhat serious problem	Serious problem
12. Worrying about the future and the possibility of serious complications?	0	1	2	3	4
13. Feelings of guilt or anxiety when you get off track with your diabetes management?	0	1	2	3	4
14. Not "accepting" your diabetes?	0	1	2	3	4
15. Feeling unsatisfied with your diabetes physician?	0	1	2	3	4
16. Feeling that diabetes is taking up too much of your mental and physical energy every day?	0	1	2	3	4
17. Feeling alone with your diabetes?	0	1	2	3	4
18. Feeling that your friends and family are not supportive of your diabetes management efforts?	0	1	2	3	4
19. Coping with complications of diabetes?	0	1	2	3	4
20. Feeling "burned out" by the constant effort needed to manage diabetes?	0	1	2	3	4

16.   Appraisal of Diabetes Scale

Developed by Michael P. Carey, Randall S. Jorgensen, Ruth S. Weinstock, Robert P. Sprofkin, Larry J. Lantinga, C. L. M. Carnike Jr., Marilyn T. Baker, and Andrew W. Meister

INSTRUMENT DESCRIPTION, ADMINISTRATION, AND SCORING GUIDELINES

The way a person appraises her/his disease as a stressor is known to influence psychological adjustment. Items for the Appraisal of Diabetes Scale (ADS) were developed from previous theory and research about the appraisal processes (Carey et al., 1991). The instrument measures the individual's appraisal of the illness in terms of her thoughts about diabetes.

ADS requires less than five minutes to complete. The score is a sum of item scores, ranging from 7 to 35 with higher scores indicating more negative appraisal (Carey et al., 1991).

PSYCHOMETRIC CHARACTERISTICS

Cronbach's alpha was .73, and test–retest reliability over one week was .85. Factor analysis showed a single factor. Results of correlational analysis with other instruments showed that higher levels of negative appraisal were associated with higher levels of anxiety, anger, depression, perceived stress, diabetes-related hassles, and moderate relationships with likelihood of adhering to diabetes regimen and poorer glycemic control, as would be expected (Carey et al., 1991). A later study showed that scores on the ADS strongly predicted diabetes quality of life and glycemic control (Trief, Grant, Elbert, & Weinstock, 1998).

CRITIQUE AND SUMMARY

Predictive validity of ADS has not yet been studied, and sensitivity to intervention must be established. A study completed by Trief and colleagues (1998) suggests that ADS would be a potentially useful first-line clinical screen among diabetics to identify individuals at risk for or currently experiencing poor quality of life. The actual use of ADS in this way could not be located and apparently remains to be done.

REFERENCES

Carey, M. P., Jorgensen, R. S., Weinstock, R. S., Sprafkin, R. P., Lantinga, L. J., Carnrike, C. L. M., Jr., Baker, M. T., & Meisler, A. W. (1991). Reliability and validity of the Appraisal of Diabetes Scale. *Journal of Behavioral Medicine, 14,* 43–51.

Trief, P. M., Grant, W., Elbert, K., & Weinstock, R. W. (1998). Family, environment, glycemic control and the psychosocial adaptation of adults with diabetes. *Diabetes Care, 21,* 241–245.

APPRAISAL OF DIABETES SCALE

People differ in their thoughts and feelings about having diabetes. We would like to know how you feel about having diabetes. Therefore, please circle the answer to each question which is closest to the way *you* feel. Please give your honest feelings—*we are interested in how you feel*, not what your doctor or family may think.

1. How upsetting is having diabetes for you?

1	2	3	4	5
not at all	slightly upsetting	moderately upsetting	very upsetting	extremely upsetting

2. How much control over your diabetes do your have?

1	2	3	4	5
none at all	slight mount	moderate amount	large amount	total amount

3. How much uncertainty do you currently experience in your life as a result of being diabetic?

1	2	3	4	5
none at all	slight amount	moderate amount	large amount	extremely large amount

4. How likely is your diabetes to worsen over the next several years? (Try to give an estimate based on your personal feelings rather than based on a rational judgment.)

1	2	3	4	5
not likely at all	slightly likely	moderately likely	very likely	extremely likely

5. Do you believe that achieving good diabetic control is due to your efforts as compared to factors which are beyond your control?

1	2	3	4	5
totally because of me	mostly because of me	partly because of me and partly because of other factors	mostly because of other factors	totally because of other factors

(continued)

6.   How effective are you in coping with your diabetes?

1	2	3	4	5
not at all	slightly effective	moderately effective	very effective	extremely effective

7.   To what degree does your diabetes get in the way of your developing life goals?

1	2	3	4	5
not at all	slight amount	moderate amount	large amount	extremely large amount

Carey, M. P., et al. (1991). Reliability and validity of the Appraisal of Diabetes Scale. *Journal of Behavioral Medicine, 14,* 43–51. Used with permission of Kluwer Academic/Plenum Publishers.

17. Barriers in Diabetes Questionnaire

Developed by E. D. Mollem, F. J. Snoek, and R. J. Heine

INSTRUMENT DESCRIPTION, ADMINISTRATION, AND SCORING GUIDELINES

One of the important determinants of self-care has proven to be the health beliefs of patients. The Barriers in Diabetes Questionnaire (BDQ) is based on the barriers element of the health belief model related to self-management of insulin-treated diabetes.

The BDQ has three subscales: I. Self-control and advice from health care providers, II. Injecting, blood glucose monitoring, and self-regulation in general, and III. Self-regulation in specific situations. Scores are the sums of the ratings with higher ratings indicating more barriers (Mollem, Snoek, & Heine, 1996).

PSYCHOMETRIC CHARACTERISTICS

BDQ was tested in 240 insulin-requiring diabetic patients. Patients with a glycosylated hemoglobin value above the median showed significantly higher scores in subscales II and III, supportive of validity. Patients perceiving more barriers reported a more negative health evaluation, also to be expected. A lower frequency of self-monitoring of blood glucose was associated with a higher score on subscale I. Cronbach's alpha for the total BDQ was .85, for subscale I, .65, subscale II, .71 and subscale III, .81 (Mollem, Snoek, & Heine, 1996).

CRITIQUE AND SUMMARY

Justification of content validity for the BDQ could not be located. The relationship between experiencing a certain barrier and the self-care behavior concerning this behavior have not been studied. Cronbach's alpha for subscale I is relatively low. The authors suggest BDQ can be used to describe patient populations as a way of finding focus points for patient education. It can also provide insight into a patient's specific problems (Mollem, Snoek, & Heine, 1996). Its sensitivity to interventions has apparently not yet been tested.

REFERENCE

Mollem, E. D., Snoek, F. J., & Heine, R. J. (1996). Assessment of perceived barriers in self-care of insulin-requiring diabetic patients. *Patient Education & Counseling, 29,* 277–281.

BARRIERS IN DIABETES QUESTIONNAIRE

	Never				Always
	1	2	3	4	5

Subscale I

1. The advice of the dietician is difficult to comprehend

2. I find it difficult to follow the advice given by the diabetes nurse

3. I find self-testing of my blood-glucose of little importance

4. Self-testing my blood-glucose costs a lot of time

5. I find it annoying to test my blood-glucose outside my home

6. I find it annoying to test my blood-glucose at night

7. Making a daily blood-glucose curve is too much trouble

8. I find it annoying to break off other activities for self-testing

9. I don't test my blood-glucose when I think it is too low, but eat at once

Subscale II

10. Self-testing my blood-glucose is painful

11. I find it difficult to inject insulin at regular intervals before meals

12. I find it annoying to inject myself out of the house

13. I'm afraid of injecting myself

14. Self-injecting is painful

15. I find it hard to maintain a normal blood-glucose level when I'm on vacation

16. I find it hard to maintain a normal blood-glucose level on weekends

17. I find it hard to maintain a normal blood-glucose level when I sleep in

18. I'm afraid to prick my finger

19. I'm afraid of getting a hypo

	Never				Always
	1	2	3	4	5

Subscale III

20. I find it hard to control my eating when I have a hypo

21. I find it difficult to feel whether my blood-glucose level is too low

22. I find it hard to adjust the amount of carbohydrates when I have a low blood-glucose level

23. I find it hard to adjust the insulin dosage when I have a low blood-glucose level

24. I find it difficult to feel whether my blood-glucose level is too high

25. I find it hard to adjust the amount of carbohydrates when I have a high blood-glucose level

26. I find it difficult to adjust the amount of carbohydrates when I exercise more

27. I find it difficult to maintain a normal blood-glucose level when I'm at a party

28. I find it difficult to maintain a normal blood-glucose level when I'm under stress

From: Mollem, E. D., Snoek, F. J., & Heine, R. J. (1996). Assessment of perceived barriers in self-care of insulin-requiring diabetic patients. *Patient Education & Counseling, 29,* 277–281. Used with permission from Elsevier Science.

18. Personal Models of Diabetes Questionnaire

Developed by Sarah E. Hampson, Russell E. Glasgow, and Deborah J. Toobert

INSTRUMENT DESCRIPTION, ADMINISTRATION, AND SCORING GUIDELINES

Personal-illness models are patients' cognitive representations of their disease and include beliefs and emotions about its cause, symptoms, course, treatment, and consequences. Patients' responses include seeking health care, complying with treatment, and performing self-care behaviors (Glasgow, Hampson, Strycker, & Ruggerio, 1997; Hampson, Glasgow, & Toobert, 1990).

Personal models are an extension of schema theory from cognitive and social psychology. They are patient generated and include those variables patients believe to be central to their experience of illness, its management, and emotional responses to the illness (Hampson, Glasgow, & Foster, 1995).

The Personal Models of Diabetes Questionnaire (PDMQ) is organized around these constructs which have emerged repeatedly across studies of both acute and chronic diseases. It is a brief eight-item, self-report instrument with a 5-point Likert scale response option. Its predecessor (PMDI) in interview format includes some open-ended items which were coded by trained raters.

PSYCHOMETRIC CHARACTERISTICS

PMDI scales and their reliabilities are: seriousness (alpha = .57), treatment effectiveness (alpha = .74), control (alpha = .53). Test–retest reliabilities over three months were .67, .70, and .56 (Hampson, Glasgow, & Strycker, 2000). PMDI has been found to significantly improve the prediction of diet and marginally improve the prediction of exercise (Hampson, Glasgow, & Toobert, 1990), and in older adults to predict dietary intake and physical activity but not blood glucose testing (Hampson, Glasgow, & Foster, 1995). In a mail survey of 2,056 U.S. adults with diabetes, treatment effectiveness as measured by PMDQ was the strongest predictor of self-reported self management (Glasgow, Hampson, Strycker, & Ruggerio, 1997) as it was in dietary management in adolescents studied by Skinner and Hampson (1998, 2001) and in other studies (Hampson, Glasgow, & Strycker, 2000).

These findings are largely supportive of PMDI validity.

CRITIQUE AND SUMMARY

Much development of PMDQ has been accomplished, moving it from a lengthy interview schedule with coding required for open-ended items, to a questionnaire format. Reliabilities remain low.

Assessing patients' personal models is likely to be valuable for individualizing education for nutrition and physical activity although no evidence could be found that verified this assumption. Adopting constructive illness representations (schema) should be helpful to coping with the demands of diabetes (Skinner, John, & Hampson, 2000). Construct validity studies of the relationships of PMDQ with other ways of conceptualizing patients' perceptions such as attitudes and health beliefs would also be helpful (Hampson, Glasgow, & Foster, 1995).

REFERENCES

Glasgow, R. E., Hampson, S. E., Strycker, L. A., & Ruggerio, L. (1997). Personal-model beliefs and social-environmental barriers related to diabetes self-management. *Diabetes Care, 20,* 556–561.

Hampson, S. H., Glasgow, R. E., & Foster, L. S. (1995). Personal models of diabetes among older adults: Relationship to self-management and other variables. *Diabetes Educator, 21,* 300–307.

Hampson, S. E., Glasgow, R. E., & Strycker, L. A. (2000). Beliefs versus feelings: A comparison of personal models and depression for predicting multiple outcomes in diabetes. *British Journal of Health Psychology, 5,* 27–40.

Hampson, S. E., Glasgow, R. E., & Toobert, D. J. (1990). Personal models of diabetes and their relations to self-care activities. *Health Psychology, 9,* 632–646.

Skinner, T. C., & Hampson, S. E. (1998). Social support and personal models of diabetes in relation to self-care and well-being in adolescents with Type 1 diabetes mellitus. *Journal of Adolescence, 21,* 703–715.

Skinner, T. C., & Hampson, S. E. (2001). Personal models of diabetes in relation to self-care, well-being and glycemic control. *Diabetes Care, 24,* 828 833.

Skinner, T. C., John, M., & Hampson, S. E. (2000). Social support and personal models of diabetes as predictors of self-care and well-being: A longitudinal study of adolescents with diabetes. *Journal of Pediatric Psychology, 25,* 257–267.

PERSONAL MODELS OF
DIABETES QUESTIONNAIRE (PMDQ)

Please circle the answer that best describes how you feel:

1. How serious is your diabetes?
    | *Not all* | *Slightly* | *Fairly serious* | *Very serious* | *Extremely* |
    | *serious* | *serious* | | | *serious* |

2. How important is following your self-care recommendations (for example, diet, exercise, and glucose testing) for controlling your diabetes?
    | *Not all* | *Slightly* | *Fairly* | *Very* | *Extremely* |
    | *important* | *important* | *important* | *important* | *important* |

3. How worried are you about developing complications of diabetes (like eye problems, foot ulcers, heart attacks)?
    | *Not all* | *Slightly* | *Fairly worried* | *Very worried* | *Extremely* |
    | *worried* | *worried* | | | *worried* |

4. How important is controlling your blood glucose level for avoiding complications from diabetes?
    | *Not all* | *Slightly* | *Fairly* | *Very* | *Extremely* |
    | *important* | *important* | *important* | *important* | *important* |

5. How frustrated do you feel when trying to take care of your diabetes?
    | *Not at all* | *Slightly* | *Fairly* | *Very* | *Extremely* |
    | *frustrated* | *frustrated* | *frustrated* | *frustrated* | *frustrated* |

6. How much has having diabetes changed your activities (such as your family and social events, work, or hobbies)?
    | *Not all* | *Slightly* | *Moderately* | *A lot* | *Completely* |

7. How much control do you feel you have over your blood glucose levels?
    | *Some control* | *Slight control* | *Moderate* | *A lot of* | *Complete* |
    | | | *control* | *control* | *control* |

Scoring

Seriousness = 1, 3, 6
Treatment effectiveness = 2, 4
Control = 5 (reversed), 7

Sarah E. Hampson, University of Surrey, UK, May 2001. Used with permission.

19. Diabetes Independence Survey (Parental Version)

Developed by Tim Wysocki, Patricia A. Meinhold, Keith C. Abrams, Martha U. Barnard, William L. Clarke, B. J. Bellando, and Michael J. Bourgeois

INSTRUMENT DESCRIPTION, ADMINISTRATION, AND SCORING GUIDELINES

Appropriate developmental expectations for the acquisition of self-care independence by children with insulin-dependent diabetes mellitus (IDDM) are an important base for teaching (Wysocki, Meinhold, Cox, & Clarke, 1990). The Diabetes Control and Complications Trial (DCCT) finding that maintenance of near-normoglycemia prevents development and slows the progression of long-term complications of IDDM makes even more important an appropriate balance between child autonomy and parental supervision that yields the tightest control. The Diabetes Independence Survey (DIS) was developed to provide data to guide parents and health professionals about this appropriate balance. Mastery of a skill is defined as the ability to complete a task correctly without verbal or physical prompting by another person.

IDS is written at grade 6–7 reading level. Score is 0–38, the number of items on which the parent has marked "yes." A copy of the instrument and age norms may be found on the following page. Age norms provide some guidance to parents, and professional/parent discrepancies can show areas of disagreement (Wysocki et al., 1992).

PSYCHOMETRIC CHARACTERISTICS

Age appropriateness of DIS was initially developed by obtaining from diabetes professionals their estimates of ages at which children typically master diabetes skills and from parents of children ages 3–19 with IDDM about whether their child had mastered each skill (Wysocki et al., 1992). Parents rated young children as more skilled and adolescents as less skilled than did health professionals (Wysocki et al., 1996b).

Composite indices of self-care autonomy and of psychological maturity were used to categorize participants as exhibiting constrained (lower tertile), appropriate (middle tertile), or excessive (higher tertile) self-care autonomy. The excessive self-care autonomy group demonstrated less favorable treatment adherence, hospitalization rates, and marginal glycemic control compared with appropriate and excessive self-care autonomy. Significant positive correlations between DIS and other measures of IDDM knowledge, skill, and responsibility are supportive of validity. Factor analysis showed a single factor (Wysocki et al., 1996a).

Cronbach's coefficient alpha was .91 and agreement between mothers and fathers, .78. DIS scores correlated .71 with age of the child with an independent measure of diabetes information, and with a measure of parent-child sharing of diabetes responsibilities.

CRITIQUE AND SUMMARY

The ultimate usefulness of DIS is to establish norms for skill acquisition that balance children's self-care autonomy with their psychological maturity. To do so requires direct, standardized evaluations of diabetes skill mastery in a large, prospective, and long-term representative sample of children with IDDM. A study of the relative merits of earlier versus later self-care autonomy (Wysocki et al., 1992) could not be located. IDS could be used to evaluate age-appropriateness of diabetes education programs (Wysocki et al., 1996a). Since diabetes care is evolving rapidly, content validity of DIS should be regularly checked. Test–retest reliability still must be checked (Wysocki et al., 1996b).

Because DIS is based on parental report, it is important to avoid overinterpretation of the scores. Although the instrument can be used for research and as a screening and program evaluation instrument in clinical sites, it should not be used alone to determine the IDDM self-care responsibilities expected of a given child (Wysocki et al., 1996a).

REFERENCES

Wysocki, T., Meinhold, P. A., Abrams, K. C., Barnard, M. U., Clarke, W. L., Bellando, B. J., & Bourgeois, M. J. (1992). Parental and professional estimates of self-care independence of children and adolescents with IDDM. *Diabetes Care, 15,* 43–52.

Wysocki, T., Meinhold, P., Cox, D. J., & Clarke, W. L. (1990). Survey of diabetes professionals regarding developmental changes in diabetes self-care. *Diabetes Care, 13,* 65–67.

Wysocki, T., Meinhold, P. M., Taylor, A., Hough, B. S., Barnard, M. U., Clarke, W. L., Bellando, B. J., & Bourgois, M. J. (1996a). Psychometric properties and normative data for the parent version of the Diabetes Independence Survey. *Diabetes Educator, 22,* 587–591.

Wysocki, T., Taylor, A., Hough, B. S., Linscheid, T. R., Yeates, K. O., & Naglieri, J. A. (1996b). Deviation from developmentally appropriate self-care autonomy. *Diabetes Care, 19,* 119–125.

DIABETES INDEPENDENCE SURVEY (DIS)
PARENT VERSION, NORMATIVE DATA

Shown for each item, the age group at which 25%, 50%, and 75% of parents of youths with IDDM answered that item affirmatively.

Does or can your child:	Yes	No	25%	50%	75%
1. Recognize symptoms of low blood sugar and tell someone else about it?			3	4	4
2. Treat low blood sugar by eating something with sugar in it?			3	4	7
3. Know when a low blood sugar reaction might happen and do something to keep it from happening?			6	7	10
4. Know that symptoms of high blood sugar may include extreme thirst, more urination than normal, nausea, vomiting, and fatigue?			6	7	9
5. Know some actions to take to lower high blood sugars?			4	7	8
6. Know when blood sugars may be going too high and do something to keep it from happening?			7	10	15
7. Know why it is important to wear some kind of diabetic identification?			3	4	7
8. Complete a urine ketone test?			6	8	14
9. Prick a finger with a lancet to get a drop of blood for blood sugar tests?			4	5	6
10. Complete a blood sugar test by reading the test strip visually?			6	8	10
11. Complete a blood sugar test using a meter?			4	6	7
12. Write down test results in a logbook?			6	7	9
13. State each type of insulin that he/she uses?			6	8	9
14. State each insulin dose that he/she uses?			7	10	10
15. State the times at which insulin is to be taken each day?			4	5	6
16. Draw up an injection of only one type of insulin?			7	8	10
17. Draw up an injection using a mixture of two types of insulin?			7	10	11

(continued)

Does or can your child:	Yes	No	25%	50%	75%
18. Give him/herself an insulin injection?			5	8	10
19. Use a different site for each insulin injection?			3	6	8
20. Write down insulin type and dose in logbook?			7	8	11
21. State the peak of action of each type of insulin that he/she uses?			10	13	> 18
22. For each type of insulin used, state how long that insulin works?			10	14	> 18
23. Adjust insulin doses according to how high or low the blood sugar is?			10	13	> 18
24. State reasons for a need to change his or her insulin dose?			7	8	12
25. Store the supply of insulin properly?			4	6	8
26. Spot bad insulin and throw it away?			10	14	> 18
27. Categorize food into food groups?			4	6	8
28. Use a meal plan?			7	9	14
29. Use a meal plan in restaurants or cafeterias?			7	10	> 18
30. Adjust how much he/she eats according to how high or low the blood sugar is?			7	9	14
31. State reasons for changing the prescribed diet?			7	10	14
32. State the role of diet in treating diabetes?			5	7	11
33. State that activities like running, swimming, cycling, and racket sports are the best kind of exercise for people with diabetes?			6	7	9
34. Plan daily exercise according to how and when meals and injections are taken?			10	12	> 18
35. Adjust amount of exercise if blood sugar is unusually high or low?			7	9	11
36. Know that exercise should be avoided if he/she is sick or has ketones in his/her urine?			6	10	15
37. State two safety precautions about exercise for people with diabetes?			8	10	16
38. State some foods which are good to eat before exercising?			6	10	10

Wysocki, T., et al. (1996). Psychometric properties and normative data for the parent version of the Diabetes Independence Survey. *The Diabetes Educator, 22,* 587–591.

20. Multidimensional Diabetes Questionnaire

Developed by Arie Nouwen, Julie Gingras, France Talbot, and Stephane Bouchard

INSTRUMENT DESCRIPTION, ADMINISTRATION, AND SCORING GUIDELINES

Research in diabetes has resulted in the development of numerous diabetes-specific measures tapping various psychosocial dimensions. Integrating these measures to define clinically meaningful subgroups of patients in terms of psychosocial adaptation will likely help to target specific interventions individualized to the pattern of coping. The Multidimensional Diabetes Questionnaire (MDQ) is theoretically linked to social learning perspectives.

The MDQ is composed of seven scales grouped into three sections: I. Perception of diabetes and related social support using 3 scales: (a) perceived interference of diabetes, (b) perceived severity of diabetes and its complications, (c) perceived social support for diabetes; II. (a) frequency of positive reinforcing behaviors, and (b) misguided support behaviors; III. (a) self-efficacy about diabetes self-care activities, and (b) outcome expectancies of self-care behavior. These factors have been consistently and significantly correlated to, or shown to predict adjustment to, diabetes.

MDQ is currently available in English and in French. A computer program has been developed that automatically scores MDQ and computes the classification statistics (Nouwen, Gingras, Talbot, & Bouchard, 1997). Section I items are summed with higher scores indicting higher levels of perceived interference, social support, and severity. For section II, higher scores indicate higher levels of positive and misguided reinforcement behaviors. Section III scores indicate level of confidence and importance. Scoring instructions may be found at the end of the questionnaire.

PSYCHOMETRIC CHARACTERISTICS

Item development was based on the experiences of diabetologists, patients, and patients' significant others. Cronbach's alpha for the various scales were: 1a .89, 1b .72, 1c .68, 2a .91, 2b .70, 3a .86, 3b .65. Confirmatory factor analysis conducted on 249 patients with NIDDM supported the instrument's construct validity. A number of psychological correlates of MDQ were found by Talbot and colleagues (1997) and support its validity. Most scales correlated significantly with levels of depressive symptoms. Higher levels of interference as well as lower levels of SE and outcome expectations were significantly related to lower levels of internal health locus of control.

Lower SE beliefs were significantly associated with lower levels of adherence to diet and exercise. Lower levels of social support and reinforcing behaviors were also significantly associated with a poorer adherence to exercise recommendations. Higher levels of interference were significantly associated with a higher number of diabetic complications. Lower levels of SE were significantly related to higher levels of glycosylated hemoglobin, indicating a less adequate metabolic control. Only the Misguided Support Behaviors scale was not correlated with any of the psychological, behavioral, or disease-related indices measured.

CRITIQUE AND SUMMARY

The MDQ was designed to provide a comprehensive assessment of diabetes-related cognitive and social factors—to go beyond multidimensional measures. It is being used as a research instrument. Three clusters of patient adaptation have been identified: adaptive copers, those with low support and not very confident in their ability to carry out self care, and those with spousal overinvolvement. Further validation of these clusters using populations other than those in hospital-based diabetes clinics and measures other than largely self report will be necessary. The interventions that might follow also need to be tested: for those with low support and confidence—support groups, problem solving skills, and SE development might be helpful and for spousal overinvolvement, development of a shared construction of the situation and realistic expectations within the couple (Nouwen, Gingras, Talbot, & Bouchard, 1997). Temporal stability of the MDQ scales and their convergent and discriminant validity remain to be studied (Talbot et al., 1997) as does its sensitivity to intervention.

REFERENCES

Nouwen, A., Gingras, J., Talbot, F., & Bouchard, S. (1997). The development of an empirical psychosocial taxonomy for patients with diabetes. *Health Psychology, 16,* 263–271.

Talbot, F., Nouwen, A., Gingras, J., Gosselin, M., & Audent, J. (1997). The assessment of diabetes-related cognitive and social factors: The Multidimensional Diabetes Questionnaire. *Journal of Behavioral Medicine, 20,* 291–312.

MULTIDIMENSIONAL DIABETES QUESTIONNAIRE

Section I

We are interested to learn more about your diabetes and the way it affects your life. For each question, *circle* the number that corresponds best to your situation.

1. To what extent does your diabetes interfere with your daily activities?

0	1	2	3	4	5	6
Not at all						Extremely

2. To what extent does your spouse (or significant other) support you with your diabetes?
    _____ Check here if you live alone

0	1	2	3	4	5	6
Not at all						Extremely

3. To what extent do you consider your diabetes to be a severe health problem?

0	1	2	3	4	5	6
Not at all						Extremely

4. To what extent does your diabetes decrease your satisfaction or pleasure from social or recreational activities?

0	1	2	3	4	5	6
Not at all						Extremely

5. To what extent do your family and friends support you or help you with your diabetes?

0	1	2	3	4	5	6
Not at all						Extremely

6. To what extent do you worry about long-term complications of diabetes?

0	1	2	3	4	5	6
Not at all						Extremely

7. To what extent does your diabetes interfere with your effectiveness at work?

0	1	2	3	4	5	6
Not at all						Extremely

8. To what extent does your diabetes interfere with your relationship with your spouse (or significant other)?
    _____ Check here if you live alone

0	1	2	3	4	5	6
Not at all						Extremely

9. To what extent do you worry about your diabetes?

0	1	2	3	4	5	6
Not at all						Extremely

(continued)

10. To what extent does your spouse (or significant other) pay attention to you because of your diabetes?

    _____ Check here if you live alone

0	1	2	3	4	5	6
Not at all						Extremely

11. To what extent does your diabetes prevent you from traveling as much as you would like?

0	1	2	3	4	5	6
Not at all						Extremely

12. To what extent does your doctor or health care team support you or help you with your diabetes?

0	1	2	3	4	5	6
Not at all						Extremely

13. To what extent does your diabetes interfere with your ability to participate in social or recreational activities?

0	1	2	3	4	5	6
Not at all						Extremely

14. To what extent does your diabetes interfere with your ability to plan your activities?

0	1	2	3	4	5	6
Not at all						Extremely

15. To what extent does your diabetes prevent you from being as active as you would like?

0	1	2	3	4	5	6
Not at all						Extremely

16. To what extent does your diabetes prevent you from having a schedule that you like (e.g., to sleep late)?

0	1	2	3	4	5	6
Not at all						Extremely

Section II

We are interested to learn about the way your spouse (or significant other) responds to you concerning your self-care program. On the scale listed below each question, *circle* the number that best indicates how often he or she responds to you in that particular way.

My spouse (or significant other):

1. Congratulates me when I follow my diet.

0	1	2	3	4	5	6
Never						Very often

2. Hassles me about my diabetes medication (pills, insulin).

    _____ Check here if you do not take medication for your diabetes

0	1	2	3	4	5	6
Never						Very often

3. Congratulates me for regularly measuring my blood glucose level.
    _____ Check here if self monitoring of blood sugar levels has *not* been recommended
0	1	2	3	4	5	6
Never						Very often

4. Hassles me about exercise.
    _____ Check here if you have been advised *not* to exercise
0	1	2	3	4	5	6
Never						Very often

5. Reminds me to take care of my feet.
    _____ Check here if foot care has *not* been recommended
0	1	2	3	4	5	6
Never						Very often

6. Congratulates me when I follow my meal schedule (meals and snacks).
0	1	2	3	4	5	6
Never						Very often

7. Reminds me to take my diabetes medication (pills, insulin).
    _____ Check here if you do *not* take medication for your diabetes
0	1	2	3	4	5	6
Never						Very often

8. Helps me to adjust my food intake when I exercise.
    _____ Check here if you have been advised *not* to exercise
0	1	2	3	4	5	6
Never						Very often

9. Hassles me about my diet.
0	1	2	3	4	5	6
Never						Very often

10. Plans family activities in a way that allows me to take my medication at the right time.
    _____ Check here if you do *not* take medication for your diabetes
0	1	2	3	4	5	6
Never						Very often

11. Hassles me about measuring my blood sugar.
    _____ Check here if self-monitoring of blood sugar levels has *not* been recommended
0	1	2	3	4	5	6
Never						Very often

12. Encourages me to exercise.
    _____ Check here if you have been advised *not* to exercise
0	1	2	3	4	5	6
Never						Very often

Section III

Treatment of diabetes involves several self-care activities (e.g., diet, exercise, etc.). People sometimes find it difficult, or do not see the importance of following one or more of these self-care activities. We like to know how this applies to you. Read each question carefully and *circle* the number that corresponds best to your situation.

1.   How confident are you in your ability to follow your diet?

/	/	/	/	/	/	/	/	/	/	/
0	10	20	30	40	50	60	70	80	90	100

Not at all   Very
confident   confident

2.   How confident are you in your ability to test your blood sugar at the recommended frequency?
            _____ Check here if measuring of blood sugar levels has **not** been recommended

/	/	/	/	/	/	/	/	/	/	/
0	10	20	30	40	50	60	70	80	90	100

Not at all   Very
confident   confident

3.   How confident are you in your ability to exercise regularly?
            _____ Check here if you have been advised **not** to exercise

/	/	/	/	/	/	/	/	/	/	/
0	10	20	30	40	50	60	70	80	90	100

Not at all   Very
confident   confident

4.   How confident are you in your ability to keep your weight under control?

/	/	/	/	/	/	/	/	/	/	/
0	10	20	30	40	50	60	70	80	90	100

Not at all   Very
confident   confident

5.   How confident are you in your ability to keep your blood sugar level under control?

/	/	/	/	/	/	/	/	/	/	/
0	10	20	30	40	50	60	70	80	90	100

Not at all   Very
confident   confident

6.   How confident are you in your ability to resist food temptations?

/	/	/	/	/	/	/	/	/	/	/
0	10	20	30	40	50	60	70	80	90	100

Not at all   Very
confident   confident

7. How confident are you in your ability to follow your diabetes treatment (diet, medication, blood sugar testing, physical activities)?

/	/	/	/	/	/	/	/	/	/	/
0	10	20	30	40	50	60	70	80	90	100

Not at all   Very
confident   confident

8. To what extent do you think that following your diet is important for controlling your diabetes?

/	/	/	/	/	/	/	/	/	/	/
0	10	20	30	40	50	60	70	80	90	100

Not at all   Very
confident   confident

9. To what extent do you think that taking your medication as recommended (pills, insulin) is important for controlling your diabetes?
    _____ Check here if you do *not* take medication for your diabetes

/	/	/	/	/	/	/	/	/	/	/
0	10	20	30	40	50	60	70	80	90	100

Not at all   Very
confident   confident

10. To what extent do you think that exercise is important for controlling your diabetes?
    _____ Check here if you have been advised *not* to exercise

/	/	/	/	/	/	/	/	/	/	/
0	10	20	30	40	50	60	70	80	90	100

Not at all   Very
confident   confident

11. To what extent do you think that measuring your blood sugar is important for controlling your diabetes?
    _____ Check here if self-monitoring of blood sugar levels has *not* been recommended

/	/	/	/	/	/	/	/	/	/	/
0	10	20	30	40	50	60	70	80	90	100

Not at all   Very
confident   confident

12. To what extent do you think that following your diabetes treatment (diet, medication, blood sugar testing, exercise) is important for controlling your diabetes?

/	/	/	/	/	/	/	/	/	/	/
0	10	20	30	40	50	60	70	80	90	100

Not at all   Very
confident   confident

(continued)

13.   To what extent do you think that following your diabetes treatment (diet, medication, blood sugar testing, exercise) is important for delaying and/or preventing long-term diabetes complications (problems related to eyes, kidneys, heart, or feet)?

/	/	/	/	/	/	/	/	/	/	/
0	10	20	30	40	50	60	70	80	90	100

Not at all   Very
confident   confident

Scoring of the MDQ:
Section I: General perceptions of diabetes and related social support
Interference: items $(1 + 4 + 7 + 8 + 11 + 13 + 14 + 15 + 16) / 9$[a]
Severity: items $(3 + 6 + 9) / 3$
Social support: items $(2 + 5 + 10 + 12) / 4$

Section II: Social incentives related to self-care activities
Positive reinforcing behaviors: items $(1 + 3 + 5 + 6 + 7 + 8 + 10 + 12) / 8$
Misguided reinforcing behaviors: items $(2 + 4 + 9 + 11) / 4$

Section III: Self-efficacy and outcome expectancies
Self-efficacy: items $(1 + 2 + 3 + 4 + 5 + 6 + 7) / 7$
Outcome expectancies: items $(8 + 9 + 10 + 11 + 12 + 13) / 6$

[a]The denominator, which reflects the number of items in that scale, will need to be adjusted if there are missing values for the summed items in a particular scale (i.e, the numerator). For example, if a patient indicated that Question 1 in Section I was not applicable or left this item blank, then the denominator of the interference scale would be 8 rather than 9, and only 8 items would be summed to form the numerator. This type of adjustment should be made for each scale that contains missing values so that a patient's score can be compared with scale norms.

21. Diabetes Self-Management Profile

Developed by Michael A. Harris, Tim Wysocki, Michelle Sadler, Karen Wilkinson, Linda M. Harvey, Lisa M. Buckloh, Nelly Mauras, and Neil H. White

INSTRUMENT DESCRIPTION, ADMINISTRATION, AND SCORING GUIDELINES

Management of Type I diabetes requires patients and their families to implement, monitor, and regulate a complex regimen of exercise, management of hypoglycemia, diet, blood glucose testing, and insulin administration and dose adjustment. Many studies show patients have difficulty consistently doing so. The most reliable and valid measure of these behaviors would require unobtrusive and continuous recording of the patient's diabetes self-management behaviors by a totally accurate observer. The Diabetes Self-Management Profile (DSMP) attempts to assess this complex regimen through semistructured interview.

To minimize response bias, sections are ordered so that management tasks for which nonadherence is more readily admitted are followed by tasks for which nonadherence may be less readily admitted. Administration time is 15–20 minutes. Total and subscale (exercise, hypoglycemia, diet, blood glucose testing, and insulin) scores are obtained (Harris et al., 2000).

PSYCHOMETRIC CHARACTERISTICS

Expert content validation was completed. DSMP was administered to 105 youths 6–15 years of age and their parents or caregivers. Internal consistency for DSMP total was .76, but since reliabilities for subscales were all less than .50 they are unreliable when used separately. Test–retest reliabilities over three months were .67 for DSMP total and less than .5 for subscales. Interrater agreement was .94 for total score with a range of .85–.97 for subscales. Concurrent validity was supported by significant correlations with diabetes quality of life and predictive validity by significant correlations with three of the subscales and glycosylated hemoglobin. Thus, more meticulous self-management was associated with better quality of life and better glycemic control, as would be expected (Harris et al., 2000).

CRITIQUE AND SUMMARY

Diabetic control is affected by genetic and biological factors and characteristics of the regimens including quality of medical management. A sound measure of diabetes self-management must capture adherence with various regimen components which are often uncorrelated and differentially stable over time. Instruments by which to measure these various elements are essential to improved control. In addition, instruments must capture recent advances in diabetes care such as insulin pump therapy, use of rapidly acting insulins, and the application of clinical algorithms for insulin dosage adjustment. DSMP is an effort to accomplish these goals. It has so far been used in research and requires training of both interviewers and raters (Harris et al., 2000).

Establishment of subscales through statistical methods and evidence of sensitivity to instruction could not be located. Reliabilities for subscales are below commonly suggested standards.

REFERENCE

Harris, M. A., Wysocki, T., Sadler, M., Wilkinson, K., Harvey, L. M., Buckloh, L. M., Mauras, N., & White, N. H. (2000). Validation of a structured interview for the assessment of diabetes self-management. *Diabetes Care, 23,* 1301–1304.

DIABETES SELF-MANAGEMENT PROFILE

Child's name:_____

Parent(s) name(s):_____

INSTRUCTIONS
For children under 11 years of age, interview child and parent(s) together. For children 11 years and older, interview child and parent(s) separately.

FOR BASELINE INTERVIEW ONLY:
Taking care of diabetes means doing a lot of different things like taking shots, doing blood sugar tests, following a meal plan, getting exercise, and dealing with low and high blood sugars. It's not easy doing all of these things exactly the way doctors and nurses might want. Very few kids with diabetes do everything exactly according to plan. Sometimes there are other things that grab your attention or you might just forget to take care of your diabetes, even though you may have wanted to. Most kids with diabetes, and their families, develop their own habits for taking care of their diabetes that are comfortable for them. What we're trying to learn in this interview is what you and your family usually do to take care of your diabetes. Your answers won't be shared with anyone else, so you can feel comfortable telling me exactly what you *do*, not just what you think you're supposed to do or what you think I want you to say. So, try to be completely honest with me about what you and your family have usually done in taking care of diabetes in the past three months.

FOR SUBSEQUENT INTERVIEWS:
Remember, that this interview is about what you and your family usually do to take care of diabetes. Again, you should know that I will not be sharing what you tell me with anyone else. Try to be as honest and accurate as you can about what you really did in the past three months.

Exercise

One part of taking care of diabetes is getting regular exercise, like running, bike riding, and swimming. Some kids manage to do this very regularly, while others have a hard time finding the time to get enough exercise. In this part of the interview, I'll be asking about your exercise habits. This could be something like taking part in sports, PE at school, or walking or riding your bike to school. Try to be as honest and accurate as you can about your exercise habits in the past three months.

What kind of exercise do you get? In the past 3 months, how often have you gotten one of those kinds of exercise for at least 20 minutes?

ADHERE #1: EXERCISE
(4) _____   > 3/wk.
(3) _____   2–3/wk.
(1) _____   1/mo.
(0) _____   < 1/mo.
ADH1 = _____ (0–4)

If you get more exercise than usual, or if you plan to get more exercise, do you makes changes in your diet or insulin?

If "yes"—what do you do?

ADHERE #2: EXERCISE, DIET, AND INSULIN
(4) ____ always eats MORE or gives LESS insulin
(3) ____ frequently eats MORE or gives LESS insulin (2–3/wk.)
(2) ____ sometimes eats MORE or gives LESS insulin (1/wk.)
(1) ____ occasionally eats MORE or gives LESS insulin (3/mo.)
(0) ____ eats LESS than usual or gives MORE insulin *or does not adjust diet or insulin*

ADH2 = ____ (0–4)

If you get less exercise than usual, or if you plan to get less exercise, do you makes changes in your diet or insulin?

If "yes"—what do you do?

ADHERE #3: EXERCISE, DIET, AND INSULIN
(4) ____ always eats LESS or gives MORE insulin
(3) ____ frequently eats LESS or gives MORE insulin (2–3/wk.)
(2) ____ sometimes eats LESS or gives MORE insulin (1/wk.)
(1) ____ occasionally eats LESS or gives MORE insulin (3/mo.)
(0) ____ eats MORE than usual or gives LESS insulin *or does not adjust diet or insulin*

ADH3 = ____ (0–4)

Hypoglycemia

Everyone with diabetes has low blood sugar reactions now and then. Your doctor and nurses have probably taught you some things to do to keep low blood sugars from happening and to take care of yourself when they do happen. This part of the interview is about what you usually do about low blood sugar reactions. Try to be as honest and accurate as you can about what you did about low blood sugar in the past 3 months.

What do you feel when you have an insulin reaction or when your sugar is too low? How do you tell when your blood sugar is too low? (check only the ones that the child mentions)

____ trembling	____ fatigue/sleepy	____ crying
____ hunger	____ headache	____ weakness
____ light-headed	____ queasy stomach	____ can't concentrate/
____ pounding heart	____ anxious/tense	difficulty paying
____ sweating	____ cranky/irritable	attention
____ other: _____		

Do you keep something handy in case you have an insulin reaction or your sugar gets too low? For example, when you are at school or at a ball game, or in the car and your sugar gets too low, do you have something handy to eat?

ADHERE #4: SUGAR AVAILABLE
1. YES ____ (1)   2. NO ____ (0)

ADH4 = ____ (0,1)

People manage low blood sugars in many different ways. What do you usually do to treat your low blood sugar reactions?

ADHERE #5: TREATING LOW BLOOD SUGAR
(4) _____ careful to quickly take the prescribed amount of carbohydrates (15gm if applicable) and test blood if possible after 10 minutes
(3) _____ take prescribed amount of carbs and goes on (does not test)
(2) _____ take carbs (not the prescribed amount) without considering how much
(1) _____ continue treatment until symptoms go away
(0) _____ ignore symptoms until he/she gets a chance to do something (waiting until it is convenient to treat symptoms)

ADH5 = _____ (0–4)

Do you wear or carry anything that identifies you as having diabetes, like a card or bracelet? If "yes"—would you show it to me?

ADHERE #6: IDENTIFICATION
(2) _____ wears necklace, bracelet, or charm
(1) _____ carries billfold identification card only
(0) _____ no diabetic identification readily available

ADH6 = _____ (0–2)

Diet

Doctors, nurses, and dieticians ask kids with diabetes to follow a meal plan and to try to eat about the same each day. Lots of things can get in the way of doing this and, even when they try their best, many kids still struggle with eating exactly according to the plan. In this part of the interview, I'll be asking about your eating habits. Try to be as honest and accurate as you can about your eating habits in the past three months.

***Do you weigh your food, count carbs or use exchanges to figure out how much you should eat, or do you generally eat the same amounts of food without using exchanges or counting carbs?If uses exchanges make sure by asking the following: *"What exchanges do you have at breakfast?"*

ADHERE #7: MEASUREMENT OF DIET
(3) _____ uses the exchange list or carb counting as a guide and weighs food or reads labels
(2) _____ uses the exchange list or carb counting as a guide, but knows diet well enough so that he/she can eat the right amounts without weighing or reading labels
(1) _____ eats about the same amounts of food each meal, but doesn't weigh or use exchange list or carb counting
(0) _____ eats the amount he/she is hungry for and doesn't follow any set patterns of types or amounts of foods

ADH7 = _____ (0–3)

It is not always possible for people to eat at the same time every day. Do you ever "delay" eating or not eat when you should? This does not include times when your sugar is too high and you need to wait before eating. For example, if you were supposed to eat at 12:00 noon and you didn't eat until 12:30 or 1:00.

In the past three months, how many times have you delayed meals when you shouldn't have delayed?

ADHERE #8: DELAY OF MEALS
(4) _____ never delays
(4) _____ seldom (1–2 times a quarter)
(3) _____ occasionally (3/mo.)
(2) _____ sometimes (1/wk)
(1) _____ frequently (2–3/wk)
(0) _____ almost always (4 or > per wk)

ADH8 = _____ (0–4)

Most people with diabetes have trouble eating all their meals. Are there ever times when you "skip" eating your meals or when you don't eat at all when you should without making adjustments in your insulin? This does not include times when your sugar is too high or when you're sick. This might be when you skip lunch, for example.

In the past three months, how many meals have you skipped?

ADHERE #9: SKIPPING MEALS
(4) _____ never skip meals
(3) _____ seldom skip meals (1 or 2)
(2) _____ occasionally skip meals (3 or 4)
(1) _____ sometimes skip meals (5 or 6)
(0) _____ frequently skip meals (more than 6)

ADH9 = _____ (0–4)

In the past three months, how many times have you made adjustments to your insulin dose when meals are skipped?

ADHERE #10: ADJUSTING INSULIN WHEN MEALS ARE SKIPPED
(4) _____ never skips without adjusting insulin
(4) _____ seldom (1–2 times a quarter) skips a meal without adjusting insulin
(3) _____ occasionally (few times a month) skips a meal without adjusting insulin
(2) _____ sometimes (1/wk) skips a meal without adjusting insulin
(1) _____ frequently (2–3/wk) skips a meal without adjusting insulin
(0) _____ almost always (4 or more times per week) skips a meal without adjusting insulin

ADH10 = _____ (0–4)

There are foods that we all should avoid such as sweets and fatty foods. Eating some of these foods is not necessarily bad for us. However, eating large amounts of sweets and/or fatty foods is not good for us. In the past three months, how often have you eaten excessive amounts (e.g., above and beyond your allotted carbs) of foods like cookies, cakes, ice cream, chips, pizza, french fries, hot dogs, or others?

ADHERE #11: EATS FOODS THAT AREN'T ON DIET PLAN
(4) _____ never or hardly ever (1–2 times a quarter)
(3) _____ occasionally (few times a month)
(2) _____ sometimes (once a week)
(1) _____ frequently (2–3 times per week)
(0) _____ almost always (4 or more times per week)

ADH11 = _____ (0–4)

Do you sometimes eat "more" food than what's on your diet plan (e.g., more carbs than allotted)? This does not include times when you should eat more when you get more exercise or when your sugar gets low. This might be when you eat because you're extra hungry or you might snack some before dinner.

In the past three months, how often have you eaten more than what is recommended for your diet plan?

ADHERE #12: EATS MORE

(4) _____ never or hardly ever (1–2 times a quarter)

(3) _____ seldom (once a month)

(2) _____ occasionally (few times each month)

(1) _____ frequently (2–3 times per week)

(0) _____ almost daily (4 or more times per week)

ADH12 = _____ (0–4)

If "yes" for eats more—If you eat more than you normally would, do you make any changes in your insulin or have you usually already given your insulin/bolus? What do you do?

ADHERE #13: EATS MORE AND CHANGES INSULIN

(1) _____ gives more insulin when eats more

(0) _____ gives less

(0) _____ does not adjust insulin

ADH13 = _____ (0–1)

Do you sometimes eat "less" food than what's on your diet plan? This does not include when your exercise changes or when you're sick or when your sugar is too high. This might be times when you just don't feel like eating everything on your plate.

In the past 3 months, how often have you eaten less than what is recommended for your diet plan?

ADHERE #14: EATS LESS

(4) _____ never or hardly ever (1–2 times a quarter)

(3) _____ seldom (once a month)

(2) _____ occasionally (few times each month)

(1) _____ frequently (2–3 times per week)

(0) _____ almost daily (4 or more times per week)

ADH14 = _____ (0–4)

If "yes" for eats less—If you eat less than you normally would, do you make any changes in your insulin or have you usually already given your insulin/bolus? What do you do?

ADHERE #15: EATS LESS AND CHANGES INSULIN

(1) _____ gives LESS insulin when eats less

(0) _____ gives MORE insulin when eats less

(0) _____ does not adjust insulin

ADH15 = _____ (0–1)

Blood Glucose Testing

Some kids do all of their blood sugar tests, but lots of other kids have trouble doing all of the tests their doctors and nurses want them to do. Next, I'll be asking about your habits when it comes to testing your blood sugar. Try to be as honest and accurate as you can about your testing habits in the past 3 months.

In the past 3 months, how often have you tested your blood?

ADHERE #16: FREQUENCY OF BLOOD TESTING

(4) _____ 4 or more times *daily*

(3) _____ 2 or 3 times *daily*

(2) _____ at least once *daily*
(1) _____ at least 4 times *a week*
(0) _____ does not test, or tests less than 4 times *weekly*

ADH16 = _____ (0–4)

How often has the doctor suggested that you test?

DOCTOR BLOOD TESTING: DOCTOR'S PRESCRIPTION OF BLOOD TESTING
(4) _____ at least 4 or more times *daily*
(3) _____ at least 2 or 3 times *daily*
(2) _____ at least once *daily*
(1) _____ at least four times a *week*
(0) _____ does not know

DBT = _____ (0–4)

TO CALCULATE ADH17 USE THE FOLLOWING TABLE: (Directions: subtract ADH16 from DBT, then use the corresponding number from ADH17 table)

DBT – ADH16:	ADH17 SCORE:
4	0
3	1
2	2
1	3
0	4

ADH17 = _____ (0–4)

In the past three months, how often have you adjusted your insulin dose, your diet, or your exercise when your blood sugar test results were running high?

ADHERE #18
(4) _____   Made an adjustment every time it was needed
(3) _____   Usually made an adjustment when needed (> 75%)
(2) _____   Sometimes made an adjustment when needed (> 50%)
(1) _____   Infrequently made an adjustment when needed (< 50%)
(0) _____   Never made an adjustment

ADH18 = _____ (0–4)

**Do you ever test your urine for ketones?
1. Yes _____   2. No _____
If "yes"—When do you test?

ADHERE #19: FREQUENCY OF URINE TESTING
(3) _____   tests when sugar is high OR when sick
(2) _____   tests only when sick
(1) _____   rarely tests
(0) _____   does not test for ketones

ADH19 = _____ (0–3)

Insulin

Taking insulin shots includes measuring the doses carefully, taking the shots on time, and maybe changing your dose depending on your blood sugar test results. This is all very complicated and takes time that many kids would prefer to spend doing other things. This part of the interview is about what you usually do about your insulin shots. Try to be totally honest when you answer my questions.

In the last three months, how often have you delayed taking your insulin? (*For Insulin Pump Users*) In the last three months, how often have you delayed a bolus when you shouldn't have delayed?

ADHERE #20: DELAYING SHOTS

(4) _____   never, always take insulin on time
(3) _____   delayed once a month or less (1–3 in a quarter)
(2) _____   delayed once a week or less
(0) _____   delayed more than once a week

ADH20 = _____ (0–4)

In the past three months, how often have you taken more than the prescribed amount of insulin? (*For Insulin Pump Users*) In the last three months, how often have you bolused more insulin than you should have bolused?

ADHERE #21: TAKING MORE THAN PRESCRIBED INSULIN

(4) _____   always took prescribed amount
(3) _____   took more than prescribed amount (1–3 times)
(2) _____   took more than prescribed amount (4–6 times)
(1) _____   took more than prescribed amount (7–10 times)
(0) _____   took more than prescribed amount more than 10 times

ADH21 = _____ (0–4)

In the past three months, how often have you taken less than the prescribed amount of insulin? (*For Insulin Pump Users*) In the last three months, how often have you bolused less than you should have bolused?

ADHERE #22: TAKING LESS THAN PRESCRIBED INSULIN

(4) _____   always took the prescribed amount
(3) _____   took less than prescribed amount (1–3 times)
(2) _____   took less than prescribed amount (4–6 times)
(1) _____   took less than prescribed amount (7–10 times)
(0) _____   took less than prescribed amount more than 10 times

ADH22 = _____ (0–4)

In the last three months, how often have you missed giving an insulin shot because you forgot or were too busy? (*For Insulin Pump Users*) In the last three months, how often have you missed a bolus because you forgot or were too busy or failed to give your basal insulin because your pump was not working or inserted?

ADHERE #23: REMEMBERING TO TAKE SHOTS

(4) _____   never forgot, always take insulin
(3) _____   forgot once a month or less (1–3 in a quarter)
(2) _____   forgot once a week or less
(0) _____   forgot more than once a week

ADH23 = _____ (0–4)

Validity and Reliability Data

Harris, M. A., Wysocki, T., Sadler, M., Wilkinson, K., Harvey, L., Buckloh, L., Mauras, N., & White, N. H. (2000). Validation of a structured interview for the assessment of diabetes self-management. *Diabetes Care, 23,* 1301–1304.

FAMILY NUMBER: _____ DATE: _____ EVALUATION: _____
RESPONDENT: YOUTH / PARENT / BOTH

Score Sheet
Diabetes Self-Management Profile (DSMP)

EXERCISE	HYPOGLYCEMIA	DIET	GLUCOSE TESTING	INSULIN
ADH1 ____ FREQ	ADH4 ____ EMERG	ADH7 ____ MEASURE	ADH16 ____ FREQ	ADH20 ____ DELAY
ADH2 ____ MORE	ADH5 ____ TREAT	ADH8 ____ DELAY	ADH17 ____ DIFFER	ADH21 ____ MORE
ADH3 ____ LESS	ADH6 ____ ID	ADH9 ____ SKIP	ADH18 ____ ADJUST	ADH22 ____ LESS
Type of Exercise	Symptoms	ADH10 ____ SKIP ADJ	ADH19 ____ KETONE	ADH23 ____ SKIP
_____	trembling	ADH11 ____ TABOO	DBT = ____ **	
_____	light headed	ADH12 ____ MORE	DBT – ADH16 = ADH17	
_____	hungry	ADH13 ____ MORE ADJ	4 0	
_____	heart pounding	ADH14 ____ LESS	3 1	
	sweating	ADH15 ____ LESS ADJ	2 2	
	weakness		1 3	
	crying		0 4	
	fatigue/sleepy			
	headache		**not added to total score	
	stomach upset			
	anxious/tense			
	cranky/irritable			
	other			

EXERCISET ____ + HYPOT ____ + DIETT ____ + GLUCOSET ____ + INSULINT ____ = ADHT ____
  (0–12)   (0–7)   (0–29)   (0–15)   (0–16)   (0–79)

22. Diabetes Empowerment Scale

Developed by Robert M. Anderson, Martha M. Funnell, James T. Fitzgerald, and David G. Marrero

INSTRUMENT DESCRIPTION, ADMINISTRATION, AND SCORING GUIDELINES

Diabetes is a self-managed disease which requires much in the way of lifestyle changes. To be successful, education should equally address blood glucose management and the psychosocial challenges of living with diabetes. The Diabetes Empowerment Scale (DES) is basically a self-efficacy scale built around a model of patient education called "empowerment," which incorporates assessing satisfaction, setting goals, solving problems, emotional coping, managing stress, obtaining support, motivating oneself, and making decisions. Scores are summed with higher scores indicating higher levels of psychosocial self-efficacy (Anderson et al., 1995; Anderson, Funnell, Fitzgerald, & Marrero, 2000).

PSYCHOMETRIC CHARACTERISTICS

Factor analysis yielded three subscales: 1) managing psychosocial aspects of diabetes (alpha = .93); 2) assessing dissatisfaction and readiness to change (alpha = .81); and 3) setting and achieving diabetes goals (alpha = .91); total scale alpha was .96. Test–retest reliability was .79. In a randomized controlled trial (RCT), the empowerment intervention group showed gains over the control group on four of the eight SE subscales, providing some evidence of scale sensitivity (Anderson et al., 1995; Anderson, Funnell, Fitzgerald, & Marrero, 2000). Description of the program did not clarify whether intervention elements known to increase SE were incorporated, thus perhaps not providing a strong test of sensitivity of DES. The intervention group also showed a modest improvement in blood glucose levels (Anderson, Funnell, Fitzgerald, & Marrero, 2000).

DES correlated positively with a measure of psychosocial adjustment to diabetes and in the expected direction with patients' self-reported comfort in asking questions of their physician and their self-reported positive adjustment to diabetes. DES had positive correlations with the self-reported Diabetes Understanding Scale (Anderson, Funnell, Fitzgerald, & Marrero, 2000). These findings support claims of validity. Via and Salyer (1999) used the final version of DES in a before and after education study with male veterans. In this study, Cronbach's alpha for the total scale was .96. Blood glucose measures were not correlated with DES but patients' self reported understanding of diabetes was.

CRITIQUE AND SUMMARY

It must be noted that this is not an SE scale for diabetes self-management, but rather for general psychosocial SE related to diabetes. The authors see its primary purpose as an outcome of successful clinical or educational interventions (Anderson, Funnell, Fitzgerald, & Marrero, 2000). Further research with different samples of diabetic patients will be required to confirm the factor structure and subscale reliability of the DES. Longitudinal studies measuring glucose control and using DES to correlate the subscales with outcomes of self management would be helpful to establish the predictive validity of the instrument (Via & Salyer, 1999). It is unusual to use a strongly agree to strongly disagree response for an SE measure.

DES is a welcome addition to instruments available to examine psychosocial factors in self-management of diabetes.

REFERENCES

Anderson, R. M., Funnell, M. M., Butler, P. M., Arnold, M. S., Fitzgerald, J. J., & Feste, C. C. (1995). Patient empowerment: Results of a randomized controlled trial. *Diabetes Care, 18,* 943–949.

Anderson, R. M., Funnell, M. M., Fitzgerald, J. J., & Marrero, D. G. (2000). The Diabetes Empowerment Scale: A measure of psychosocial self-efficacy. *Diabetes Care, 23,* 739–743.

Via, P. S., & Salyer, J. (1999). Psychosocial self-efficacy and personal characteristics of veterans attending a diabetes education program. *Diabetes Educator, 25,* 727–737.

DIABETES EMPOWERMENT SCALE

PLEASE ANSWER THE FOLLOWING QUESTIONS

BACKGROUND:

1. Sex: Male ❏   Female ❏
2. How old are you? _____ years old
3. How long ago were you told by a doctor that you had diabetes? _____ years
4. Which type of diabetes did your doctor say that you have?
   ❏ insulin-dependent diabetes, also called juvenile or Type 1 diabetes
   ❏ non insulin-dependent diabetes, also called adult onset or Type 2 diabetes (some people with non insulin-dependent diabetes take insulin)
5. How often does your diabetes prevent you from doing your normal daily activities (could not work or go to school)? Circle one number.

   Never   Frequently
   1   2   3   4   5   6   7

6. Have you ever attended a diabetes patient education program (a series of classes)?
   ❏ No   ❏ Yes (If "Yes," how many years ago? ____)
7. How would you rate your understanding of diabetes and its treatment? Circle one number.

   Poor   Excellent
   1   2   3   4   5   6   7

8. How much schooling have you *completed*?
   ❏ 8th grade or less
   ❏ some high school
   ❏ high school graduate
   ❏ some college or technical school
9. Are you now taking diabetes pills? ❏ Yes   ❏ No
10. Are you now taking insulin? ❏ Yes   ❏ No
11. Have you *always* treated your diabetes with insulin? ❏ Yes   ❏ No
12. What is your height? _____ feet _____ inches
13. How much do you weigh? _____ pounds
14. Please circle the number that indicates how able you are to fit diabetes into your life in a positive manner.

    Not At All   Very
    Able   Able
    1   2   3   4   5   6   7

15. Please circle the number that indicates how comfortable you feel asking your doctor questions about diabetes.

    Not At All   Very
    Comfortable   Comfortable
    1   2   3   4   5   6   7

Attitudes Toward Diabetes—DES

	Strongly Agree	Agree	Neutral	Disagree	Strongly Disagree
In general, I believe that I:					
1. . . . know what part(s) of taking care of my diabetes that I am **satisfied** with.	( )	( )	( )	( )	( )
2. . . . know what part(s) of taking care of my diabetes that I am **dissatisfied** with.	( )	( )	( )	( )	( )
3. . . . know what part(s) of taking care of my diabetes that I am ready to change.	( )	( )	( )	( )	( )
4. . . . know what part(s) of taking care of my diabetes that I am **not** ready to change.	( )	( )	( )	( )	( )
5. . . . can choose realistic diabetes goals.	( )	( )	( )	( )	( )
6. . . . know which of my diabetes goals are most important to me.	( )	( )	( )	( )	( )
7. . . . know the things about **myself** that either help or prevent me from reaching my diabetes goals.	( )	( )	( )	( )	( )
8. . . . can come up with good ideas to help me reach my goals.	( )	( )	( )	( )	( )
9. . . . am able to turn my diabetes goals into a workable plan.	( )	( )	( )	( )	( )
10. . . . can reach my diabetes goals once I make up my mind.	( )	( )	( )	( )	( )
11. . . . know which **barriers** make reaching my diabetes goals more difficult.	( )	( )	( )	( )	( )
12. . . . can **think** of different ways to overcome barriers to my diabetes goals.	( )	( )	( )	( )	( )

	Strongly Agree	Agree	Neutral	Disagree	Strongly Disagree
13. . . . can try out different ways of overcoming barriers to my diabetes goals.	( )	( )	( )	( )	( )
14. . . . am able to decide which way of overcoming barriers to my diabetes goals works best for me.	( )	( )	( )	( )	( )
15. . . . can tell how I'm feeling about **having** diabetes.	( )	( )	( )	( )	( )
16. . . . can tell how I'm feeling about **caring** for my diabetes.	( )	( )	( )	( )	( )
17. . . . know the ways that having diabetes causes stress in my life.	( )	( )	( )	( )	( )
18. . . . know the **positive** ways I cope with diabetes-related stress.	( )	( )	( )	( )	( )
19. . . . know the **negative** ways I cope with diabetes-related stress.	( )	( )	( )	( )	( )
20. . . . can cope well with diabetes-related stress.	( )	( )	( )	( )	( )
21. . . . know where I can get support for having and caring for my diabetes.	( )	( )	( )	( )	( )
22. . . . can ask for support for having and caring for my diabetes when I need it.	( )	( )	( )	( )	( )
23. . . . can support myself in dealing with my diabetes.	( )	( )	( )	( )	( )
24. . . . know what helps me stay motivated to care for my diabetes.	( )	( )	( )	( )	( )
25. . . . can motivate myself to care for my diabetes.	( )	( )	( )	( )	( )
26. . . . know enough about diabetes to make self-care choices that are right for me.	( )	( )	( )	( )	( )

(continued)

	Strongly Agree	Agree	Neutral	Disagree	Strongly Disagree
27. . . . know enough about myself as a person to make diabetes care choices that are right for me.	( )	( )	( )	( )	( )
28. . . . am able to figure out if it is worth my while to change how I take care of my diabetes.	( )	( )	( )	( )	( )

Thank you very much for completing this questionnaire.

Diabetes Empowerment Scale (DES) Scoring Key

The DES measures the patient's self-efficacy related to:
Subscales & Items

I.   Managing the psychosocial aspects of diabetes (9 items)   (18, 20–27)

II. Assessing dissatisfaction and readiness to change (9 items)   (1–4, 15–17, 19, 28)

III. Setting and achieving diabetes goals (10 items)   (5–14)

The scoring of the DES is straightforward and is based on completed items. An item checked "strongly agree" receives 5 points; "agree" — 4 points; "neutral" — 3 points; "disagree" — 2 points; and "strongly disagree" receives 1 point. The numerical values for a set of items in a particular subscale (for example: items 5–14 in the "Goal Setting" subscale) are added and the total is divided by the number of items (in this case 10) in the subscale. The resulting value is the score for that subscale. An overall score for the DES can be calculated by adding all of the item scores and dividing by 28.

Robert D. Anderson, Martha M. Funnell, Thomas Fitzgerald. University of Michigan, Diabetes Research and Training Center. Used with permission.

Section C

Arthritis and Other Rheumatic Diseases

Like other chronic disorders, rheumatic diseases including arthritis require a strong sense of patient self-efficacy. The Arthritis SE Scale is perhaps the most widely studied and tested instrument in this book and has served as a model for similar instruments with other chronic diseases.

---

23. Rheumatology Attitudes Index

Developed by Leigh Callahan, Health Report Services

INSTRUMENT DESCRIPTION, ADMINISTRATION, AND SCORING GUIDELINES

The Rheumatology Attitudes Index (RAI) is a revision of the Arthritis Helplessness Index (AHI), originally established to measure motivational, cognitive, and emotional deficits found in individuals who are forced to deal with stressful situations, in this case rheumatic disease. The largely unpredictable nature of the remissions and exacerbations in rheumatic disease may contribute to uncertainty, feelings of helplessness, passive resignation, and a sense of loss of control. Helplessness generally refers to a psychological state in which individuals expect that their efforts will be ineffective (DeVellis & Callahan, 1993).

Although the constructs of learned helplessness, health locus of control (expectation about whether one's health is controlled by one's own behavior or by external forces), self-esteem (evaluation of self-worth), and self-efficacy (beliefs regarding one's own capabilities in specific situations) appear related in most patients, they are, in part, independent. Further research is needed to better understand distinctions among them and associations of specific constructs with specific disease status measures (Callahan, Brooks, & Pincus, 1988).

The RAI is a modification on the AHI in which the items have been reworded to be applicable to rheumatic diseases more generally instead of rheumatoid arthritis specifically and a fifth, neutral response option has been added to the original four options. The RAI consists of 15 belief statements, scored on a 5-point Likert scale: strongly disagree (1), disagree (2), do not agree or disagree (3), agree (4), or strongly agree (5). Scores are reversed for items 2, 3, 5, 6, 8, 9, 11, 13, and 15, summed, and can range from 15 to 75. A higher score indicates a greater sense of control (Callahan et al., 1988).

PSYCHOMETRIC PROPERTIES

The original development study of the AHI showed a Cronbach's alpha of .69, a test–retest reliability of .52 over a 1-year period, and a unidimensional scale. It was later shown to be composed of two relatively independent subscales of internality and personal helplessness. Tests of the AHI found greater perceived helplessness correlated with greater age, lesser education, lower self-esteem, lower internal health locus of control, higher anxiety, depression, and impairment in performing activities of daily living. Changes in AHI scores were strongly correlated with changes in difficulty scores in individual patients, reflecting overall disease severity. The AHI was thought to be useful in clinical evaluation and screening of patients who might benefit from psychosocial interventions, such as education to promote independence and better coping skills (Nicassio, Wallston, Callahan, Herbert, & Pincus, 1985).

In yet another study, perceived helplessness as measured by the AHI and disease severity were the two best predictors of physical functioning cross-sectionally and longitudinally, accounting for 35% to 59% of the variance in physical functioning (Lorish, Abraham, Austin, Bradley, & Alarcon, 1991).

The modified renamed scale (RAI) was found to have an alpha reliability coefficient of .68, an indication that the RAI and the AHI provide similar information. There was support for external criterion validity in significant correlations between RAI scores and physical measures of disease status including joint count, grip strength, walking time, and button test, and self-report scores for difficulty, dissatisfaction, and pain in activities of daily living (Callahan et al., 1998).

A study of the factor structure of the RAI was based on 1,420 individuals with rheumatoid arthritis in 11 cities, with a mean formal education of 12.5 years. The study found two relatively independent scales, which tap separate constructs. One scale measures more of an arthritis specific internal locus of control dimension (items 2, 3, 5, 6, 8, and 9, with a Cronbach's alpha of .75 and a stability coefficient of .59 over 6 months) and a helplessness scale (items 1, 10, 12, 13 reverse scored, and 14, with a Cronbach's alpha of .63 and a stability coefficient of .64 over 6 months). The helplessness subscale is the more clinically useful, associated with greater adjustment difficulties including measures of noncompliance with recommended treatment regimens, greater use of passive pain coping behaviors, and higher impairment in functional status. This scale also appears to be sensitive to changes over time, showing distinct differences in psychological functioning, and behavior and symptom severity 2 years after the original assessment (Stein, Wallston, & Nicassio, 1988).

The helplessness scale by itself has been found to be more significantly related to grip strength; button-test time; 25-foot walking time; joint tenderness, swelling, limited motion, deformity, total joint count, and erythrocyte sedimentation rate than was the entire RAI. The authors believe this scale constitutes an acceptable measure of helplessness for research and for screening purposes. Because there is no widely accepted measure of general helplessness, it is difficult to show concurrent validity between the general concept and the rheumatology-specific measures (DeVellis & Callahan, 1993).

Although development of the RAI was accomplished with patients with rheumatoid arthritis, subsequent studies have provided information about its measurement characteristics with patients with systemic lupus erythematosis. As with studies cited previously, Cronbach's alpha was .70, and there were significant correlations with self-reported physical disability, dissatisfaction, and pain scores (Engle, Callahan, Pincus, & Hochberg, 1990).

Burckhardt, Mannerkorpi, Hedenberg, and Bjelle (1994) used RAI in a trial of education and education with physical training for women with fibromyalgia (FMS). Classes included information on FMS, the role of stress in the development and maintenance of symptoms, coping strategies, problem-solving techniques, assertiveness training, relaxation strategies, and the importance of physical conditioning. After each educational session, the second experimental group was given an additional hour of physical training. Although the control group did not change significantly on the index, the education group changed significantly in a positive direction.

Burkhardt and Bjelle (1996) found the Swedish version of RAI to have acceptable reliability (Cronbach's alpha from .64–.78, test–retest at 4 weeks during which disease severity remained stable at .69–.79), evidence of validity in the relationship with ability to control pain and perceived quality of life, two distinct factors (internality and helplessness) on factor analysis, and evidence of sensitivity to change related to an educational strategy designed to increase patient ability to self-manage their symptoms.

Recently, a group of investigators studied psychometric characteristics of the RAI in Asian patients with systemic lupus erythematosis (SLE). Factor analysis corresponded to internality and helplessness factors found in the original factor analysis with patients with rheumatoid arthritis with Cronbach's alpha of .77 for the internality scale and .64 for the helplessness scale, and .74 for the RAI. Test–retest after 8 days found clinically insignificant differences. Construct validity was supported (Thumboo et al., 1999).

CRITIQUE AND SUMMARY

Considerable evidence of the RAI's psychometric characteristics has been accumulated by study of American, Swedish, and Asian patients. One potential use of the RAI would be to identify patient subgroups who are more likely to benefit from patient education. Because the reliabilities are at the low end of the acceptable range, the scales may be adequate, at present, for research or general screening purposes but should not be used by themselves for making individual clinical judgments. In addition, the items did not factor as clearly as one might hope, raising concerns about validity (DeVellis & Callahan, 1993). Because rheumatic diseases are painful and often unpredictable, obtaining a sense of control over symptoms is a difficult but important task for patients. The lack of correlations between RAI and objective disease severity measures suggests that the painful tender points of fibromyalgia and the inflammation of rheumatoid arthritis exist independent of a patient's sense of personal control or feelings of helplessness (Burckhardt & Bjelle, 1996).

REFERENCES

Burckhardt, C. S., & Bjelle, A. (1996). Perceived control: a comparison of women with fibromyalgia, rheumatoid arthritis and systemic lupus erythematosis using a Swedish version of the Rheumatology Attitudes Index. *Scandinavian Journal of Rheumatology, 25,* 300–306.

Burckhardt, C. S., Mannerkorpi, K., Hedenberg, L., & Bjelle, A. (1994). A randomized controlled clinical trial of education and physical training for women with fibromyalgia. *Journal of Rheumatology, 21,* 714–720.

Callahan, L. F., Brooks, R. H., & Pincus, T. (1988). Further analysis of learned helplessness in rheumatoid arthritis using a "Rheumatology Attitudes Index." *Journal of Rheumatology, 15,* 418–425.

DeVellis, R. F., & Callahan, L. F. (1993). A brief measure of helplessness in rheumatic disease: The helplessness subscale of the Rheumatology Attitudes Index. *Journal of Rheumatology, 20,* 866–869.

Engle, E. W., Callahan, L. F., Pincus, T., & Hochberg, M. C. (1990). Learned helplessness in systemic lupus erythematosis: Analysis using the Rheumatology Attitudes Index. *Arthritis and Rheumatism, 33,* 281–286.

Lorish, C. D., Abraham, N., Austin, J., Bradley, L. A., & Alarcon, G. S. (1991). Disease and psychosocial factors related to physical functioning in rheumatoid arthritis. *Journal of Rheumatology, 18,* 1150–1157.

Nicassio, P. M., Wallston, K. A., Callahan, L. F., Herbert, M., & Pincus, T. (1985). The measurement of helplessness in rheumatoid arthritis: The development of the Arthritis Helplessness Index. *Journal of Rheumatology, 12,* 462–467.

Stein, M. J., Wallston, K. A., & Nicassio, P. M. (1988). Factor structure of the Arthritis Helplessness Index. *Journal of Rheumatology, 15,* 427–432.

Thumboo, J., et al. (1999). The Rheumatology Attitudes Index and its helplessness subscale are valid and reliable measures of learned helplessness in Asian patients systemic lupus erythematosis. *Journal of Rheumatology, 26,* 1512–1517.

RHEUMATOLOGY ATTITUDES INDEX

Question	Strongly disagree	Disagree	Do not agree or disagree	Agree	Strongly agree
1.* My condition is controlling my life.	1	2	3	4	5
2.* Managing my condition is largely my own responsibility.	1	2	3	4	5
3.† I can reduce my pain by staying calm and relaxed.	1	2	3	4	5
4.† Too often, my pain just seems to hit me from out of the blue.	1	2	3	4	5
5.* If I do all the right things, I can successfully manage my condition.	1	2	3	4	5
6.* I can do a lot of things myself to cope with my condition.	1	2	3	4	5
7.* When it comes to managing my condition, I feel I can only do what my doctor tells me to do.	1	2	3	4	5
8.* When I manage my personal life well, my condition does not flare as much.	1	2	3	4	5
9.† I have considerable ability to control my pain.	1	2	3	4	5
10.* I would feel helpless if I couldn't rely on other people for help with my condition.	1	2	3	4	5
11.* Usually, I can tell when my condition will flare.	1	2	3	4	5
12.† No matter what I do, or how hard I try, I just can't seem to get relief from my pain.	1	2	3	4	5
13.* I am coping effectively with my condition.	1	2	3	4	5
14.* It seems as though fate and other factors beyond my control affect my condition.	1	2	3	4	5
15.* I want to learn as much as I can about my condition.	1	2	3	4	5
Total Score					

*The word "condition" is used in the RAI in lieu of "arthritis" in the Arthritis Helplessness Index.
†The statement is identical in the RAI and Arthritis Helplessness Index.
From Callahan, L. F., Brooks, R. H., & Pincus, T. (1988). Further analysis of learned helplessness in rheumatoid arthritis using a "Rheumatology Attitudes Index." *Journal of Rheumatology, 15,* 418–425.
Used with permission: Health Services Report.

24. Patient Knowledge Questionnaire in Rheumatoid Arthritis

Developed by J. Hill, H. A. Bird, R. Hopkins, C. Lawton, and V. Wright

INSTRUMENT DESCRIPTION, ADMINISTRATION, AND SCORING GUIDELINES

In therapy of rheumatoid arthritis (RA), patients must adjust daily exercise regimens, rest/activity periods, and drug regimens according to the changing activity of their disease. The authors believe that knowledge of the disease and its treatment is necessary to carry out these self-care tasks. Scoring is indicated on the test. Total score is 30, with a maximum score of 9 on the general knowledge section, 7 for questions on drugs, and 7 for questions on exercise (Hill, Bird, Harmer, Wright, & Lawton, 1994).

In one administration (Hill, Bird, Hopkins, Lawton, & Wright, 1991), some patients thought that nonsteroidal anti-inflammatory drugs (NSAIDs) stopped the disease from progressing, two people thought exercise could cure RA, and patients had difficulty in distinguishing between joint protection and energy conservation.

PSYCHOMETRIC PROPERTIES

Topics in the Patient Knowledge Questionnaire in Rheumatoid Arthritis (PKQ) included those which patients had identified as important: general knowledge including etiology, symptoms, and tests; drugs and how to take them; exercise regimens; joint protection; and pacing and priorities. After three revisions, the PKQ was considered suitable for piloting with 40 patients, after which items with an index of difficulty of more than .75 were removed or altered to avoid ceiling effects. It was then repiloted with 29 patients with a mean score of 15.2 and range of 5 to 24. The Kuder Richardson for internal consistency was .72 and for test–retest reliability .81, with a 4-week interval (Hill et al., 1994).

Seventy randomly selected patients with RA in the outpatient clinic of a large teaching hospital completed the PKQ. There was a wide variation in total scores ranging from 3 to 28 out of 30, with a mean of 16 (Hill et al., 1991). A later study (Hill et al., 1994) showed a significant increase in PKQ scores after instruction, especially for those cared for by a rheumatology nurse practitioner (mean score = 22) as opposed to those cared for in a clinic (mean score = 16.2).

Subsequent use of the PKQ compared scores among patients who had the disease for a year or less and a group who had it 10 years or more and found no statistically significant differences. Mean values may be found in Barlow, Cullen, and Rowe (1999).

CRITIQUE AND SUMMARY

More explicit establishment of the content of the domains of knowledge to be tested and expert and patient judgment about the representativeness of the items would be helpful. It would also be helpful to test the notion that this knowledge is important for carrying out self-care regimens. Theory would suggest that items testing problem-solving skills in using the knowledge would be more predictive than would the factual knowledge tested in the PKQ. In view of Barlow, Cullen, and Rowe's (1999) findings, it would be helpful to check differences on the PKQ of groups who ought to show differences on a basis other than length of disease.

REFERENCES

Barlow, J. H., Cullen, L. A., & Rowe, I. F. (1999). Comparison of knowledge and psychological well-being between patients with short disease duration (less than or equal to 1 year) and patients with more established rheumatoid arthritis (greater than or equal to ten years duration). *Patient Education and Counseling, 38,* 195–203.

Hill, J., Bird, H. A., Harmer, R., Wright, V., & Lawton, C. (1994). An evaluation of the effectiveness, safety and acceptability of a nurse practitioner in a rheumatology outpatient clinic. *British Journal of Rheumatology, 33,* 283–288.

Hill, J., Bird, H. A., Hopkins, R., Lawton, C., & Wright, V. (1991). The development and use of a patient knowledge questionnaire in rheumatoid arthritis. *British Journal of Rheumatology, 30,* 45–49.

RHEUMATISM RESEARCH UNIT
UNIVERSITY OF LEEDS
KNOWLEDGE QUESTIONNAIRE

This questionnaire has been devised to help us find out how arthritis affects your life.
All your answers will remain strictly confidential.
Could you please answer the questions by circling the letter opposite your answer as in the example below.

1.   What is the name of the type of arthritis you have?
      A.   Ankylosing Spondylitis
      Ⓑ.   Rheumatoid Arthritis
      C.   Fibrositis
      D.   Osteoarthritis

IT IS IMPORTANT TO TRY TO ANSWER ALL THE QUESTIONS

1.   Can you choose TWO true statements from the following list?

Rheumatoid Arthritis

      A.   is inherited from your parents.
      B.   starts after a joint has been damaged.
      C.   is caused by cold damp weather.
      D.   the cause is not known.
      E.   may be triggered by a bacteria or virus.
      F.   Don't know

2.   Can you choose TWO true statements from the following list?
      Rheumatoid Arthritis

      A.   affects only the bones of the body.
      B.   occasionally affects the lungs, eyes, or other tissues.
      C.   is most common in old age.
      D.   is a long-term disease.
      E.   is curable.
      F.   Don't know

3.   Can you choose THREE symptoms which can be caused by Rheumatoid Arthritis?

      A.   Anaemia.
      B.   Nodules.
      C.   Overweight.
      D.   Hair loss.
      E.   High blood pressure.
      F.   Fatigue.
      G.   Don't know

4. Can you choose TWO blood tests which are used to assess how active your arthritis is?

    A. Cholesterol level (CL).
    B. Erythrocyte sedimentation rate (ESR).
    C. Blood group.
    D. Plasma viscosity (PV).
    E. Plasma protein.
    F. Don't know

5. Can you choose TWO true statements about non-steroidal anti-inflammatory drugs?

    A. They stop the disease from progressing.
    B. They take many weeks to start working.
    C. They reduce pain, swelling, and stiffness.
    D. They need only be taken when the pain is bad.
    E. They should be taken with food.
    F. Don't know

6. Can you choose the ONE most common side effect that non-steroidal anti-inflammatory tablets can cause?

    A. Itching of the skin.
    B. Indigestion.
    C. Bruising.
    D. Dry mouth.
    E. Loss of taste.
    F. Don't know

7. Can you choose TWO "long-term drugs" which can put the disease into remission?

    A. D-penicillamine also called Distamine, Pendramine.
    B. Diclofenac also called Voltarol.
    C. Indomethacin also called Indocid, Indocid "R," Imbrilon.
    D. Sulphasalazine also called Salazopyrin, E/C Salazopyrin.
    E. Ibuprofen also called Brufen, Fenbid, Nurofen.
    F. Don't know

8. Can you choose TWO true statements about pain killing tablets?

    Pain killers

    A. are not addictive.
    B. should only be taken when pain is severe.
    C. should be taken before carrying out an activity which you know causes you pain.
    D. should be taken when pain starts to build up.
    E. should always be taken with food.
    F. Don't know

9. Can you choose TWO correct answers about exercise and Rheumatoid Arthritis?

    A. It is unnecessary to exercise if you are normally active.
    B. Exercise will cure rheumatoid arthritis.

(continued)

    C.   Exercise weakens damaged joints.

    D.   Move your joint to the point of pain and then a bit further.

    E.   Exercise can reduce the chance of a joint deforming.

    F.   Don't know

10.   Can you choose the TWO most suitable ways for someone with Rheumatoid Arthritis to take regular exercise?

    A.   Muscle tightening exercises.

    B.   Gentle jogging.

    C.   Walking.

    D.   Yoga.

    E.   Shopping trips.

    F.   Don't know

11.   Can you choose ONE activity which you should carry out when all your joints are painful and stiff?

    A.   Refrain from all exercise.

    B.   Rest in bed for most of the day.

    C.   Carry out your usual range of movement exercises.

    D.   Exercise quite vigorously.

    E.   Don't know

12.   Can you choose TWO treatments which would be most suitable if your wrists are becoming more than usually painful, swollen, and stiff?

    A.   Rest them by putting on wrist splints.

    B.   Reduce the stiffness by vigorous exercise.

    C.   Use them as much as possible.

    D.   Avoid movement by keeping them in one position as much as possible.

    E.   Put the joints through a full range of movement several times a day.

    F.   Don't know

13.   Can you choose TWO sentences from this list?

The most practical way to protect your joints from strain is to

    A.   use them quickly.

    B.   use the larger joints rather than the smaller ones where possible.

    C.   slide objects rather than lift them.

    D.   do as little as possible.

    E.   carry on as though you did not have arthritis.

    F.   Don't know

14.   Can you choose the ONE most suitable activity when you have a busy day planned but realize you're feeling tired?

    A.   Take the day off and do more tomorrow.

    B.   Do everything you had planned to do.

    C.   Take a short rest and then do all the things you had planned.

    D.   Do essentials and leave the rest.

    E.   Spend the day resting in bed.

    F.   Don't know

15. Can you choose TWO suitable methods of conserving your energy?

    A. Sit down whilst ironing.
    B. Plan activities to balance work and rest periods.
    C. Wear splints.
    D. Use the strongest and largest muscles possible.
    E. Use both hands to carry objects such as full saucepans.
    F. Don't know

16. Can you choose TWO methods of joint protection?

    A. Grip objects tightly.
    B. Use a dish cloth rather than a sponge.
    C. Use the palm of your hands not your fingers when opening a jar.
    D. Apply heat or ice to the joint.
    E. Having power assisted steering on your car.
    F. Don't know

THANK YOU FOR ANSWERING THIS QUESTIONNAIRE

CORRECT ANSWERS

    1. d, e
    2. b, d
    3. a, b, f
    4. b, d
    5. c, e
    6. b
    7. a, d
    8. c, d
    9. d, e
    10. a, c
    11. c
    12. a, e
    13. b, c
    14. d
    15. a, b
    16. c, e

From Hill, J., Bird, H. A., Hopkins, R., Lawton, C., & Wright, V. (1994). An evaluation of the effectiveness, safety and acceptability of a nurse practitioner in a rheumatology outpatient clinic. *British Journal of Rheumatology, 30,* 45–49. Used with permission of Oxford University Press.

25. Arthritis Self-Efficacy Scale

Developed by Kate Lorig, Robert L. Chastain, Elaine Ung, Stanford Shoor, and Halsted R. Holman

INSTRUMENT DESCRIPTION, ADMINISTRATION, AND SCORING GUIDELINES

This scale was developed to measure patient perceived self-efficacy (SE) to cope with the consequences of chronic arthritis. SE appears to be particularly important for patients with rheumatoid arthritis (RA) because the unpredictable fluctuations of RA symptoms may contribute to feelings of helplessness. Patients who feel helpless report more psychological distress and pain than do their less helpless counterparts (Buescher et al., 1991). Patients rate the strength of their perceived ability to perform each item on a scale ranging from 10 to 100 in steps in 10. Item scores are then summed, with a higher score indicating greater SE. A spousal version of this instrument that asks how confident the spouse is that the patient could perform the specific behaviors (Keefe and others, 1997) has also been developed.

PSYCHOMETRIC PROPERTIES

Based on a national conference on outcomes measures, specific behaviors of controlling pain and disability were identified as important, translated into items, and refined in patient groups through item analysis.

Patients were recruited for the Arthritis Self-Management Course (ASMC) ($N = 97$) by means of public service announcements and referrals from health professionals. Subjects for the concurrent validation and reliability group were past ASMC participants who had not previously completed the efficacy scale questionnaire. Two factors were identified through factor analysis: self-efficacy for physical function (FSE) and self-efficacy for controlling other arthritis symptoms (OSE) (Lorig, Chastain, Ung, Shoor, & Holman, 1989).

Construct validity was upheld by a finding of significant correlations between baseline SE and baseline health status, between baseline SE and health status 4 months later, and between 4-month SE and 4-month health status, congruent with SE theory. FSE was most highly related to function (disability); OSE was most highly related to depression. A test of concurrent validity of the FSE showed a moderately high correlation (.61) between performance as perceived by patients and actual performance as measured by blinded trained observers. Such findings are consistent with self-efficacy theory (Lorig, Chastain, Ung, Shoor, & Holman, 1989).

A factor analysis from a replication study ($N = 144$ new subjects) showed three SE subscales: an FSE scale of 9 items (coefficient alpha = .89), an OSE scale of 6 items (coefficient alpha = .87), and a pain-management self-efficacy scale (PSE) of 5 items (coefficient alpha = .76), presented at the end of this description. The three subscales were then applied to data from the initial 97-person sample used for development of the instrument. Coefficient alpha estimates of internal reliability were .90 for FSE, .87 for OSE, and .75 for PSE. A test–retest reliability study with a third sample of 91 subjects showed subscale reliabilities of .85 for FSE, .90 for OSE, and .87 for PSE. Patients in these studies were largely female, with a mean age of 63 to 65 years and average education of 14 years (Lorig, Chastain, Ung, Shoor, & Holman, 1989).

Outcome data show that levels of pain and depression at 4 months declined significantly from baseline, whereas perceived SE for pain and for other symptoms rose significantly from baseline levels for the experimental group that received the ASMC, but not for the control group. Mean baseline scores for the experimental group were FSE, 73.27; OSE, 55.62; and PSE, 52.04 (Lorig, Chastain, Ung, Shoor, & Holman, 1989).

In a small ($N = 15$, experimental; $N = 15$, control), related study using efficacy-enhancing methods (individual goals, specific instructions and practice, self-relaxation with guided imagery, contracting, modeling, and reinterpretation of physiological symptoms), even greater gains in perceived SE and larger correlations with health outcomes in pain, disability, and functioning were found. Experimental patients learned psychological pain-management strategies including relaxation with guided imagery, attention refocusing, vivid imagery, dissociation, relabeling, and self-encouragement; strategies were tailored for use during specific painful activities such as climbing stairs, carrying groceries, and mopping floors. Control patients received copies of The Arthritis Helpbook (as did experimental patients) containing much relevant information for managing arthritis; this group achieved little or no change in SE or health outcomes. Mean subscale scores for the treatment group were PSE: 52.67, pretest; 63.40, posttest; FSE: 56.2, pretest; 64.27, posttest; and OSE: 52.53, pretest; 66.86, posttest. Mean subscale scores for the control group were PSE: 54.33, pretest; FSE: 63.64, pretest; 57.44, posttest; and OSE: 55.7, pretest; 58.33, posttest (O'Leary, Shoor, Lorig, & Holman, 1988). In an independent study, pain coping skills training was found to be superior on similar outcomes than traditional education (Keefe et al., 1996). Intentions to increase use of adaptive, and decrease use of maladaptive, pain coping strategies could also be helpful. Ignoring pain sensation and coping self-statements were related to higher SE and catastrophizing to lower SE (Keefe et al., 1997). These findings suggest building strong efficacy-enhancing methods into psychosocial interventions for patients with arthritis and shows Arthritis Self-Efficacy Scale sensitivity to intervention.

Other studies provide further evidence supporting validity of the Arthritis SE Scale. In patients with rheumatoid arthritis, those who reported higher SE exhibited fewer pain behaviors measured by pain behavior ratings. Although the effects were small, this relationship held true for all three subscales. Mean scores for FSE were 54.5; for PSE, 51.6; and for OSE, 59.3 (Buescher et al., 1991). Smarr and colleagues (1997) tested a stress-management intervention with rheumatoid arthritis patients and found total SE scores associated with decreased depression and lower pain. And Riesma and colleagues (1998) found the scales were strongly related to fatigue as well as to pain, in persons with rheumatoid arthritis.

The Arthritis Self-Efficacy Scale is also available in other languages. A Swedish version of the scale was tested for validity by Lomi and Nordholm (1992). Scores on the three subscales were correlated with indicators of present pain status, with scores on the Multidimensional Health Locus of Control Scales, and for FSE negatively with disease duration, all in the direction predicted by self-efficacy theory. The scales also discriminated between a group of patients with chronic pain and the rheumatology group, evidence of discriminant validity. Internal consistency was .82 to .91, and test–retest reliability .81 to .91 for the various subscales. The scale has also been translated into Spanish with preliminary psychometric testing to assess whether it is understood and easily administered to Spanish-speaking groups of varied national origin and living in different regions of the United States. The translated scale and results of validity and reliability studies on it may be found in Gonzalez, Stewart, Ritter, and Lorig (1995). The Spanish version of the scales showed an internal consistency alpha of .92, a test–retest reliability of .69, and item-to-scale correlations ranging from .65 to .83. The pain and other subscales have been tested in the United Kingdom. Factor structure was confirmed and internal consistency reliabilities were .82 to .85 for pain subscale and .89 to .91 for other symptoms subscale. Concurrent and predictive validity were partially supported (Barlow, Williams, & Wright, 1997).

The scales have also been used to test the effects of instructions for home exercise for persons with RA, with a finding of improved OSE, increased capacity in most functional tasks, and increased joint activity among other findings (Stenstrom, 1994).

In patients with fibromyalgia, when scores on the Arthritis Self-Efficacy Scale were high, patients exhibited fewer pain behaviors, although the amount of variance in pain behavior accounted for by SE ranged from only 10% to 14% (Buckelew et al., 1994). In an intervention study of 86 patients with fibromyalgia, those who received education or education plus physical training showed significantly higher scores than did those in the control group (Burckhardt, Mannerkorpi, Hedenberg, & Bjelle, 1994).

CRITIQUE AND SUMMARY

There has been more study of these scales than of most other instruments in this book. Findings from validity studies support hypotheses that there is an association between perceived SE and both present and future health status related to arthritis, that SE can be changed by educational interventions, and growth in SE is associated with improvement in health status and a decrease in health care costs, consistent with construct validity of the instrument (Lorig et al., 1989).

SE is an important variable clinically. For example, Beckham, Burker, Rice, and Talton (1995) found that patient SE expectations regarding RA symptoms explained a significant proportion of variance in measures of caregiver burden and optimism. These results suggest the importance of assessing patient psychological status in evaluating caregiver responses.

REFERENCES

Barlow, J. H., Williams, B., & Wright, C. C. (1997). The reliability and validity of the arthritis self-efficacy scale in a UK context. *Psychology, Health & Medicine, 2,* 3–17.

Beckham, J. C., Burker, E. J., Rice, J. R., & Talton, S. L. (1995). Patient predictors of caregiver burden, optimism, and pessimism in rheumatoid arthritis. *Behavioral Medicine, 20,* 171–178.

Buckalew, S. P., Parker, J. C., Keefe, F. J., Deuser, W. E., Crews, T. M., Conway, R., Kay, D. R., & Hewett, J. E. (1994). Self-efficacy and pain behavior among subjects with fibromyalgia. *Pain, 59,* 377–384.

Buescher, K. L., Johnson, J. A., Parker, J. C., Smarr, K. L., Buckelew, S. P., Anderson, S. K., & Walker, S. E. (1991). Relationship of self-efficacy to pain behavior. *Journal of Rheumatology, 18,* 968–972.

Burckhardt, C. S., Mannerkorpi, K., Hedenberg, L., & Bjelle, A. (1994). A randomized, controlled clinical trial of education and physician training for women with fibromyalgia. *Journal of Rheumatology, 21,* 714–720.

Gonzalez, V. M., Stewart, A., Ritter, P. L., & Lorig, K. (1995). Translation and validation of arthritis outcome measures into Spanish. *Arthritis and Rheumatism, 38,* 1429–1446.

Keefe, F. J., Caldwell, D. S., Baucom, D., Salley, A., Robinson, E., Timmons, K., Beaupre, P., Weisberg, J., & Helms, M. (1996). Spouse-assisted coping skills training in the management of osteoarthritic knee pain. *Arthritis Care & Research, 9,* 279–291.

Keefe, F. J., Kashikar-Zuck, S., Robinson, E., Salley, A., Beaupre, P., Caldwell, D., Baucom, D., & Haythornwaite, I. (1997). Pain coping strategies that predict patients' and spouses' ratings of patients' self-efficacy. *Pain, 73,* 191–199.

Lomi, C., & Nordholm, L. A. (1992). Validation of a Swedish version of the Arthritis Self-Efficacy Scale. *Scandinavian Journal of Rheumatology, 21,* 231–237.

Lorig, K., Chastain, R. L., Ung, E., Shoor, S., & Holman, H. R. (1989). Development and evaluation of a scale to measure perceived self-efficacy in people with arthritis. *Arthritis and Rheumatism, 32,* 27–34.

O'Leary, A., Shoor, S., Lorig, K., & Holman, H. R. (1988). A cognitive-behavioral treatment for rheumatoid arthritis. *Health Psychology, 7,* 527–544.

Riesma, R. P., Rasker, J. J., Taal, E., Griep, E. N., Wouters, J. M. G. W., & Wiegman, O. (1998). Fatigue in rheumatoid arthritis: The role of self-efficacy and problematic social support. *British Journal of Rheumatology, 37,* 1042–1046.

Smarr, K. L., Parker, J. C., Wright, G. E., Stucky-Ropp, R. C., Buckelew, S. P., Hoffman, R. W., O'Sullivan, F. X., & Hewett, J. E. (1997). The importance of enhancing self-efficacy in rheumatoid arthritis. *Arthritis Care and Research, 10,* 18–26.

Stenstrom, C. H. (1994). Home exercises in rheumatoid arthritis functional class II: Goal setting versus pain attention. *Journal of Rheumatology, 21,* 627–634.

ARTHRITIS SELF-EFFICACY SCALE*

Self-efficacy pain subscale

In the following questions, we'd like to know how your arthritis pain affects you. For each of the following questions, please circle the number which corresponds to your certainty that you can *now* perform the following tasks.

1. How certain are you that you can decrease your pain *quite a bit*?
2. How certain are you that you can continue most of your daily activities?
3. How certain are you that you can keep arthritis pain from interfering with your sleep?
4. How certain are you that you can make a *small-to-moderate* reduction in your arthritis pain by using methods other than taking extra medication?
5. How certain are you that you can make a *large* reduction in your arthritis pain by using methods other than taking extra medication?

Self-efficacy function subscale

We would like to know how confident you are in performing certain daily activities. For each of the following questions, please circle the number which corresponds to your certainty that you can perform the tasks as of *now*, *without* assistive devices or help from another person. Please consider what you *routinely* can do, not what would require a single extraordinary effort.

AS OF NOW, HOW CERTAIN ARE YOU THAT YOU CAN:

1. Walk 100 feet on flat ground in 20 seconds?
2. Walk 10 steps downstairs in 7 seconds?
3. Get out of an armless chair quickly, without using your hands for support?
4. Button and unbutton 3 medium-size buttons in a row in 12 seconds?
5. Cut 2 bite-size pieces of meat with a knife and fork in 8 seconds?
6. Turn an outdoor faucet all the way on and all the way off?
7. Scratch your upper back with both your right and left hands?
8. Get in and out of the passenger side of a car without assistance from another person and without physical aids?
9. Put on a long-sleeve front-opening shirt or blouse (without buttoning) in 8 seconds?

Self-efficacy other symptoms subscale

In the following questions, we'd like to know how you feel about your ability to control your arthritis. For each of the following questions, please circle the number which corresponds to the certainty that you can *now* perform the following activities or tasks.

1. *How certain* are you that you can control your fatigue?
2. *How certain* are you that you can regulate your activity so as to be active without aggravating your arthritis?
3. *How certain* are you that you can do something to help yourself feel better if you are feeling blue?
4. As compared with other people with arthritis like yours, *how certain* are you that you can manage arthritis pain during your daily activities?

5. *How certain* are you that you can manage your arthritis symptoms so that you can do the things you enjoy doing?
6. *How certain* are you that you can deal with the frustration of arthritis?

*Each question is followed by the scale:

10	20	30	40	50	60	70	80	90	100
very uncertain				moderately uncertain					very certain

Each subscale is scored separately, by taking the mean of the subscale items. If one-fourth or less of the data are missing, the score is a mean of the completed data. If more than one-fourth of the data are missing, no score is calculated. (The authors invite others to use the scale and would appreciate being informed of study results.)

From Lorig, K., Chastain, R. L., Ung, E., Shoor, S., & Holman, H. R. (1989). Development and evaluation of a scale to measure perceived self-efficacy in people with arthritis. *Arthritis and Rheumatism, 32,* 37–44. Copyright, American College of Rheumatology. Used with permission.

26. Parent's Arthritis Self-Efficacy Scale

Developed by J. H. Barlow, K. L. Shaw, and C. C. Wright

INSTRUMENT DESCRIPTION, ADMINISTRATION, AND SCORING GUIDELINES

Parents of children with chronic illnesses such as juvenile idiopathic arthritis (JIA) are at increased risk for psychosocial dysfunction and prior research suggests that maternal competence is one of the most important influences in the psychosocial adjustment of children with JIA. For both of these reasons, development of a parent's arthritis self-efficacy scale to measure perceived ability to carry out the courses of action that produce desired outcomes for children with JIA was seen as important.

Scores are obtained by summing items on the subscales, with higher scores indicating stronger self-efficacy (Barlow, Shaw, & Wright, 2000).

PSYCHOMETRIC CHARACTERISTICS

Generation of items for the Parents' Arthritis Self-Efficacy Scale (PASE) was aided by focus groups with parents, health professionals, and children with JIA. Many of the issues identified (such as management of children's pain, fatigue, sadness) paralleled those covered in the Arthritis Self-Efficacy Scale, which was designed for adults and is reviewed above. Some items were adapted from this scale. PASE was pilot tested for comprehensibility and ease of use.

A two-factor structure was identified: "symptom" and "psychosocial," each with seven items. Significant positive correlations between PASE subscales and measures of generalized SE and children's hope supported construct validity. Significant negative correlations between PASE subscales and mothers' anxious and depressed moods supported concurrent validity. In addition, mothers' ratings of the child's symptoms were associated with both SE subscales in the expected direction, as was children's functional status, indicating that greater SE was associated with better functioning (Barlow, Shaw, & Wright, 2000).

Cronbach's alphas were .92 (symptom subscale) and .96 (psychosocial subscale) for mothers, and .89 and .93 for fathers (Barlow, Shaw, & Wright, 2000).

CRITIQUE AND SUMMARY

PASE has so far been used with middle-class families and needs to be tested with broader population groups. In addition, the pattern of correlations between fathers' SE and children's well-being was weaker than that found for mothers.

Test–retest reliability, predictive and discriminant validity, and sensitivity to interventions known to improve SE remain to be completed and are important before the instrument can be used to evaluate psychosocial interventions. Comparison between the PASE and actual performance of management behaviors is needed to further examine concurrent validity. Further exploration of the utility of this scale seems warranted, given the increasing recognition of the importance of the family unit rather than considering the child in isolation (Barlow, Shaw, & Wright, 2000).

REFERENCE

Barlow, J. H., Shaw, K. L., & Wright, C. C. (2000). Development and preliminary validation of a self-efficacy measure for use among parents of children with juvenile idiopathic arthritis. *Arthritis Care & Research, 3,* 227–236.

THE PARENT'S ARTHRITIS SELF-EFFICACY SCALE (PASE)

For each of the following questions, please *CIRCLE* the *number* that corresponds to your certainty that *you* can perform each of the following tasks *at the present time*. If any question has no relevance to you, please tick the "not applicable" box to the right of the page.

How certain are you that you can . . .   not applicable

| Decrease your child's pain quite a bit? | very uncertain   very certain
 1   2   3   4   5   6   7 | ❐ |

Decrease your child's pain quite a
bit?
very uncertain   very certain   ❐
1   2   3   4   5   6   7

Decrease your child's stiffness quite
a bit?
very uncertain   very certain   ❐
1   2   3   4   5   6   7

Help ease your child's swollen
joints?
very uncertain   very certain   ❐
1   2   3   4   5   6   7

Keep arthritis pain from interfering
with your child's sleep?
very uncertain   very certain   ❐
1   2   3   4   5   6   7

Make a *small to moderate* reduction
in your child's arthritis pain by using
methods other than taking extra
medication?
very uncertain   very certain   ❐
1   2   3   4   5   6   7

Control your child's arthritis-related
fatigue?
very uncertain   very certain   ❐
1   2   3   4   5   6   7

Regulate your child's activity so that
they can be active without
aggravating their arthritis?
very uncertain   very certain   ❐
1   2   3   4   5   6   7

Do something to help your child feel
better when their arthritis makes them
feel sad?
very uncertain   very certain   ❐
1   2   3   4   5   6   7

Do something to help your child feel
better when their arthritis makes them
feel lonely?
very uncertain   very certain   ❐
1   2   3   4   5   6   7

Do something to help your child
deal with the frustration of arthritis?
very uncertain   very certain   ❐
1   2   3   4   5   6   7

Manage your child's arthritis
symptoms so that they can take
pleasure from the things that they
enjoy?
very uncertain   very certain   ❐
1   2   3   4   5   6   7

Manage your child's arthritis so that
they can participate fully in school
activities?
very uncertain   very certain   ❐
1   2   3   4   5   6   7

How certain are you that you can . . .								not applicable
Manage your child's arthritis so that they can participate fully in activities with friends?	very uncertain			very certain				❐
	1	2	3	4	5	6	7	
Manage your child's arthritis so that they can participate fully in family activities?	very uncertain			very certain				❐
	1	2	3	4	5	6	7	

From: Barlow, J. H., Shaw, K. L., & Wright, C. C. (2000). Development and preliminary validation of a self-efficacy measure for use among parents of children with juvenile idiopathic arthritis. *Arthritis Care & Research, 13,* 227–236. © 2000. Used with permission of John Wiley & Sons, Inc.

27. Arthritis Community Research and Evaluation Unit Rheumatoid Arthritis Knowledge Inventory

Developed by Sydney C. Lineker, Elizabeth M. Bradley, E. Ann Hughes, and Mary J. Bell

INSTRUMENT DESCRIPTION, ADMINISTRATION, AND SCORING GUIDELINES

Since rheumatoid arthritis (RA) is a chronic disease characterized by flares and remissions with no curative treatment, teaching patients self-management strategies is essential.

A score is derived by assigning one point to each correct answer and summing, with a higher score indicating more knowledge and a total possible score of 31. Nineteen items require a positive response (1, 2, 4, 5, 7–13, 16, 22, 23, 25, 26, 28, 29, 31) (Lineker, Bradley, Hughes, & Bell, 1997).

PSYCHOMETRIC CHARACTERISTICS

Items were generated using focus groups with patients and health professionals and covering domains of prognosis (8 items), pain management (3 items), medications (2 items), joint protection (5 items), energy conservation (2 items), exercise (2 items), and coping strategies (9 items).

Cronbach's alpha was .76. Test–retest reliability over 6.7 days was .92. Individuals in the focus groups scored higher than ambulatory or clinic patients. These findings are supportive of validity. Change in the instrument scores was significantly greater for those receiving a teaching intervention than for those in a control group, supporting its sensitivity to intervention. The effect size for the education group was .55, suggesting a clinically important increase in knowledge (Lineker, Bradley, Hughes, & Bell, 1997; Bell, Lineker, Wilkins, Goldsmith, & Bradley, 1998) and extending to one year (Lineker, Bell, Wilkins, & Bradley, 2001).

CRITIQUE AND SUMMARY

This instrument was developed for use in community-based rehabilitation programs for people with rheumatoid arthritis. One of its strengths is that items were based on the learning issues identified as important by individuals with RA.

REFERENCES

Bell, M. J., Lineker, S. C., Wilkins, A. L., Goldsmith, C. H., & Bradley, E. M. (1998). A randomized controlled trial to evaluate the efficacy of community-based physical therapy in the treatment of people with rheumatoid arthritis. *Journal of Rheumatology, 25,* 231–237.

Lineker, S. C., Bell, M. J., Wilkins, A. L., & Bradley, E. M. (2001). Improvements following short-term home-based physical therapy are maintained at one year in people with moderate to severe rheumatoid arthritis. *Journal of Rheumatology, 28,* 165–168.

Lineker, S. C., Bradley, E. M., Hughes, E. A., & Bell, M. J. (1997). Development of an instrument to measure knowledge in individuals with rheumatoid arthritis: The ACREU Rheumatoid Arthritis Knowledge Questionnaire. *Journal of Rheumatology, 24,* 647–653.

ARTHRITIS COMMUNITY RESEARCH AND EVALUATION UNIT (ACREU) RHEUMATOID ARTHRITIS KNOWLEDGE INVENTORY

STRONGLY AGREE (1), AGREE (2), UNCERTAIN/DON'T KNOW (3), DISAGREE (4), STRONGLY DISAGREE (5)

Examples:

1. Aspirin sometimes causes stomach upset. (*example indicates response option "strongly agree"*) This person strongly agrees that aspirin causes stomach upset.
2. Cows get arthritis as often as humans. (*example indicates response option "uncertain/don't know"*) This person is not sure whether or not cows can get arthritis.

QUESTIONS:

1. For some people, rheumatoid arthritis causes very few problems
2. Meeting other people with rheumatoid arthritis in a group can teach you many things
3. When you are feeling well, you should reduce your arthritis medications
4. The presence of rheumatoid arthritis often results in family stress
5. Splints should be worn if you have pain in your wrists when you work with your hands
6. Ice treatments often make the joints swell
7. Many people with rheumatoid arthritis are scared about the future
8. To save energy, people with rheumatoid arthritis should sit when working instead of standing
9. Anger is a common reaction when someone is first told they have rheumatoid arthritis
10. If you have rheumatoid arthritis, the arches in your feet may need extra support
11. It is common to feel depressed when you have rheumatoid arthritis
12. You can protect the joints in your hands by using the palms of your hands instead of your fingers to do chores
13. People with rheumatoid arthritis often lose confidence in themselves
14. A damaged joint hurts more when you rest it
15. Most people with rheumatoid arthritis have to quit their jobs
16. The pharmacist is a good source of information about your arthritis medications
17. Rheumatoid arthritis affects only the joints
18. There is no relationship between stress and rheumatoid arthritis
19. Your doctor will tell you everything you need to know about your rheumatoid arthritis
20. When you are in a flare, you should stop all exercise
21. Most people with rheumatoid arthritis end up in a wheelchair
22. It's good for your feet to wear supportive shoes in the house instead of slippers

23. The cause of rheumatoid arthritis is not known
24. It is easy for your family/friends to tell when you are in pain
25. If you have rheumatoid arthritis, the ability to fully straighten and bend your joints can be lost quickly
26. Rheumatoid arthritis sometimes goes away
27. When you're having a good day, you should get all your chores done
28. Rheumatoid arthritis is different in everyone
29. Neck pain can be caused by a poor sleep position
30. All people with rheumatoid arthritis get "crooked joints"
31. Talking about your rheumatoid arthritis with someone you trust can make you feel better

---

From: Lineker, S. C., Bradley, E. M., Hughes, E. A., & Bell, M. J. (1997). Development of an instrument to measure knowledge in individuals with rheumatoid arthritis: The ACREU Rheumatoid Arthritis Knowledge Questionnaire. *Journal of Rheumatology, 24,* 647–653. Used with permission.

28. Ankylosing Spondylitis: What Do You Know?

Developed by E. Lubrano, P. Helliwell, P. Moreno,
B. Griffiths, P. Emery, and D. Veale

INSTRUMENT DESCRIPTION, ADMINISTRATION, AND SCORING GUIDELINES

Ankylosing spondylitis (AS) is a chronic inflammatory disease, which, if left untreated, may progress to bony ankylosis of the entire spine.

Instrument content is based on the Arthritis and Rheumatism Council's leaflet and examines four areas: A) general knowledge including etiology, symptoms, and blood tests; B) immunogenetic tests and inheritance; C) general management including drug treatment and physical therapy, and D) joint protection, pacing, and priorities. Score is the sum of correct answers with a total possible score of 25, 8 in area A, 3 in area B, 9 in area C and 5 in area D. Analysis of readability showed the instrument to be easier than standard writing. Scores of a group of 62 patients with AS may be found in Lubrano and colleagues (1998).

PSYCHOMETRIC CHARACTERISTICS

The instrument was written in consultation with professional experts. Internal consistency reliability was .85, test–retest reliability after 4 weeks was .77 (Lubrano et al., 1998).

CRITIQUE AND SUMMARY

The instrument is based on Hill et al.'s Knowledge Questionnaire in Rheumatoid Arthritis, presented on page 122. It shares weaknesses of that instrument in needing patient verification of the content domain, and in testing the notion that this knowledge is important in carrying out self-care regimens. Theory would suggest that testing problem-solving skills in using the knowledge would be more predictive than the factual knowledge tested in this instrument.

The authors indicate that the instrument can be used to detect changes in knowledge from educational initiatives (Lubrano et al., 1998); however, no evidence of such sensitivity was included in their analysis.

REFERENCE

Lubrano, E., Helliwell, P., Moreno, P., Griffiths, B., Emery, P., & Veale, D. (1998). The assessment of knowledge in ankylosing spondylitis patients by a self-administered questionnaire. *British Journal of Rheumatology, 37,* 437–441.

ANKYLOSING SPONDYLITIS: WHAT DO YOU KNOW?

1. Can you choose **the two true** statements from the following list:
   Ankylosing Spondylitis:
   a. is an infectious disease
   b. the cause is not known
   c. occasionally more than one member of a family gets the disease
   d. is most common in old age
   e. is caused by athletic activity or injury
   f. don't know

2. Can you choose **the two true** statements from the following list:
   Ankylosing Spondylitis:
   a. is an inflammation in the joints of the spine
   b. in a few cases the first complaint may not be in the back at all
   c. gets worse in the cold weather
   d. is a curable disease
   e. don't know

3. Can you choose **the two true** statements from the following list:
   Ankylosing Spondylitis:
   a. sometimes involves the eye and the heel bone
   b. increases the risk of heart attacks or stroke
   c. causes aching and stiffness in the back
   d. increases the risk of cancer
   e. don't know

4. Can you choose **the two blood tests** which are used to assess how active your
   spondylitis is?
   a. cholesterol levels (CL)
   b. ESR (erythrocyte sedimentation rate)
   c. full blood count
   d. CRP (C reactive protein)
   e. don't know

5. Can you choose **the blood test** which is used to assess the tendency to develop
   ankylosing spondylitis?
   a. urea
   b. HLA-B27
   c. HLA-DR4
   d. plasma viscosity
   e. don't know

6. Can you choose **the two correct** answers about the medical approach for ankylosing
   spondylitis:
   a. pain killers are helpful in pain relief
   b. drug therapy is the only approach in controlling the disease
   c. no drugs are able to control the disease

(continued)

    d.   several anti-inflammatory drugs give a good quality night's sleep and sufficient freedom from pain to do exercise

    e.   don't know

7. Can you choose **the two true** statements from the following list:

    a.   every patient will return to normal, even when the exercises are followed

    b.   the symptoms may come and go over a long period

    c.   it is most important to maintain a good posture

    d.   AS doesn't interfere with your work and physical activity

    e.   don't know

8. Can you choose **the two correct** answers about **rest** for ankylosing spondylitis:

    a.   rest in bed for most of the day is the best approach when your back is painful and stiff

    b.   a spell off work or in hospital may be necessary when the disease is very active

    c.   lie all night on the back

    d.   lie on your front some time before going to bed and before rising in the morning

    e.   don't know

9. Can you choose **the two correct** answers about the **ideal bed** for patients with ankylosing spondylitis:

    a.   every bed is suitable

    b.   the bed should be firm

    c.   a sheet of plywood below the mattress is ideal

    d.   a soft mattress is more helpful when the back is stiff

    e.   don't know

10. Can you choose **the two correct** answers about **exercise treatment** for ankylosing spondylitis:

    a.   exercise is an important part of treatment for ankylosing spondylitis

    b.   exercise will cure ankylosing spondylitis

    c.   exercise weakens damaged joints

    d.   regular daily exercise is a wise approach to keep active

    e.   don't know

11. Can you choose **the two most** suitable activities for someone with ankylosing spondylitis:

    a.   shopping trips

    b.   swimming

    c.   cross-country running

    d.   football

    e.   muscle strengthening exercise

    f.   don't know

12. Can you choose **the one activity** which you **should** carry out when all your joints are painful and stiff, i.e., when in acute flare?

    a.   refrain from all exercise

    b.   rest in bed for most of the day

    c.   carry out range of movement exercises within your pain-free limits

    d.   exercise quite vigorously

    e.   don't know

13. Can you choose **the one** correct sentence from the list:
    a. manipulation of the spine can help the disease
    b. acupuncture can cure the disease
    c. exercise in the pool can help movement
    d. exercise in the pool can deteriorate the disease, because the water and humidity can damage the joints
    e. don't know

14. Can you choose **the two** correct sentences describing how ankylosing spondylitis can affect the family?
    a. parents with AS have a high chance of having children with AS
    b. parents with AS have a low chance of having children with AS
    c. the HLA-B27 test will give the answer as to whether the patient's children will develop the disease
    d. the HLA-B27 test will not give the answer as to whether the patient's children will develop the disease
    e. don't know

The letters in bold represent the correct answers.

From: Lubrano, E., Helliwell, P., Moreno, P., Griffiths, B., Emery, P., & Veale, P. (1998). The assessment of knowledge in ankylosing spondylitis patients by a self-administered questionnaire. *British Journal of Rheumatology, 37,* 437–441, by permission of Oxford University Press.

Section D

Asthma

A wide range of measurement instruments for both children and adults is available for clinical and research use in asthma. Besides the knowledge and self-efficacy instruments usual for management of a chronic illness, this field has a rich variety of instruments dealing with changing lifestyles and perceived control.

---

29. Asthma Autonomy Preference Scale

Developed by Peter G. Gibson, Phillipa I. Talbot, Ruth C. Toneguzzi, and The Population Medicine Group 91C

INSTRUMENT DESCRIPTION, ADMINISTRATION, AND SCORING GUIDELINES

Management guidelines emphasize increased autonomy for persons with asthma through patient education and written patient-initiated action plans. These are meant to facilitate the early detection and treatment of an exacerbation and to minimize the risk of hospitalization and death. The extent to which patients wish to be well-informed participants in the management of their illness is largely unknown. Studies of other illnesses have shown that although most patients actively sought information about their condition, few preferred to have the major role in decision making (Gibson, Talbot, Toneguzzi, & The Population Medicine Group, 1995).

The Asthma Autonomy Preference Scale (AAPS) examines preferences of patients for information about their condition and for decision making in asthma exacerbations of varying severity. The instrument takes about 10 minutes to administer. Strongest preferences in favor of decision making or information seeking by the patient are assigned scores of 5, with the weakest score 1. Overall preference is determined by adding the scores in the respective scales. Final scores were linearized to range from 1 to 100 and for each scale to a range of 0 to 10, with the lowest scores corresponding to a preference for the physician to take complete control, midrange indicating equally shared responsibility, and the highest scores for the patient to take complete control of decision making (Gibson et al., 1995).

146

PSYCHOMETRIC PROPERTIES

This tool was adapted to asthma using the published guidelines for management of this disease from the Autonomy Preference Index (API) (Ende, Kazis, Ash, & Moskowitz, 1989). Items for the original index were developed from a Delphi study of clinical medical sociologists and ethicists. It was tested in a study of 312 patients from a hospital-based primary care clinic. Factor analysis supported a scale on information seeking and one on decision making. Test–retest reliability for the scales was .83 and .84, and Cronbach's alpha for each was .82. Responses to a global item about amount of control of patient and physician correlated significantly with decision-making scores on the API, supporting concurrent validity. Scores on the decision-making scale administered to persons with diabetes adept on self-care and home monitoring were significantly higher than were scores from the general population, supporting convergent validity. Studies using the API found that although patients wanted information, their preferences for decision making were frequently weak, especially as they were asked to consider increasingly severe illnesses (Ende, Kazis, Ash, & Moskowitz, 1989).

The AAPS consists of two scales: information-seeking preferences (8 items) and decision-making preferences (18 items). Authors of the AAPS indicated that its structure had been previously validated, based on the work done on the API. It was administered to 85 adults purchasing albuterol inhalers for asthma from community pharmacies as well as to 38 persons recently hospitalized for acute, severe asthma. Both groups indicated high preferences for information seeking (mean values over 90 out of a possible of 100), with preferences for decision making significantly lower (mean of 51 and 52, respectively). Scores on items related to the scenarios may be found in Gibson and colleagues (1995).

Although, on average, preferences for participation declined even further with severe exacerbation of asthma, one-third of participants indicated they still would prefer equal or greater participation in decision making under these circumstances. Quality of life in asthma was not associated with patient preference for autonomy. It is important to note that results were similar to those found with the API (Gibson et al., 1995).

CRITIQUE AND SUMMARY

The AAPS describes patient attitudes rather than the specific behaviors of patients with asthma. Although the expected results of these attitudes, namely, failure to initiate self-management in asthma exacerbations, have been documented to occur in several settings, no evidence of predictive validity could be located either for the AAPS or for the API. The number of subjects involved in studies of the AAPS is limited. In addition, no estimates of reliability and validity (apart from those that exist for API) could be located. A recent study of 293 low-income Australian patients using the AAPS showed that lower preference for autonomy in asthma management decisions was associated with increased hospitalizations (Adams, Smith, & Ruffin, 2000).

Several implications for patient care and new research flow from the findings to date. First, many of the patients tested so far do not conform to the model of strong patient decision-making autonomy assumed in guidelines for asthma self-management, in that only a minority have action plans to use for management of deteriorating asthma. Studies of asthma deaths and severe asthma exacerbations frequently indicate delay in using medication or seeking help as potentially reversible factors. Programs designed to improve self-management can be shown to decrease morbidity as well as decrease health care costs. Why does this occur? Do physicians not provide management plans (Gibson et al., 1995)? Do patient education programs focus solely on information about the disease and not provide explicit skill building to the point of mastery in how to manage exacerbations? Will adequate patient programs shift the decision-making autonomy preference? If, after adequate education, patients are still resistant to strong decision-making roles, perhaps a different system of caregiving must be constructed. Is the AAPS useful in identifying individuals who are at risk for poor asthma control? This is important since this group uses a disproportionate amount of health care costs (Adams, Smith, & Ruffin, 2000).

Second, and not surprising, because patients differ in their preferences for decision-making autonomy, it would be useful to know up front who prefers strong or weak decision-making responsibility. Particularly if these preference tools show predictive validity with actual self-management behaviors, it would be possible to identify individuals who need backup systems to deal with serious exacerbations of their illness.

REFERENCES

Adams, R. J., Smith, B. J., & Ruffin, R. E. (2000). Factors associated with hospital admissions and repeat emergency department visits for adults with asthma. *Thorax, 55,* 566–573.

Ende, J., Kazis, L., Ash, A., & Moskowitz, M. A. (1989). Measuring patients' desire for autonomy. *Journal of General Internal Medicine, 4,* 23–30.

Gibson, P. G., Talbot, P. I., Toneguzzi, R. C., & The Population Medicine Group. (1995). Self-management, autonomy, and quality of life in asthma. *Chest, 107,* 1003–1008.

THE ASTHMA AUTONOMY PREFERENCE INDEX

I.   Decision-making preference scale.

A.   General items for decision-making preferences. Scored using 5-point Likert scale, with scores ranging from "strongly agree" to "strongly disagree."

1. The important medical decisions about your asthma should be made by your physician, not you.
2. You should go along with your physician's advice even if you disagree with it.
3. When hospitalized for asthma, you should not be making decisions about your own care.
4. You should feel free to make decisions about everyday problems with your asthma.
5. If you were sick, as your asthma became worse you would want your physician to take greater control.
6. You should decide how frequently you need a check-up for your asthma.

B.   Scenarios. Subjects respond to each item on a 5-point scale. Choices are "you alone," "mostly you," "the doctor and you equally," "mostly the doctor," "the doctor alone."

Stable Asthma:
Suppose you have visited your physician for a routine check-up of your asthma and to obtain prescriptions for your asthma medicines. Who should make the following decisions?

7. When the next visit to check your asthma should be.
8. Whether you should buy a peak flowmeter and use this to monitor your asthma.
9. Whether you should be seen by a specialist.
10. What action you should take if your asthma gets worse.

Mild Exacerbations:
For the last 4 days you have been feeling more wheezy and breathless than usual, and you have found it increasingly difficult to get on with your everyday activities. Last night you were awakened twice because of asthma and you found it difficult to get back to sleep. Today you wake earlier than usual and are feeling very wheezy and breathless. Who should make the following decisions?

11. Whether you should be seen by the physician.
12. Whether you should take more albuterol (Ventolin, Respolin) terbutaline (Bricanyl)/fenoterol (Berotec).
13. Whether you should increase your preventive asthma inhalers (beclomethasone [Becotide, Becloforte], cromolyn [Intal], budesonide [Pulmicort]).
14. Whether you should take prednisone or cortisone tablets.

Severe Asthma in Hospital:
Suppose you had an attack of severe asthma that was not relieved by your inhaler, frightening you enough so that you went to the hospital emergency (casualty) department. In the emergency department, physicians treat your asthma and you are taken up to the intensive care unit. Who should make the following decisions?

(continued)

15. How often the nurses should wake you up to check your temperature and blood pressure.
16. Whether you may have visitors aside from your immediate family.
17. When you are able to be discharged.
18. Whether the nurses should wake you from sleep to give you the nebulizer.

II.   Information-seeking preference scale.

   A.   Items for information-seeking preferences. Responses presented as a 5-point Likert scale with choices ranging from "strongly agree" to "strongly disagree."

19. As you become sicker, you should be told more and more about your asthma.
20. You should understand what is happening inside your body as a result of asthma.
21. Even if the news is bad, you should be well informed about your asthma.
22. Your physician should explain the purpose of your laboratory tests.
23. You should be given information about your asthma only when you ask.
24. It is important for you to know all the side effects of your asthma medication.
25. Information about asthma is as important as treatment.
26. When there is more than one method to treat asthma, you should be told about each one.

From Gibson, P. G., Talbot, P. I., Toneguzzi, R. C., and The Population Medicine Group. (1995). Self-management, autonomy, and quality of life in asthma. *Chest, 107,* 1003–1008.

30. Asthma Opinion Survey

Developed by James M. Richards, Jr., Jeffrey J. Dolce, Richard A. Windsor, William C. Bailey, C. Michael Brooks, and Seng-jaw Soong

INSTRUMENT DESCRIPTION, ADMINISTRATION, AND SCORING GUIDELINES

Poor self-management appears to contribute significantly to unnecessary morbidity and perhaps mortality in adults with asthma. The Asthma Opinion Survey (AOS) was designed to measure attitudes relevant to self-management in adult outpatients. Prior research has confirmed that psychological characteristics are related to effectiveness of asthma self-management. In addition to a similar tool focused on inpatient treatment, development of the AOS was guided by the Health Belief Model and by the PRECEDE diagnostic model for patient education. Thus, it includes items designed to tap predisposing (knowledge, attitudes, beliefs, and values); enabling (skills in self-management); and reinforcing factors (effects of self-management on symptoms and social support) (Richards et al., 1989).

PSYCHOMETRIC PROPERTIES

Items fall into 11 clusters: general vulnerability, specific vulnerability, attitudes toward patient knowledge, recognition of airway obstruction, accessibility of health care, panic-fear, belief in treatment efficacy, staff-patient relationships, sense of control, personal impact, and social impact (Richards et al., 1989). Because the reliability levels of these clusters vary from .48 to .87, it is suggested that future research with the AOS should rely mainly on the three factor scores: vulnerability (alpha = .87), perceived quality of care (alpha = .76), and recognition and control (alpha = .71). In a separate study (Vazquez, 2000), alpha of .85 was found for vulnerability and alpha .69 for perceived quality of care.

The AOS has been tested with one group of 132 adults receiving outpatient treatment in a teaching hospital in Birmingham. The full range of age, severity, and duration of asthma was present in this group, and it closely reflected racial characteristics in the Birmingham, Alabama community. AOS scores correlated with the Asthma Symptoms Checklist in ways supporting construct validity. Higher scores on the vulnerability factor were associated with use of the more intense forms of health care, and higher scores on the recognition and control factor were associated with use of an emergency room. No scores could be located in published sources.

CRITIQUE AND SUMMARY

Evidence is needed both with respect to the extent to which scores on the AOS predict self-management behaviors and outcomes, and with respect to whether or not scores on the survey change in response to interventions (Richards et al., 1991). In addition, the instrument needs to be tested with more subjects in other sites because the way in which care is delivered clearly will affect responses on some items.

REFERENCES

Richards, J. M., Jr., Dolce, J. J., Windsor, R. A., Bailey, W. C., Brooks, C. M., & Soong, S. (1989). Patient characteristics relevant to effective self-management: Scales for assessing attitudes of adults toward asthma. *Journal of Asthma, 26,* 99–108.

Vazquez, M. I. (2000). Relationships between psychological variables relevant to asthma and patients' quality of life, *Psychological Reports, 86,* 31–33.

ASTHMA OPINION SURVEY

NAME: _____ DATE: _____

Instructions: We want to learn more about your opinions concerning your asthma and the quality of care you currently are receiving from the clinic, hospital, physician, etc., where you go for asthma treatment. Please draw a circle around the number beside each of the following statements to indicate the extent to which you agree or disagree with it.

		Strongly Disagree				Strongly Agree
1.	I have asthma attacks quite often.	1	2	3	4	5
2.	People with asthma do better if they learn a lot about their disease.	1	2	3	4	5
3.	I can tell when I'm about to have an asthma attack from how I feel inside.	1	2	3	4	5
4.	When I get short of breath, I often get too upset to do much about it.	1	2	3	4	5
5.	Patients here would get a lot better treatment for their asthma somewhere else.	1	2	3	4	5
6.	I know some things to do that will help when I get short of breath.	1	2	3	4	5
7.	I would be more successful if I didn't have so many breathing problems.	1	2	3	4	5
8.	I always have to wait a long time here before I get to see the doctor.	1	2	3	4	5
9.	I generally know if I'm about to have a breathing problem.	1	2	3	4	5
10.	My asthma interferes with my social life quite a bit.	1	2	3	4	5
11.	Patients have very little to say about what happens to them here.	1	2	3	4	5
12.	When I get short of breath, I can tell if it's going to get worse from how I feel inside.	1	2	3	4	5
13.	I often worry about getting a serious disease such as cancer or a heart attack.	1	2	3	4	5
14.	The doctors, nurses, and other staff here are quite nice to patients.	1	2	3	4	5

(continued)

		Strongly Disagree				Strongly Agree
15.	If an asthma attack starts to get worse, I know some things that will help me if I do them.	1	2	3	4	5
16.	Because I have asthma, I am always going to have some breathing problems.	1	2	3	4	5
17.	The doctors here are too busy to give enough time to their asthma patients.	1	2	3	4	5
18.	I usually can feel it when my chest begins to get tight from asthma.	1	2	3	4	5

Scoring instructions. The current version has been reduced to 18 items. Subjects respond in terms of a 5-point scale ranging from 1 to 5. Scores are computed for three factors by summing the items that loaded on that factor in the study reported in the *Journal of Asthma* article. The factors and the items that should be included are listed below. The scoring for some items is reversed in computing the total score on the factor. These items are identified by an asterisk (*).

> Factor A—Vulnerability
>   Items 1, 4, 7, 10, 13, 16
>
> Factor B—Perceived Quality of Care
>   Items 2, 5*, 8*, 11*, 14, 17*
>
> Factor C—Recognition and Control
>   Items 3, 6, 9, 12, 15, 18

This scale was developed at the Lung Health Center, University of Alabama at Birmingham, with research funding from the Division of Lung Diseases, National Heart, Lung, and Blood Institute Grant HL 31481-02 to William C. Bailey, MD.

31. Asthma Knowledge Questionnaire

Developed by John Kolbe, Marina Vamos, Frances James, Gail Elkind, and Jeffrey Garrett

INSTRUMENT DESCRIPTION, ADMINISTRATION, AND SCORING GUIDELINES

Traditionally, asthma education has focused on teaching patients the pathophysiology of asthma, identification and modification of triggers, and the mechanism of drug action. The effects of such programs on hospital admissions, emergency room visits, and urgent physician visits are modest. Practical knowledge of how to self-manage acute asthma focuses on recognition and assessment of the severity of an asthma attack, pharmacologic and nonpharmacologic means of abating the attack, and when and how to seek medical help if such strategies are not effective. The increase in asthma deaths and severe life-threatening attacks makes such skills all the more important (Kolbe, Vamos, James, Elkind, & Garrett, 1996).

The Asthma Knowledge Questionnaire (AKQ) uses scenarios for slow onset (7 days) and rapid onset (1 hour) attacks (Kolbe, Vamos, James, Elkind, & Garrett, 1996). The scoring guide, weighted for strategies considered to be most important in aborting an attack or potentially lifesaving, is attached. The total score for each scenario is 25. Respiratory physicians considered a score of 15 or greater to indicate a satisfactory level of asthma self-management knowledge (Kolbe, Vamos, James, Elkind, & Garrett, 1996).

PSYCHOMETRIC CHARACTERISTICS

The scoring system is based on Thoracic Society consensus statements and patient behaviors (Kolbe, Vamos, Fergusson, Elkind, & Garrett, 1996). Intra- and inter-rater reliability was 80% or better. Scores for the slow-onset attack were predicted by the score for the rapid-onset attack, and vice versa, and by the interviewer's overall rating of management ability, supporting validity (Kolbe, Vamos, James, Elkind, & Garrett, 1996).

Kolbe, Vamos, Fergusson, Elkind, and Garrett (1996) studied the relation of AKQ scores and reported behavior during an actual asthma attack. A higher level of formal education was associated with using theoretical knowledge during an actual attack and with possession of a PEF meter, a written action plan, and a supply of corticosteroids—features associated with appropriate asthma education and good medical care.

CRITIQUE AND SUMMARY

Most studies of deaths from asthma or severe life-threatening attacks of asthma have identified a variety of management errors by the patient or doctor during the attack and have frequently concluded that most attacks of slow onset are theoretically preventable by currently available strategies. Thus, the cutoff score on Practical Knowledge needs to be empirically validated. Despite considerable traditional asthma education, patients were quite poor at applying knowledge to action in the scenarios (Kolbe, Vamos, James, Elkind, & Garrett, 1996).

REFERENCES

Kolbe, J., Vamos, M., James, F., Elkind, B., & Garrett, J. (1996). Assessment of practical knowledge of self-management of acute asthma. *Chest, 109,* 86–90.

Kolbe, J., Vamos, M., Fergusson, W., Elkind, G., & Garrett, J. (1996). Differential influences on asthma self-management knowledge and self-management behavior in acute severe asthma. *Chest, 110,* 1463–1468.

ASTHMA KNOWLEDGE QUESTIONNAIRE

Asthma Knowledge

Hypothetical Asthma Attacks

Now I am going to ask you some questions about the kind of experiences that some people with asthma may have and I would like you to talk about the sorts of things you would do if they were to happen to you.

I will begin by describing to you a short scene about a particular situation. Then I will ask you some questions and then go on to the next scene.

Some of your answers may cover all the stages. I must read you every scene so if that happens just repeat anything that relates to that particular scene.

I will tape our conversation because writing slows things down. If there is anything you do not understand, tell me and I will go over it again.

A. Slow-Onset Attack

(Days 1 to 3)
For the last 2 days you have been feeling a little more wheezy and breathless than usual, but not enough to interfere with your everyday activities. Last night you woke up once because of asthma, but were able to get to sleep again easily. This morning you again woke up feeling more wheezy and breathless than usual.
What would you do?
Prompt—
  (i)   Would you do anything else? (or anything after that?)
  (ii) Would you take any extra medication?

(Days 4 to 5)
It is now for 3 days that you have been more short of breath and wheezy. Your breathing got slightly worse over the next 2 days and you found it increasingly difficult to get on with your everyday activities. Last night you were wakened twice because of asthma and you found it difficult to get back to sleep. Today you wake earlier than usual and are feeling very wheezy and breathless.
What would you do?
Prompt—
  (i)   Would you do anything else? (or anything else after that?)
  (ii) Would you take any extra medications?

(Days 6 to 7)
It is now 5 days that you have been more short of breath and wheezy. Your wheezing and breathlessness got worse over the next day. Last night you wakened three times because of asthma and the last time you could not get back to sleep. It is now morning and you are so wheezy and breathless that you find it difficult to speak or walk across the room.
What would you do?
Has anything like this ever happened to you? (Yes/No)

(continued)

B.   Rapid-Onset Attack

(Start)

   You woke this morning feeling perfectly well and spent the day doing your usual activities. At 7 o'clock in the evening you sit down to relax and notice you are feeling a little wheezy and breathless.

What would you do?

Prompt—
   (i)   Would you do anything else? (or anything after that?)
   (ii) Would you take any extra medication?

(30 min)

   Over the next half hour the wheezing and breathlessness get worse and you find it a little difficult to walk to the kitchen for a drink.

What would you do?

Prompt—
   (i)   Would you do anything else? (or anything else after that?)
   (ii) Would you take any extra medication?

(1 h)

   It has now been about 1 h and your breathing continues to get worse and by 8 o'clock you are so wheezy and breathless that you find it difficult to speak or get up from your chair.

What would you do?

Has anything like this ever happened to you? (Yes/No)

Scoring (Amended)

A.   Slow-Onset Attack

   (i)   Take peak expiratory flow rate (PEFR) reading   2
         Use β-agonist   2
         Repeat measure of PEFR/monitor more closely   1
         Increase regular steroids (inhaled or oral)   2
         (Nil for oral steroids)
         (Nil for going to doctor)
   (ii) Take PEFR reading   2
         Use (+ regular) β-agonist   2
         Increase inhaled steroids   3 ⎫
         Take oral steroids/action plan   4 ⎬
         Consult general practitioner (GP), emergency medical services (EMS) or ED 2 ⎭
         (within 24 to 48 h) (< 24 hours if no steroids)
   (iii) Call ambulance—ED   4 ⎫
         Call GP (to see at home)   2 ⎬
         Go to ED, EMS, GP, or Asthma Clinic (private transport) (Score 0 if drive 1 ⎭
         themselves)

Take oral steroids/action plan (only if not already taken)	2
Continue β-agonist therapy	1
Maximum total	25

B. *Rapid-Onset Attack*

(i) Take PEFR reading	2
Take extra β-agonist	
Repeat measure of PEFR/check response	1
Take increased dose of inhaled steroids	1
(ii) Take PEFR reading	2
Action plan:	
Oral steroids and/or	6 ⎫
Call GP (home visit or urgent appointment) and/or	⎬
Go immediately to ED	⎭
Use β-agonist	2
Increase inhaled steroids	1
(iii) Call for ambulance	7 ⎫
Call GP (home visit)	2 ⎬
Go to ED, EMS, or GP (private transport) (Score 0 if drive themselves)	1 ⎭
Take oral steroids/action plan (only if not already taken)	3
Use β-agonist	1
Maximum total	25

*Braces indicate mutually exclusive scores.

From: Kolbe, J., Vamos, M., James, F., Elkind, G., & Garrett, J. (1996). Assessment of practical knowledge of self-management of acute asthma. *Chest, 109*, 86–90. Used with permission.

32. Asthma General Knowledge Questionnaire for Adults

Developed by Rae M. Allen, Michael P. Jones, and Brian Oldenburg

INSTRUMENT DESCRIPTION, ADMINISTRATION, AND SCORING GUIDELINES

Good control of asthma symptoms is believed to be a realistic goal for most asthmatic patients. It requires both good medical treatment and good self-management with one of the basic building blocks of the latter being knowledge.

The Asthma General Knowledge Questionnaire (AGKQ) was developed to assess knowledge of asthma concepts covered in an educational program. Content areas tested included etiology, pathophysiology, medications, assessment of severity, and symptoms management, including trigger minimization and exercise. Score is the total of correct answers. The instrument is written at the fifth to sixth grade level.

PSYCHOMETRIC CHARACTERISTICS

Content and face validity were assessed and found to be adequate by respiratory physicians, patients, and asthma educators involved in program development. Factor analysis suggested the scale was unidimensional (Allen & Jones, 1998). Discriminant validity was supported by significantly higher scores obtained by study participants than by those who did not have asthma and had never been involved in its management. In a randomized controlled trial (RCT), intervention group participants who attended four weekly educational sessions had significantly better scores than did those in the control group, and this improvement was maintained 12 months later (Allen, Jones, & Oldenbert, 1995). In another RCT, the Asthma General Knowledge Questionnaire for Adults (AGKQA) scores were not significantly different at 6 months postintervention, although this study suffered low rates of participation in the educational intervention (Abdulwadud, Abramson, Forbes, James, & Walters, 1999).

Internal consistency reliability was .56 at baseline, .80 immediately postintervention, and .75 twelve months later. Test–retest reliability was .72. Similar psychometric results were obtained when AGKQA was used in the training of asthma educators (Allen, Abdulwadud, Jones, Abrmason, & Walters, 2000).

CRITIQUE AND SUMMARY

Because AGKQA closely follows the content of one asthma self-management program, it would be useful to have outside experts, including patients, judge the content and implicit objectives inherent in the instrument. A true–false format carries the liability that successful guessing can inflate scores, especially in this case because whenever possible, wording was consistent with that used in the program manual received by each participant (Allen & Jones, 1998).

REFERENCES

Abdulwadud, O., Abramson, M., Forbes, A., James, A., & Walters, E. H. (1999). Evaluation of a randomized controlled trial of adult education in a hospital setting. *Thorax, 54*, 493–500.

Allen, R. M., Abdulwadud, O. A., Jones, M. P., Abramson, M., & Walters, H. (2000). A reliable and valid asthma general knowledge questionnaire useful in the training of asthma educators. *Patient Education & Counseling, 39*, 237–242.

Allen, R. M., & Jones, M. P. (1998). The validity and reliability of an asthma knowledge questionnaire used in the evaluation of a group asthma education self-management program for adults with asthma. *Journal of Asthma, 35*, 537–545.

Allen, R. M., Jones, M. P., & Oldenberg, B. (1995). Randomised trial of an asthma self-management programme for adults. *Thorax, 50*, 731–738.

ASTHMA GENERAL KNOWLEDGE QUESTIONNAIRE
FOR ADULTS WITH ASTHMA

Here are some questions about asthma in general. Circle T, if you think the statement is true; F, if you think that the statement is false; NS, if you are not sure or do not know whether the statement is true or false.

Item		Correct Response	
1.	Left untreated, asthma will eventually go away.	T	F
2.	Asthma is a nervous or psychological illness.	T	F
3.	Asthma is a breathing problem that may be triggered by strong emotions.	T	F

During an asthma attack: . . .

4.	. . . the muscles around the airtubes tighten and the tubes become narrow.	T	F
5.	. . . more mucus is produced in the airtubes.	T	F
6.	. . . the lining of the airtubes becomes swollen.	T	F
7.	. . . the changes in the airtubes make it difficult to get the air out of the lungs.	T	F
8.	. . . the airtubes collapse.	T	F
9.	. . . the changes in the airtubes make it difficult to get the air into the lungs.	T	F
10.	Medication returns the airtubes to normal and no permanent damage usually occurs.	T	F
11.	You can become addicted to asthma medications if you use them all the time.	T	F
12.	Asthma medications do not work as well if you use them all the time.	T	F
13.	Although it cannot be cured, asthma can usually be controlled by taking the correct medication.	T	F
14.	Side-effects are less likely with inhaled medication than with tablets because inhaled medication is not absorbed into the body.	T	F
15.	Syrups and tablets work about as quickly as inhaled medications.	T	F
16.	If you get a cold or flu, you should increase your asthma medications.	T	F
17.	A doctor is best able to measure how bad asthma is by listening to the chest with a stethoscope.	T	F
18.	Measuring the amount of air in the lungs with a peak flow meter or spirometer is the most accurate way of measuring how bad asthma is.	T	F
19.	Most asthma deaths could have been prevented.	T	F
20.	If a person has died from an asthma attack, it usually means that the attack must have begun so quickly that there was no time to start treatment.	T	F
21.	You may have fewer asthma attacks if you can identify and avoid things that trigger them.	T	F
22.	When asthma is well controlled by medication it is not triggered so easily.	T	F

When you know that you are going to be exposed to something that triggers your asthma, . . .

Item	Correct Response	
23. ... you should take medication just before exposure.	T	F
24. ... you should wait until you develop symptoms before taking medication.	T	F
25. Regular exercise such as swimming can cure asthma.	T	F
26. Exercise can help keep you fit and well and better able to cope with asthma.	T	F
27. Exercising until you become breathless can damage the heart and/or lungs.	T	F
28. You should not exercise if exercise brings on even the occasional asthma attack.	T	F
29. Some medications taken 10 minutes before exercising can stop you getting asthma when you exercise.	T	F
30. Some medications can be used during exercise if you get asthma.	T	F
31. Only a doctor can call an ambulance for you.	T	F

From Allen, R. M., & Jones, M. P. (1998). The validity and reliability for asthma knowledge questionnaire used in the evaluation of a group asthma self-management program for adults with asthma. *Journal of Asthma, 35,* 537–545. Used with permission.

Answers: 1. F; 2. F; 3. T; 4. T; 5. T; 6. T; 7. T; 8. F; 9. T; 10. T; 11. F; 12. F; 13. T; 14. T; 15. F; 16. T; 17. F; 18. T; 19. T; 20. F; 21. T; 22. T; 23. T; 24. F; 25. F; 26. T; 27. F; 28. F; 29. T; 30. T; 31. F

33. Asthma Decisional Balance Questionnaire and Asthma Readiness to Change Questionnaire

Developed by Karen B. Schmaling, Niloofar Afari, and Arthur W. Blume

INSTRUMENT DESCRIPTION, ADMINISTRATION, AND SCORING GUIDELINES

Studies have found that about half of adult asthmatics take 50% or less of the prescribed amount of inhaled medications. The Asthma Decisional Balance Questionnaire (DBQ) and Asthma Readiness to Change Questionnaire (RTC) flow from the widely used Cognitive-Behavioral models, the Health Belief Model and the Transtheoretical Model. Both emphasize the usefulness of assessing patient perception of advantages and disadvantages of taking a health action (in this case use of asthma medication).

In the DBQ, participants are asked to indicate their level of agreement from strongly disagree (−3) to strongly agree (+3). Pro and con subscale scores are the average of all pro and con item scores (sum of scores divided by 16), respectively. Positive scores on the pro scale indicate more reasons for using asthma medications as prescribed. A total scale or decisional balance score (DB) is obtained by subtracting the con from the pro subscale score. A positive value for DB indicates more reasons for using asthma medications as prescribed.

The Asthma Readiness to Change Questionnaire was developed to classify individuals into one of five stages of change regarding optimal medication use. The first part yields the stage of change, and the medication use behavior score is the total of all affirmative answers (Schmaling, Afari, & Blume, 2000).

PSYCHOMETRIC CHARACTERISTICS

DBQ items reflecting positive and negative aspects of optimal asthma medication use were generated by a group of asthma patients and researchers. They were based on several decisional categories: gains and losses expected for self; gains and losses expected for other; self-approval and disapproval of the target behavior; and approval and disapproval of the behavior by others. Cronbach's alpha for the pro subscale was .88, for the con subscale .71, and for the total scale .83. Scores on the pro and con subscale were not significantly correlated with each other, as would be expected. Intraclass correlations for the pro, con, and total DB scales respectively over a 1–4 week period were .86, .77, and

.86. The internal consistency reliability coefficient for the RTC Questionnaire was .73 (Schmaling, Afari, & Blume, 2000).

A number of associations support validity of the subscale. Cons for taking medications as prescribed outweighed pros for those subjects in the precontemplation, contemplation, and preparation stages. Pros and cons were roughly equivalent in the action stage, but pros outweighed cons for those participants in the maintenance stage. This pattern of data is consistent with the association between decisional balance and stage of change postulated by the transtheoretical model. Second, the total number of affirmative medication use behaviors was significantly correlated with RTC stage of change. Third, increased ratings of readiness and confidence were associated with increasingly more committed RTC stages of change. Fourth, objective measures of medication adherence were significantly correlated with RTC stages of change. Subjects in more committed stages of change (action and maintenance) took more of the daily and P.R.N. medications than did those in the preparation stage. Participants who rated themselves as more ready to use medications were more likely to actually use them. Schmaling, Blume, and Afari (2001) completed a randomized controlled trial with a small number of participants which showed DBQ to be sensitive to interventions of education and motivational interviewing.

CRITIQUE AND SUMMARY

The DBC and RTC assess psychological factors important to adherence with medication regimens. Items on DBQ were actually generated in part by patients!

Work remaining to be done includes studying the temporal relationship between decisional balance, stage of change, and actual behavior. The authors believe that DBQ and RTC along with SE measures could form the basis for preintervention assessment (Schmaling, Afari, & Blume, 2000).

REFERENCES

Schmaling, K. B., Afari, N., & Blume, A. W. (2000). Assessment of psychological factors associated with adherence to medication regimens among adult asthmatic patients. *Journal of Asthma, 37,* 335–343.

Schmaling, K. B., Blume, A. W., & Afari, N. (2001). A randomized controlled pilot study of motivational interviewing to change attitudes about adherence to medications for asthma. *Journal of Clinical Psychology in Medical Settings, 8,* 167–172.

ASTHMA DECISIONAL BALANCE QUESTIONNAIRE

The following questionnaire lists some of the reasons why people with asthma take or don't take their asthma medications as they were prescribed by their doctor. Please read each statement carefully and circle the number that best matches how much you agree or disagree with each statement.

		Strongly Disagree	Somewhat Disagree	Disagree a Little	Agree a Little	Somewhat Agree	Strongly Agree
P	1. Taking my medications as prescribed gives me a feeling of control over my asthma.	−3	−2	−1	1	2	3
P	2. My asthma medications help me handle the *outdoors* more easily (like cold weather, temperature changes, exercise).	−3	−2	−1	1	2	3
C	3. I don't like how the asthma medications make me feel when I take them.	−3	−2	−1	1	2	3
P	4. Using my asthma medications as prescribed lets me *do things more easily* than when I'm having trouble breathing (like eat, work, concentrate, have sex).	−3	−2	−1	1	2	3
C	5. I'm too busy to go to the pharmacy to get refills of my asthma medications.	−3	−2	−1	1		3
C	6. I don't like taking medications in general.	−3	−2	−1	1	2	3
P	7. Taking my asthma medications as prescribed may help to prevent some of my asthma flare-ups.	−3	−2	−1	1	2	3
C	8. I really don't know how to use my asthma medications.	−3	−2	−1	1	2	3
C	9. I just don't need to use my asthma medications as often as my doctor has told me to.	−3	−2	−1	1	2	3
P	10. Any side effects from asthma medications are worth the benefit I get.	−3	−2	−1	1	2	3

		Strongly Disagree	Somewhat Disagree	Disagree a Little	Agree a Little	Somewhat Agree	Strongly Agree
C	12. I don't like doing things according to a schedule, like taking medications.	−3	−2	−1	1	2	3
P	13. Other people (family, friends) would suffer if I became ill from asthma.	−3	−2	−1	1	2	3
C	14. The asthma medications just don't make that much difference.	−3	−2	−1	1	2	3
P	15. Regular use of my asthma medications lets me *do more things* that I want to do.	−3	−2	−1	1	2	3
P	18. Regular use of my asthma medications lets me be more active.	−3	−2	−1	1	2	3
C	19. My partner/family/friends don't approve of me using my asthma medications.	−3	−2	−1	1	2	3
P	20. It's easier to take my asthma medications than go to the doctor or hospital.	−3	−2	−1	1	2	3
C	21. The asthma medications are too bulky to carry around.	−3	−2	−1	1	2	3
C	22. I don't need conventional medications for my asthma.	−3	−2	−1	1	2	3
P	23. I like myself better when I use my asthma medications as prescribed.	−3	−2	−1	1	2	3
C	24. I should be able to control my asthma with willpower.	−3	−2	−1	1	2	3
P	26. My health could probably improve if I used my asthma medications as prescribed.	−3	−2	−1	1	2	3
C	27. It's embarrassing to use my asthma medications in public.	−3	−2	−1	1	2	3
C	28. My partner/family/friends don't like the fact that I have asthma.	−3	−2	−1	1	2	3

(continued)

	Strongly Disagree	Somewhat Disagree	Disagree a Little	Agree a Little	Somewhat Agree	Strongly Agree
P 29. I could be more energetic if I used my asthma medications as prescribed.	-3	-2	-1	1	2	3
P 30. My asthma medications help me breathe more easily.	-3	-2	-1	1	2	3
C 31. Asthma medications are too expensive.	-3	-2	-1	1	2	3
P 32. Using my asthma medications as prescribed makes me feel better about myself.	-3	-2	-1	1	2	3

Your special reasons:

I don't use my asthma medications as my doctor has told me to because _____

I use my asthma medications as my doctor has told me to because _____

Asthma Readiness to Change Questionnaire

Please choose only one of the items below that best describes how you use your asthma medications **now**.

☐ I have not been taking my asthma medications as prescribed in the past month, and do not intend to do so in the next month.

☐ I have not been taking my asthma medications as prescribed in the past month, but am thinking about doing so in the next month.

☐ I have not been taking my asthma medications as prescribed in the past month, but plan to do so in the next month.

☐ I am taking my asthma medications as prescribed.

☐ I have been taking my asthma medications as prescribed in the past month, and plan to continue doing so in the next month.

34. Children with Asthma: Parent Knowledge, Attitude, Self-Efficacy, and Management Behavior Survey

Developed by Ilse Mesters, R. Meertens,
H. Crebolder, and G. Parcel

INSTRUMENT DESCRIPTION, ADMINISTRATION, AND SCORING GUIDELINES

Most children with asthma experience symptoms before they reach 5 years of age and account for a considerable number of hospitalizations resulting from the disease. Erroneous beliefs and attitudes held by parents were found using questionnaires and focus groups, and presumably affected their ability to care for their children. For example, preventive medication was considered ineffective because children still suffered from asthma symptoms. Parents were disappointed when the amount of medication was increased despite all their efforts and were afraid of addiction, not understanding that doses were likely to increase because of fast growth in children. Some thought that symptoms should not be suppressed but allowed to come out so that the child could get used to them and grow out of asthma. Some parents delayed the use of medicines as long as possible and tried several alternative treatments (Mesters, Pieterse, & Meertens, 1991).

Parents wanted objective indicators of the child's physical well-being and criteria by which to monitor the progress of an asthma episode, especially important because their child was too young to express verbally how and what he or she felt. The focus groups revealed that parents' knowledge appeared to be insufficient and incoherent, especially about medication, signs preceding an attack, and preventive activities. Parents also appeared to have an inadequate understanding of how to apply the information they received and a lack of confidence in their ability to do so. Warning signs of an asthma attack were not considered to be cues to action when the symptoms were mild to moderate.

This needs assessment led to development of the surveys reviewed here. Questionnaires are available in both Dutch and English. Item scores are summed. An educational protocol consisting of 16 modules has also been developed and tested (Mesters, Meertens, Crebolder, & Parcel, 1993). In a pilot sample of U.S. middle-income families, Horner (1998) found mean scores on the Management Behavior Survey much higher (3.39) than had Mesters and colleagues (2.42).

PSYCHOMETRIC PROPERTIES

The questionnaire was pretested for readability and uniform interpretation with 10 mothers of young children with asthma. The knowledge questionnaire was constructed to test an understanding of basic concepts about the nature of asthma and general management procedures and had an alpha of .81. The attitude survey was based, in part, on an earlier instrument and showed an alpha of .59. The self-efficacy survey (SE) focused on prevention, treatment and monitoring of asthma symptoms and showed an alpha of .93. The management behavior survey inquired about the extent to which self-management activities were performed and showed an alpha of .92 (Mesters et al., 1993).

Parents participating in the education program had significantly more knowledge (mean score pretest, 38.64; posttest, 58.96); a more favorable attitude toward asthma (mean score pretest, 26.12; posttest, 35.83); and a higher SE score. Also, they reported performing self-management behaviors more frequently than they had before the program. A similar study but with a randomized trial found mean posttest scores for the treatment group ($N = 31$) of 56.74 for knowledge, 34.66 for attitudes, .94 for SE, and 3.13 for self-management, all higher than scores of the control group ($N = 32$). Changes were sustained at one year. The treatment group was found to have decreased its emergency and nonemergency use of the physician's office and a reduction in reported asthma severity. Gain in knowledge was the best predictor of gain in (reported) self-management behavior, followed by gain in SE. This finding is congruent with social learning theory, which suggests that behavioral capability (which includes knowledge of what to do and how to do it) and SE mediate behavior. Alpha levels for all scales were above .80 except for the attitude scale, which was .33 (Mesters, Meertens, Kok, & Parcel, 1994). Thus, the tools were sensitive to an appropriate intervention.

CRITIQUE AND SUMMARY

Development and testing of these tools has occurred in The Netherlands, with small and nonrandom numbers of more highly educated parents. Although results of the needs assessment provide some assurance of content validity, structured description of the domains of knowledge, attitudes, and self-efficacy tasks were not found, nor were other studies of validity. Reliability of the attitude scale is problematic.

Goals of asthma self-management programs are increased adherence to prescribed medication, increased ability and confidence in managing asthma attacks, and decreased anxiety and disruptions of daily life. Although the educational program for which these instruments were developed was targeted at the parents of preschool children, they may be usable with parents of older children.

REFERENCES

Horner, S. D. (1998). Using the Open Airways curriculum to improve self-care for third-grade children with asthma. *Journal of School Health, 68,* 329–333.

Mesters, I., Meertens, R., Crebolder, H., & Parcel, G. (1993). Development of a health education program for parents of preschool children with asthma. *Health Education Research, 8,* 53–68.

Mesters, I., Meertens, R., Kok, G., & Parcel, G. S. (1994). Effectiveness of a multidisciplinary education protocol in children with asthma (0–4 years) in primary health care. *Journal of Asthma, 31,* 347–359.

Mesters, I., Pieterse, M., & Meertens, R. (1991). Pediatric asthma, a qualitative and quantitative approach to needs assessment. *Patient Education and Counseling, 17,* 23–34.

PARENT KNOWLEDGE QUESTIONNAIRE

Categories: true or false for each item

A.   Most children who have asthma:
   1.   need to be dressed more warmly than children without asthma
   2.   have both physical and psychological problems
   ③.   can normally take part in any activity requiring some physical exercise
   4.   cannot go on a holiday

B.   When a child has asthma:
   5.   the heart sometimes doesn't work right
   6.   the lungs sometimes do not work right
   ⑦.   the air tubes in the lungs are very sensitive to certain things
   8.   something is wrong with the child's blood

C.   Asthma attacks can be caused by:
   ⑨.   different things in different people
   10. spicy foods like hot peppers and lots of salt
   ⑪. things you are allergic to like dust, pollen, animals
   ⑫. virus infections like flu
   ⑬. irritants (paint, fumes, perfume, smoke, pollution)
   ⑭. emotions (laughing too hard, getting upset)
   15. drinking too much liquid
   ⑯. temperature difference
   ⑰. bacterial infections
   ⑱. physical exercise like running

D.   Preventing asthma symptoms:
   19. is never possible
   ⑳. might be possible by removing those things that cause symptoms
   ㉑. might be possible by staying away from those things that cause symptoms
   ㉒. may be helped by performing warming-up exercises before physical exercise
   23. is something only a child's doctor can do anything about
   ㉔. may be helped by taking preventive medication

E.   Children with asthma:
   ㉕. have less chance of getting symptoms when they are in good physical condition
   26. can be cured with medication
   ㉗. have a greater chance of keeping symptoms when the severity is worse
   ㉘. will remain sensitive

F.   When asthmatic children have an attack or asthma symptoms:
   ㉙. they have most trouble getting air out of the lungs
   ㉚. they have shortness of breath
   31. the air tubes inside their lungs become wider
   32. the muscles in the air tubes are paralyzed
   ㉝. the air passages in the lungs become filled with mucus
   ㉞. the tissue of the air tubes gets swollen
   ㉟. the muscles in the air tubes go into spasm and tighten

G. Some asthma medication:
- (36). can be used to prevent an attack or symptoms
- 37. causes addiction
- (38). can be used to remedy an attack or symptoms
- 39. requires increasing dosages
- 40. causes damaging side effects even in low doses

H. Children with allergic asthma:
- (41). react differently than other people do to the same substance
- (42). respond especially with their airways
- 43. only react immediately after contact with triggers
- (44). have a genetic tendency toward allergy
- (45). symptoms are triggered by the release of substances in the body after contact with a trigger

I. If children with asthma are starting to have an asthma attack:
- 46. there is no way one can tell an attack is going to happen
- (47). they might notice a tight feeling in their chest before the wheezing starts
- (48). one could give medicine before the wheezing starts
- 49. one should give medicine only after the wheezing starts
- (50). the degree to which expiration is prolonged might indicate the severity of the attack
- 51. they breathe very slowly taking long breaths
- (52). sucking in the skin of the chest might indicate the severity of the attack (retractions)
- (53). using a peakflow meter might indicate the severity of the attack

J. When the child has a moderate attack/symptoms:
- 54. the parent can do nothing to try and stop the attack
- 55. the parent must rush to the hospital before doing anything else
- (56). the parent can give medicine to stop the wheezing
- (57). it is important the child rests and tries to relax
- 58. the parent should try not to pay any attention to the wheezing and hope that it will go away
- (59). the child should drink lots of liquids
- (60). the parent should call the doctor if breathing does not get better shortly after taking medicine
- 61. always wait at least a day before calling the doctor to give medicine time to work

K. Children with hyperreactive airways:
- (62). react sooner and longer to a substance than other people
- (63). might get out of breath during and after exercise
- (64). can trigger an attack by yelling
- (65). have more symptoms in the early morning due to the low levels of hormones in the blood

L. Adapting the environment focuses on:
- (66). making the home as dustproof as possible
- 67. increasing the humidity in the home
- (68). improving ventilation in the home
- (69). removing material the child is allergic to

M. When using:
- 70. a dry-powder inhaler, the powder needs to be inhaled by taking a slow and deep breath

(continued)

. an aerosol, the child needs to inhale the spray the moment the spray is released
72. a peakflow meter, the cursor needs to be moved with a single puff of breath
73. inhalers, the child needs to hold his/her breath for a few seconds after inhalation

True answers are circled; others are false.

ASTHMA ATTITUDE SURVEY

Categories: strongly agree (1), agree a little (2), uncertain (3), disagree a little (4), strongly disagree (5)

1. My observations of my child's asthma symptoms are important in helping to get the asthma under control
2. Missing a dose of medication won't hurt
3. Asthma is a problem, even when my child has no symptoms
4. I consider it important to do things that can prevent my child from getting asthma symptoms
5. My child is like most other kids, except that he/she has asthma
6. I don't believe it is necessary to adapt my home because of my child's asthma
7. It is important to take asthma medicines on time
8. Early detection of asthma symptoms is important for getting them under control
9. Every asthma attack needs to be treated with medication
10. I think it is important to find out which triggers cause symptoms in my child
11. I have little control over my child's asthma symptoms
12. Eating properly and/or healthy food can help my child's asthma
13. Taking asthma medication during longer periods of time isn't good for children
14. People with asthma can be successful
15. When taking medicine the advantages outweigh the disadvantages
16. The more I know about asthma the better I can help my child
17. I don't believe that medicines really help to make symptoms go away
18. Children with asthma should be disciplined pretty much like other children
19. It is important to keep my child away from triggers
20. Asthma attacks generally do not happen just like that
21. It is important to let my child get used to triggers
22. I consider it important to be able to help my child when she/he has an attack
23. It is no use asking other people to take account of the fact that my child has asthma
24. The fact that asthma symptoms can disappear during puberty is no reason not to treat asthma

Scoring for the following items is reversed: 2, 3, 6, 11, 13, 17, 21, 23

PARENT SELF-EFFICACY SURVEY

Categories: very well (1), quite well (2), uncertain (3), rather poorly (4), very poorly (5), not applicable (6)

1. Imagine giving your child medicines: HOW well can you determine the dosage?
2. Imagine your child having a mild or moderate attack: HOW well can you treat this attack?

3. Imagine your child having a severe attack: HOW well can you treat this attack?
4. Imagine your child having asthma symptoms: HOW well can you estimate the moment to start giving medicines?
5. Imagine your child having a mild or moderate attack: HOW well can you estimate the severity of the attack?
6. Imagine your child having a mild or moderate attack: HOW well can you estimate the severity from wheezing?
7. Imagine your child having a mild or moderate attack: HOW well can you estimate the severity from retractions?
8. Imagine your child having a mild or moderate attack: HOW well can you estimate the severity from your child's breathing frequency?
9. Imagine your child having a mild or moderate attack: HOW well can you estimate the severity from the relative duration of breathing in and out?
10. Imagine your child having a severe attack: HOW well can you estimate the severity of the attack?
11. Imagine your child having a severe attack: HOW well can you estimate the severity from wheezing?
12. Imagine your child having a severe attack: HOW well can you estimate the severity from retractions?
13. Imagine your child having a severe attack: HOW well can you estimate the severity from your child's breathing frequency?
14. Imagine your child having a severe attack: HOW well can you estimate the severity from the relative duration of breathing in and out?
15. HOW well can you avoid asthma symptoms?
16. Imagine the symptoms of your child become worse: HOW well can you make the right choice of medicines?
17. Imagine the symptoms of your child become less severe: HOW well can you make the right choice of medicines?
18. Imagine your child having asthma symptoms: HOW well can you judge whether the medication works?
19. HOW well can you indicate what triggers cause asthma problems in your child?
20. HOW well can you decide when to call in the help from others (primary or clinical physician)?

HOW well can you cope with triggers inside the home such as:

21. dust/housemites?
22. animal dander?
23. molds?
24. pollen from trees, grasses, and weeds?
25. change in temperature?
26. dampness?
27. cigarette/cigar smoke?
28. smells of detergents, paint, spray, or glue?

HOW well can you cope with triggers outside the home such as:

29. fog, rain, humidity?
30. air pollution?
31. HOW well can you influence your child's physical resistance?
32. HOW well can you relax your child during an attack (distracting attention away from attack)?

MANAGEMENT BEHAVIOR SURVEY

Categories: never (1), seldom (2), sometimes (3), often (4), always (5), not applicable (6)

To what extent do you take the following actions to avoid asthma symptoms in your child?

1. Give medication
2. Avoid allergic triggers outside the home
3. Avoid allergic triggers inside the home
4. Avoid chemicals (like smoke, perfumes)
5. Avoid foods my child is sensitive to
6. Ventilate the home correctly
7. Decrease the degree of humidity in the home
8. Dustproof the home
9. Pay attention to composition of furniture and textiles
10. Stimulate physical activity of my child

To what extent do you take the following actions to treat asthma symptoms in your child?

11. Give medication
12. Give liquids
13. Relax the child
14. Remove triggers
15. Let the child rest

To what extent do you take the following actions to estimate the severity of an attack?

16. Control breathing frequency
17. Control the duration of breathing in and breathing out
18. Control presence of wheezing
19. Inspect the skin around the chest
20. Use peakflow meter

STATE-ANXIETY QUESTIONNAIRE

Categories: not at all, a little, much, very much

When my child has an asthma attack:

1. I feel calm
2. I am tense
3. I feel at ease
4. I feel certain
5. I feel nervous
6. I am indecisive
7. I am relaxed
8. I am worried

From Mesters, I., Meertens, R., Crebolder, H., & Parcel, G. Development of health education program for parents of pre-school children with asthma, Table A1. *Health Education Research, 16*(1), 53–68. Reprinted with permission.

35. Parent Barriers to Managing Asthma, Parent Asthma Self-Efficacy, Parent Belief in Treatment Efficacy, and Child Asthma Self-Efficacy Scales

Developed by Brenda Bursch, Lenore Schwankovsky, Jean Gilbert, and Robert Zeiger

INSTRUMENT DESCRIPTION, ADMINISTRATION, AND SCORING GUIDELINES

This cluster of instruments was developed to assess the impact of intervention and to help explain variance in self-management behaviors of children with asthma and their parents. The Parent Barriers to Managing Asthma (PBMA) was designed to measure a range of perceived barriers to managing asthma, the Parent Asthma Self-Efficacy Scale (PASE) to measure parent self-efficacy (SE) regarding preventing or managing asthma, the Parent Belief in Treatment Efficacy Scale (PBTE) to measure parents' belief in treatment efficacy, and Child Asthma Self-Efficacy Scale (CASE) to measure the child's SE regarding attack prevention and management (Bursch, Schwankovsky, Gilbert, & Zeiger, 1999). Scales are summed.

PSYCHOMETRIC CHARACTERISTICS

Items were developed from the literature and information interviews with asthma patients and parents and tested on asthmatic children age 7–15 and their parents. Evidence in support of validity follows. PBMA scores were positively related to emergency department use, asthma symptoms, and impact of the child's illness on the family. PASE subscales of attack prevention and management were positively related to health states and child SE and negatively related to asthma symptoms and impact on the family. PBTE scores were negatively associated with emergency department use, perceived barriers, and asthma symptoms, and were positively related to parent and child SE. CASE subscales on attack prevention and management were positively related to health status and child age, and negatively related to emergency department use and asthma symptoms. For the most part, these findings support construct validity.

Internal consistency reliability was PBMA .79; PASE .87 with attack prevention subscale (items 1–6) .77 and attack management subscale (items 7–13) .82; PTE .76; and CASE .87 with subscales attack prevention (items 1–8) .75 and attack management (items 9–14) .82 (Bursch, Schwankovsky, Gilbert, & Zeiger, 1999).

CRITIQUE AND SUMMARY

Further research is needed to examine the relationships between the measures and varying types of health care utilization based on the notion that inappropriate utilization of services will decrease as barriers decrease and as parent belief in treatment efficacy and child SE increase. In addition, the instruments were developed and tested in a group practice prepaid health plan, offering a set of barriers that might not be the same in a fee-for-service model. Also, the usefulness of these measures in assessing the impact of intervention and adherence to treatment schedules should be studied (Bursch, Schwankovsky, Gilbert, & Zeiger, 1999).

REFERENCE

Bursch, B., Schwankovsky, L., Gilbert, J., & Zeiger, R. (1999). Construction and validation of four childhood asthma self-management scales: Parent barriers, child and parent self-efficacy and parent belief in treatment efficacy. *Journal of Asthma, 36,* 115–128.

PARENT BARRIERS TO MANAGING ASTHMA

How much do the following make it hard for you to help your child to manage his/her asthma?

		Not hard at all	Slightly hard	Moderately hard	Quite hard	Extremely hard
1.	Getting my child to take the medications	1	2	3	4	5
2.	Reaching clinic staff here to ask questions	1	2	3	4	5
3.	Waiting for a long time before getting an appointment with the asthma doctor	1	2	3	4	5
4.	The staff are too busy to answer my questions	1	2	3	4	5
5.	Not having a way to get to appointments	1	2	3	4	5
6.	Clinic hours don't fit my work schedule	1	2	3	4	5
7.	Bad effects of medications	1	2	3	4	5
8.	Waiting for a long time in the waiting room before seeing the doctor	1	2	3	4	5
9.	Long-term effects of medications	1	2	3	4	5

PARENT ASTHMA SELF-EFFICACY

	Not at all sure	A little bit sure	Fairly sure	Quite sure	Completely sure	Does not apply
1. How sure are you that you can get your child to take his/her medications?	1	2	3	4	5	8
2. How sure are you that you can use the medication correctly?	1	2	3	4	5	8
3. How sure are you that you can get your child to a doctor's appointment?	1	2	3	4	5	8
4. How sure are you that you can follow the directions for giving medications to your child?	1	2	3	4	5	8
5. How sure are you that you can help your child avoid things he/she is allergic to?	1	2	3	4	5	8
6. How sure are you that you can help your child prevent a serious breathing problem?	1	2	3	4	5	8
7. How sure are you that you can have inhalers with you if your child has a serious breathing problem?	1	2	3	4	5	8
8. How sure are you that you can control a serious breathing problem at home rather than take your child to the ER?	1	2	3	4	5	8
9. How sure are you that you can keep the asthma from getting worse if your child starts to wheeze or cough?	1	2	3	4	5	8

	Not at all sure	A little bit sure	Fairly sure	Quite sure	Completely sure	Does not apply
10. How sure are you that you can help your child stay calm during a serious breathing problem?	1	2	3	4	5	8
11. How sure are you that you would know which medications to use when your child is having a serious breathing problem?	1	2	3	4	5	8
12. How sure are you that you know when your child's breathing problem can be controlled at home?	1	2	3	4	5	8
13. How sure are you that you know when to take your child to the emergency room during a serious breathing problem?	1	2	3	4	5	8

(continued)

PARENT BELIEF IN TREATMENT EFFICACY

	Not helpful	Slightly helpful	Moderately helpful	Quite helpful	Extremely helpful	Does not apply
1. How helpful is *avoiding things that cause allergic reactions* in preventing asthma attacks?	1	2	3	4	5	8
2. How helpful is *seeing a doctor regularly* in helping control asthma?	1	2	3	4	5	8
3. How helpful are *inhalers* in controlling a serious breathing problem?	1	2	3	4	5	8
4. How helpful is *keeping a child calm* in stopping a serious breathing problem?	1	2	3	4	5	8
5. How helpful is *calling the clinic* for advice for a serious breathing problem?	1	2	3	4	5	8

CHILD ASTHMA SELF-EFFICACY SCALE

	Not at all sure	A little bit sure	Fairly sure	Quite sure	Completely sure	NA
1. How sure are you that you can have inhalers with you the next time you have a serious breathing problem?	1	2	3	4	5	8
2. How sure are you that you can use your inhaler correctly?	1	2	3	4	5	8
3. How sure are you that you can prevent a serious breathing problem?	1	2	3	4	5	8
4. How sure are you that you can get to your next doctor's appointment?	1	2	3	4	5	8
5. How sure are you that you can slow yourself down to prevent serious breathing problems?	1	2	3	4	5	8
6. How sure are you that you can avoid things you are allergic to?	1	2	3	4	5	8
7. How sure are you that you can learn the skills you need to control your asthma?	1	2	3	4	5	8
8. If someone near you was smoking, how sure are you that you could ask them to stop?	1	2	3	4	5	8
9. How sure are you that you can control a serious breathing problem yourself rather than go to the emergency room?	1	2	3	4	5	8

(continued)

	Not at all sure	A little bit sure	Fairly sure	Quite sure	Completely sure	NA
10. How sure are you that you can keep your asthma from getting worse if you start to have symptoms such as wheezing or coughing?	1	2	3	4	5	8
11. How sure are you that you can stay calm during a serious breathing problem?	1	2	3	4	5	8
12. How sure are you that you know which medications to use during a serious breathing problem?	1	2	3	4	5	8
13. How sure are you that you can tell when a serious breathing problem can be controlled at home?	1	2	3	4	5	8
14. How sure are you that you know when you should go to the emergency room during a serious breathing problem?	1	2	3	4	5	8

From: Bursch, B., Schwankovsky, L., Gilbert, J., & Zeiger, R. (1999). Construction and validation of four childhood asthma self-management scales: Parent barriers, child and parent self-efficacy, and parent belief in treatment efficacy. *Journal of Asthma, 36,* 115–128. Used with permission.

36. Child's Perception of Asthma Medication Scale and Parents' Perception of Asthma Medication Scale

Developed by Laura M. DePaola, Michael C. Roberts, Michael S. Blaiss, Paul J. Frick, and Rodney E. McNeal

INSTRUMENT DESCRIPTION, ADMINISTRATION, AND SCORING GUIDELINES

Because the most commonly prescribed medical treatment for asthma is at-home medication use, the premise of the Child's Perceptions of Asthma Medications Scale (C-PAM) is that successful education of the child depends in part on understanding her perception of the medication. The health belief model (HBM) with its focus on perceived susceptibility to a particular illness, perception of severity of the illness, and the benefits and drawbacks of the recommended health behavior, forms the framework for C-PAM. Although research has been generally supportive of the HBM in adults, markedly less research has investigated the applicability of HBM or other health belief models in children and has produced more equivocal results.

Children's perceptions of medication, especially those with possible immediate and distressing side effects, are especially believed to be important to home treatment (DePaola, Roberts, Blaiss, Frick, & McNeal, 1997). Because medication use at home is usually controlled by parents, their perceptions are also studied (Parent's Perceptions of Asthma Medications Scale; P-PAM).

These instruments use three elements of the HBM (perceived severity, drawbacks, and benefits). C-PAM is written at the fourth-grade reading level and P-PAM at the seventh-grade level. C-PAM is completed by the child who has asthma or by her mother who predicts her answers. Responses are summed and averaged for each of the factors identified below (DePaola, Roberts, Blaiss, Frick, & McNeal, 1997).

PSYCHOMETRIC CHARACTERISTICS

Items were generated from mother/child interviews and reviewed by medical experts. Participants in this study were 162 children with asthma and their mothers, one-third of the group being Black. Through factor analysis two subscales were identified for each instrument: child or parent drawbacks (alpha = .85, .85) and child or parent benefits (alpha = .72, .84). Findings confirmed the drawbacks and benefits components of the HBM, although a significant portion of influence on asthma medications was not discovered by the model. Corresponding parent and child components were significantly related. Test–retest reliabilities were .87 (P-PAM) and .81 (C-PAM) (DePaola, Roberts, Blaiss, Frick, & McNeal, 1997).

CRITIQUE AND SUMMARY

Development and study of psychometric characteristics of these instruments were accomplished by a single team of researchers at one site. The authors suggest that it would be fruitful to alter any inaccurate perceptions of drawbacks of the medication and develop alternatives such as information about management of side effects, to overcome reality-based drawbacks.

REFERENCE

DePaola, L. M., Roberts, M. C., Blaiss, M. S., Frick, P. J., & McNeal, R. E. (1997). Mothers' and children's perceptions of asthma medications. *Children's Health Care, 26,* 265–283.

CHILDREN'S PERCEPTIONS OF ASTHMA MEDICATION

HI! This is *not* a test! I just want to know what you think about your asthma medicine. Please choose the number that best shows your thoughts about the sentence and put it on the line next to the sentence. For example: I like ice cream. <u>5</u> I answered with a 5 because I really do like ice cream.

1	2	3	4	5
Really	Sort of	Don't	Sort of	Really
Do not	Do not	Know	Agree	*Do*
Agree	agree			Agree

1. Taking the asthma medicine wastes a lot of time. _____

2. The asthma medicine makes me want to laugh and play more than usual. _____

3. If I don't take the asthma medicine, I will get an asthma attack. _____

4. The asthma medicine keeps me from having to go to the hospital. _____

5. My asthma is very bad. _____

6. My asthma medicine keep me from getting sick with asthma problems. _____

7. I can play more outside when I use my asthma medicine. _____

8. When I get an asthma attack, I usually end up in the hospital. _____

9. Even when I take my asthma medicine, I get sick with asthma anyway. _____

10. When I have an asthma attack, I usually have to go to the doctor's office. _____

11. When I take my asthma medicine, I can sleep through the night without waking up coughing or wheezing. _____

12. I don't miss as many days of school because I use my asthma medicine and it keeps me feeling well. _____

13. If I don't take my medicine, I will have an asthma attack sometime this week. _____

14. I fuss a lot when I have to take the asthma medicine. _____

15. My asthma medicine makes me act weird. _____

16. If I start to have asthma problems and I *don't* take the asthma medicine, then the asthma problems will get worse. _____

17. I don't want to take my asthma medicine when I'm at school. _____

18. My asthma medicine will keep my asthma from getting any worse than it is now. _____

19. Sometimes my asthma medicine makes me sick and makes me miss school. _____

20. My asthma medicine puts me in a bad mood. _____

21. My friends treat me like I'm weird because I use asthma medicine. _____

22. I *don't* want to use the asthma medicine when I'm out in public, like if I'm at the mall or something. _____

23. The asthma medicine makes me feel sick. _____

(continued)

24. The asthma medicine costs a lot of money. _____

25. The asthma medicine tastes good. _____

26. I feel better when I have the asthma medicine with me. _____

27. I don't like to have to take any medicine. _____

28. Taking the medicine at school is hard to do. _____

29. I would rather be like other kids and not have to take any asthma medicine. _____

30. Because I use asthma medicine, I can get out of doing stuff I don't want to do. _____

31. Taking the asthma medicine gets me a lot of attention. _____

32. I cough or wheeze a lot. _____

33. The asthma medicine makes me tired. _____

34. I can't do stuff I want to do because I use asthma medicine. _____

35. The asthma medicine makes it hard for me to think. _____

36. The asthma medicine tastes bad. _____

37. My friends treat me better than other kids because I take asthma medicine. _____

38. The asthma medicine makes it hard for me to do my schoolwork. _____

39. Because I use asthma medicine, I can get to do more of the stuff I want to do. _____

40. My asthma is: (Circle one)
     1. not very bad
     2. sort of bad
     3. very bad

Do you want me to know anything else about your asthma medicine that I haven't asked you?

PARENT'S PERCEPTIONS OF ASTHMA MEDICATION

Dear Parent, please choose the number that tells how you feel about that statement, and put it on the line next to it. For example: I like ice cream. 5 I chose a 5 because I really do like ice cream.

1	2	3	4	5
Really	Sort of	Don't	Sort of	Really
Do not	Do not	Know	Agree	*Do*
Agree	agree			Agree

1. Giving the asthma medicine to my child is very disruptive to our family's schedule. _____

2. My child's asthma medicine makes him/her hyperactive. _____

3. My child will get an asthma attack if he/she *does not* take the asthma medication. _____

4. The asthma medicine will keep my child out of the hospital most of the time. _____

5. If my child has an asthma attack at home this week I will be able to handle it at home, without a trip to the doctor. _____

6. My child's asthma is very serious. _____

7. My child will end up very sick with asthma if I *do not* give the asthma medicine. _____

8. My child's asthma medicine is a financial burden to our family. _____

9. The asthma medicine will keep my child well most of the time. _____

10. My child can exercise more when he/she uses the asthma medicine. _____

11. We have insurance that covers most of the cost of the medicine. _____

12. My child's asthma medicine is good at preventing attacks. _____

13. My child dislikes the asthma medicine. _____

14. Having to remember to give my child his/her asthma medicine is a burden. _____

15. If my child has an attack this week we will end up in the emergency room. _____

16. My child can sleep through the night better when on the asthma medicine. _____

17. My child misses *fewer* days of school because the asthma medicine makes his/her asthma better. _____

18. I am afraid that my child will have health problems in the future because of the asthma medicine he/she takes now. _____

19. My child fusses when taking the medicine. _____

20. Sometimes I skip giving the medicine because my child fusses. _____

21. My child experiences bad side effects because of the asthma medicine. _____

22. Getting my child to take the medicine when out in public is difficult. _____

23. The school has been cooperative with my child's asthma medicine schedule. _____

24. The medicine will keep my child's asthma from getting worse. _____

25. Deciding when to give my child the medicine (other than at routine times) is difficult. _____

26. My child has mood swings and I think it's because of the asthma medicine. _____

27. My child misses school because of the medicine's side effects. _____

28. My child is embarrassed because he/she uses asthma medicine. _____

29. My child says the asthma medicine tastes bad. _____

30. My child gets away with things more than he/she should because he/she is on asthma medicine. _____

31. My child's asthma medicine keeps him/her from getting other illnesses besides asthma. _____

32. My child's asthma medicine makes him/her act strangely. _____

33. My child's asthma medicine makes him/her gain weight. _____

34. Having the asthma medicines around gives me peace of mind. _____

35. Other children treat my child differently because he/she uses asthma medicine. _____

36. Getting my child to take his/her asthma medicine at school is difficult. _____

37. Adults treat my child differently because he/she uses asthma medicine. _____

(continued)

38. If we were out somewhere and discovered that I hadn't brought the asthma medicine with us, I would be very worried. _____

39. My child will probably have an asthma attack within the next mouth *even if I do* give him/her the asthma medicine. _____

40. My child's asthma is: (circle one)
    Mild   Moderate   Severe

From: DePaola, L. M., Robert, M. C., Blaiss, M. S., Frick, P. J., & McNeal, R. E. Used with permission.

37. Asthma Self-Regulatory Development Interview

Developed by Barry J. Zimmerman, Sebastian Bonner, David Evans, and Robert B. Mellins

INSTRUMENT DESCRIPTION, ADMINISTRATION, AND SCORING GUIDELINES

The Asthma Self-Regulatory Development Interview (ASRDI) was developed to test a model of self-regulatory development in which families' cognitive beliefs and behavioral skills for managing asthma symptoms emerge in four successive phases as described on page 194. Significant numbers of families are unresponsive to self-regulatory training perhaps because it requires changes in entrenched patterns of health beliefs and behavioral styles of coping, including self-perceptions of vulnerability and perceived efficacy for coping with symptoms (Zimmerman, Bonner, Evans, & Mellins, 1999).

ASRDI is a structured interview of family members available in both Spanish and English. Items 1–4 are designed to measure asthma acceptance (phase 2), items 5–7 asthma compliance (phase 3), and items 8–11 phase 4 (self-regulation). Scoring on items is pass/fail with failure to score at phase 2 level resulting in a phase 1 classification (asthma symptom avoidance) (Zimmerman, Bonner, Evans, & Mellins, 1999).

PSYCHOMETRIC CHARACTERISTICS

Interscorer agreement was .81. Factor analysis indicated a high level of sequentiality in ASRDI phase scores corresponding to the three item groups. A negative linear trend was found between family phase and the frequency of wheezing, sleep disturbance, home restriction, emergency department visits, and activity restrictions. Management/prevention behaviors, self-efficacy, and resourcefulness increase as family self-regulatory phase increases, supportive of validity (Zimmerman, Bonner, Evans, & Mellins, 1999).

CRITIQUE AND SUMMARY

ASRDI is currently a research instrument, developed and used at a single hospital with a largely Latino, lower socioeconomic status, inner-city population. The authors found that only two percent of the families studied could self-regulate on their own.

Self-regulatory theory undergirding ASRDI suggests that self-regulating asthma should be envisioned as a complex developmental process rather than a simple educational one. An optimal educational intervention especially for lower phase families probably requires a family coordinator to work families through the phases (Zimmerman, Bonner, Evans, & Mellins, 1999). Although much further testing of content and compiling other evidence of validity and reliability remain to be done, the instrument does address a crucial area. Analysis shows decrease in asthma severity across the four phases and increase in asthma regulatory practices.

REFERENCE

Zimmerman, B. J., Bonner, S., Evans, D., & Mellins, R. B. (1999). Self-regulating childhood asthma: A developmental model of family change. *Health Education and Behavior, 26,* 55–71.

ASTHMA SELF-REGULATORY
DEVELOPMENT INTERVIEW (ASRDI)

Phase	Item	
2	1.	Do you ever worry that you may not be able to get to the doctor or hospital in time to get the care your child needs for an attack? Why or why not? *Responses that fail to indicate worry about asthma are not credited with passing; any mention of worry is scored as passing.*
2	2.	How much do you feel that your child's asthma restricts daily activities or prevents him or her from being able to do the things he or she would like to do? *Responses that fail to indicate asthma restrictions are not credited with passing; any mention of restrictions is scored as passing.*
2	3.	How serious can your child's asthma be? *Responses that fail to indicate that asthma is potentially life threatening for the child or that asthma has potential long-term consequences are not credited with passing; responses that mention limitation in lives or long-term consequences are scored as passing.*
2	4.	Do you feel that your child's asthma could possibly be life threatening if nothing is done to treat it? Why or why not? *Disagreement that asthma can be life threatening is not credited with passing; agreement is scored as passing.*
3	5.	How important is it for your child to have regularly scheduled appointments with the doctor for his or her asthma? Why? *Responses that fail to indicate that the child keeps regularly scheduled doctor visits for asthma are not credited with passing; responses that indicate that the child keeps regularly scheduled doctor visits are scored as passing.*
3	6.	How important is it to take all the medicines at the exact dosage that the doctor has prescribed? Why? *Responses that fail to indicate adherence to the prescribed pharmacotherapy are not credited with passing; responses that indicate adherence are scored as passing.*
3	7.	If the asthma medicine that the doctor prescribes doesn't seem to help your child, how important is it to continue giving it? Why? *Responses that fail to indicate consultation with the doctor before changing asthma medication are not credited with passing; responses that indicate consultation with the doctor for alterations of pharmacotherapy are scored as passing.*
4	8.	Do you have any special method to check for early signs of an oncoming asthma attack? What is it? *Responses that fail to specify early symptoms of an attack are not credited with passing; responses that specify early symptoms are scored as passing.*

(continued)

Phase	Item

4   9.   Do you have a special procedure that you follow starting at the first sign of an asthma attack? What is it?
           Procedures that fail to specify the rescue medicines that must be administered at the first sign of an attack are not credited with passing; procedures that specify the rescue medicines are scored as passing.

4   10. Do you have a systematic plan to adjust your child's medicine if his or her pattern of symptoms gets better or worse? What is it?
           Responses that indicate the failure to work out a stepped pharmacological plan with the doctor are not credited with passing; stepped plans that have been worked out with the doctor are scored passing.

4   11. Do you have any special procedure for observing changes in your child's symptoms after you give him or her asthma medicine? What is it?
           Responses that fail to indicate the necessity of personally monitoring specific symptoms are not credited with passing; responses that indicate the necessity of personally monitoring specific symptoms are scored as passing.

Family Characteristics by Phase of Asthma Self-Regulation

Phase 1   *Asthma symptom avoidance.* The patient or family may perceive a periodic cough or wheeze, but they do not attribute these symptoms to an inherent physiological vulnerability with serious health-threatening outcomes if untreated. They try to avoid asthma symptoms nonmedically through activity restrictions and emotional calming.

Phase 2   *Asthma acceptance.* The patient or family accepts asthma as a serious health-threatening disease, but they respond to asthma only reactively (nonpreventively), primarily by using bronchodilators. Their main pharmacological efforts are toward a rescue from acute episodes, and they are resigned to the recurrence of exacerbations.

Phase 3   *Asthma compliance.* The patient or family seeks to prevent and control asthma symptoms by following the physician's treatment recommendations and is therefore less likely to need emergency treatment. However, they lack the confidence to self-regulate asthma because they are unskilled at preventively altering medications.

Phase 4   *Asthma self-regulation.* The patient or family develops an adaptable medical plan in consultation with the physician. They monitor lung functioning with peak flow meters or symptom recognition and can identify early warning signs of inflammation. They adjust their medical regimens on the basis of self-monitored signs, symptoms, or contact with triggers and are confident of their efficacy in implementing the plan and in contacting their doctor when modifications are needed.

From: Zimmerman, B. J., Bonner, S., Evans, D., & Mellins, R. B. (1999). Self-regulatory childhood asthma: A developmental model of family change. *Health Education & Behavior, 26,* 55–71. Used with permission.

Section E

Cardiovascular Illness

Many more instruments are available for cardiac than for vascular illnesses. This group includes assessment of learning needs and information but fewer more integrative instruments that could approximate active daily problem solving for self management.

---

38. Representation of Heart Attack Symptoms Questionnaire

Developed by Julie Johnson Zerwic

INSTRUMENT DESCRIPTION, ADMINISTRATION, AND SCORING GUIDELINES

Because acute myocardial infarction (AMI) is the leading cause of death in America and minimization of delay is important in successful treatment, it is important to understand why patients may delay seeking care. One explanation for delayed behavior is that individuals have expectations about the symptoms of AMI that are not consistent with what they experience. Leventhal's common sense model of illness provides the theoretic structure for the instrument.

The Representation of Heart Attack Symptoms Questionnaire (RHAS) requires response by degree of likelihood (4 = very likely to, 1 = very unlikely to) particular symptoms. A single item asks for a rating about intensity of the discomfort from 0 (no discomfort) to 10 (the most discomfort imagined) (Zerwic, 1998).

PSYCHOMETRIC CHARACTERISTICS

In prior studies, expectations concerning the location, quality, and intensity of discomfort and other associated symptoms were crucial to delay. Content validity was also supported by expert review. Test–retest reliability at two weeks was 88% for the subscale of associated symptoms, 90% for the quality and location subscales, and .81 for expectation of intensity (Zerwic, 1998).

CRITIQUE AND SUMMARY

Understanding symptom expectations held by the public is essential to develop educational interventions that might reduce delay. Interventions to date have ranged from negligible effect to modest improvement perhaps because they have targeted an area (insufficient knowledge of classic AMI symptoms) that was not contributing to the delay behavior. Use of RHAS is seen as a way to improve the precision of such interventions (Zerwic, 1998).

Only very beginning psychometric data are available for RHAS—additional validity and reliability studies should be completed. It does, however, address a critical issue, and initial trial of it showed subjects overwhelmingly expecting the discomfort of AMI to be severe instead of the range that it can be. Prospective designs are needed to determine the aspects of inaccurate expectations that adversely affect delay (Zerwic, 1998).

REFERENCE

Zerwic, J. J. (1998). Symptoms of acute myocardial infarction: Expectations of a community sample. *Heart & Lung, 27,* 75–81.

REPRESENTATION OF HEART ATTACK
SYMPTOMS QUESTIONNAIRE

Directions:

I am interested in learning what you believe are the symptoms commonly experienced during a heart attack. I am going to ask you a series of questions and I would like you to rate how likely or unlikely you would have expected that particular item to be associated with a heart attack. The possible responses are very likely, somewhat likely, somewhat unlikely, very unlikely, or unsure.

1. Please indicate how likely you believe a person having a heart attack would have any of the following symptoms.

$$4 = \text{very likely}$$
$$3 = \text{somewhat likely}$$
$$2 = \text{somewhat unlikely}$$
$$1 = \text{very unlikely}$$
$$0 = \text{unsure}$$

						Ranking of "likely" symptoms
Nausea	4	3	2	1	0	_____
Shortness of breath	4	3	2	1	0	_____
Headache	4	3	2	1	0	_____
Dizziness	4	3	2	1	0	_____
Fainting	4	3	2	1	0	_____
Sweating	4	3	2	1	0	_____
Palpitations/irregular heart beats	4	3	2	1	0	_____
Tired	4	3	2	1	0	_____
Coughing	4	3	2	1	0	_____
Chest pain	4	3	2	1	0	_____
Loss of appetite	4	3	2	1	0	_____
Unable to move arms or legs	4	3	2	1	0	_____
Confusion	4	3	2	1	0	_____
Fear	4	3	2	1	0	_____
Vomiting	4	3	2	1	0	_____
Chills	4	3	2	1	0	_____
Stomach ache	4	3	2	1	0	_____

©Julie Zerwic (2001). Used with permission.

(continued)

						Ranking of "likely" symptoms

Please list and rate any other symptoms you would expect with a heart attack.

_____   4   3   2   1   0   _____

_____   4   3   2   1   0   _____

1.b.   You have listed _____ (read symptoms designated as very or somewhat likely) as likely symptoms to experience during a heart attack. Of these symptoms which one did you think was **the most likely** symptom of a heart attack (place the number one under ranking column). What did you think was the **second most likely** symptom of a heart attack. (Continue until the top 5 likely symptoms are ranked.)

2.   Please indicate for each locations how likely or unlikely you believe it would be for an individual who was having a heart attack to have discomfort in this location.

         4 = very likely
         3 = somewhat likely
         2 = somewhat unlikely
         1 = very unlikely
         0 = unsure

						Ranking of "likely" locations
Ears	4	3	2	1	0	_____
Cheeks	4	3	2	1	0	_____
Jaw	4	3	2	1	0	_____
Teeth	4	3	2	1	0	_____
Throat/neck	4	3	2	1	0	_____
Left side of chest	4	3	2	1	0	_____
Middle of chest	4	3	2	1	0	_____
Right side of chest	4	3	2	1	0	_____
Upper back	4	3	2	1	0	_____
Lower back	4	3	2	1	0	_____
Upper abdomen	4	3	2	1	0	_____
Lower abdomen	4	3	2	1	0	_____
Left shoulder	4	3	2	1	0	_____
Left arm	4	3	2	1	0	_____
Right shoulder	4	3	2	1	0	_____
Right arm	4	3	2	1	0	_____
Left leg	4	3	2	1	0	_____
Right leg	4	3	2	1	0	_____

2.b.   You have listed _____ (read locations designated as very or somewhat likely) as likely locations to experience the symptoms for a heart attack. Of these locations which one did you think was **the most likely** location of heart attack symptoms (place the number one under ranking column). What was the **second most likely** location of a heart attack. (Continue until the top 5 likely locations are ranked.)

3.   Listed below are a variety of words people use to describe different types of pain or discomfort. Please indicate how likely you believe each word would be used to describe the discomfort during a heart attack.

$$4 = \text{very likely}$$
$$3 = \text{somewhat likely}$$
$$2 = \text{somewhat unlikely}$$
$$1 = \text{very unlikely}$$
$$0 = \text{unsure}$$

						Ranking of "likely" descriptors
Sharp	4	3	2	1	0	_____
Pressure	4	3	2	1	0	_____
Heaviness	4	3	2	1	0	_____
Cold	4	3	2	1	0	_____
Aching	4	3	2	1	0	_____
Stabbing	4	3	2	1	0	_____
Crushing	4	3	2	1	0	_____
Knife-like	4	3	2	1	0	_____
Burning	4	3	2	1	0	_____
Constricting	4	3	2	1	0	_____
Hot	4	3	2	1	0	_____
Tightness	4	3	2	1	0	_____
Cutting	4	3	2	1	0	_____

Please list and then rate any other words you would use to describe the discomfort of a heart attack.

_____	4	3	2	1	0	_____
_____	4	3	2	1	0	_____

3.b.   You have listed _____ (read descriptors designated as very or somewhat likely) as likely words to describe the discomfort associated with a heart attack. Of these words which one did you think was **the best word** to describe the discomfort of heart attack symptoms (place the number one under ranking column). What word was the **second best** word to describe the discomfort of a heart attack. (Continue until the top 5 likely words are ranked.)

(continued)

4. How intense or severe do you believe the discomfort of a heart attack would be? Please make a check on the line below. 0 = no discomfort and 10 = the most discomfort you can imagine.

0	1	2	3	4	5	6	7	8	9	10

No   Maximum
Discomfort   Discomfort

39. Cardiac Knowledge Questionnaire

Developed by John G. Maeland and Odd E. Havik

INSTRUMENT DESCRIPTION, ADMINISTRATION, AND SCORING GUIDELINES

The Cardiac Knowledge Questionnaire (CKQ) was developed to measure knowledge about: (a) the cardiovascular system and nature of coronary heart disease (Basic Cardiac Knowledge Scale; BCKS), (b) behavioral aspects of the cause and consequences of a heart attack (Cardiac Lifestyle Knowledge Scale; CLKS), and (c) prognostic implications of a heart infarction (Cardiac Misconceptions Scale). Together, the Basic Cardiac Knowledge Scale and the Cardiac Lifestyles Knowledge Scale form a Total Cardiac Knowledge Scale. The Cardiac Misconceptions Scale has been separate, with a high score indicating the patient has few unwarranted frightening beliefs about the heart attack. In each scale a score is calculated as percentage of correct items of all items in the scale, with "don't know" counted as an incorrect answer (Maeland & Havik, 1987).

PSYCHOMETRIC CHARACTERISTICS

Content validity including correct answers was supported by health care professionals and patients although the misconceptions scale was not. Internal consistency for the CLKS was .69, for the CMS .74, and for the BCKS .84 (Maeland & Havik, 1987). In a subsequent study, the BCKS Cronbach's alpha was .78, CMS .50, and CLKS .48 (Lidell & Fridlund, 1996).

For most items, nurses were better informed than were patients, those working in cardiac specialty better informed than those who did not, and more experienced nurses better informed than less experienced (known groups) (Newens, McColl, Bond, & Priest, 1996).

A short educational course for heart patients resulted in improved average scores in all three scales, indicating their sensitivity to intervention. Also, Lidell and Fridlund (1996) found that patients who had attended a comprehensive rehabilitation program had more basic cardiac knowledge and knowledge about misconceptions than those who had not.

CRITIQUE AND SUMMARY

CKQ is expected to be useful in studies of cardiac rehabilitation (Newens, McColl, & Bond, 1997) and as evaluation of the effectiveness of patient education (Maeland & Havik, 1987). Because these scales were developed some time ago, content should be reviewed for currency. Internal consistencies are frequently low in knowledge tests which must be diverse to test the domain.

REFERENCES

Lidell, E., & Fridlund, B. (1996). Long-term effects of a comprehensive rehabilitation programme after myocardial infarction. *Scandinavian Journal of Caring Sciences, 10*, 67–74.

Maeland, J. G., & Havik, O. E. (1987). Measuring cardiac health knowledge. *Scandinavian Journal of Caring Sciences, 1*, 23–31.

Newens, A. J., McColl, E., & Bond, S. (1997). Changes in reported dietary habit and exercise levels after an uncomplicated first myocardial infarction in middle-aged men. *Journal of Clinical Nursing, 6*, 153–160.

Newens, A. J., McColl, E., Bond, S., & Priest, J. F. (1996). Patients' and nurses' knowledge of cardiac-related symptoms and cardiac misconceptions. *Heart & Lung, 25*, 190–199.

CARDIAC KNOWLEDGE QUESTIONNAIRE

T = true, F = false

1.	The blood is circulated through the heart by the arteries.	(F)
2.	The blood supply to the heart is delivered from the heart chamber.	(F)
3.	The blood is delivered to the heart through a separate vascular system.	(T)
4.	Hardening of the arteries (arteriosclerosis) is caused by too much calcium in the blood.	(F)
5.	In hardening of the arteries (arteriosclerosis) calcium is deposited on the outside of the arteries causing constriction.	(F)
6.	Hardening of the arteries begins with the accumulation of fat deposits within the arterial wall.	(T)
7.	The arteries of the heart (the coronary arteries) may be subject to arteriosclerosis.	(T)
8.	A heart infarction usually lasts only a few minutes.	(F)
9.	A heart infarction is usually caused by changes in the arteries of the heart (the coronary arteries).	(T)
10.	A heart infarction is caused by the blocking of the blood flow to a part of the heart.	(T)
11.	A heart infarction results from a spasm or cramp in the heart muscle.	(F)
12.	A heart infarction is caused by a blood clot inside the heart chamber blocking the blood stream.	(F)
13.	In a heart infarction a part of the heart gets too little oxygen.	(T)
14.	A heart infarction results in damage of the heart muscle.	(T)
15.	A heart infarction is relieved in a few minutes by rest.	(F)
16.	Nitroglycerin is of great help in a heart infarction.	(F)
17.	A patient with a heart infarction should seek hospitalization as soon as possible.	(T)
18.	A heart infarction is better tolerated if physical fitness is good.	(T)
19.	Angina pectoris usually occurs during physical exertion.	(T)
20.	Angina pectoris is usually caused by changes in the arteries of the heart (the coronary arteries).	(T)
21.	Angina pectoris results from a spasm or cramp in the heart muscle.	(F)
22.	Angina pectoris is caused by a blood clot inside the heart chamber blocking the blood stream.	(F)
23.	In angina pectoris a part of the heart gets too little oxygen.	(T)
24.	Angina pectoris results in damage of the heart muscle.	(F)
25.	Angina pectoris is relieved in a few minutes by rest.	(T)
26.	Angina pectoris usually lasts only a few minutes.	(T)
27.	Nitroglycerin is a great help in angina pectoris.	(T)

(continued)

T = true, F = false

28. A patient with angina pectoris should seek hospitalization as soon as   (F)
    possible.

29. Angina pectoris will result in a weak area in the heart wall that can easily   (F)
    rupture.

30. Physical training can reduce the symptoms in angina pectoris.   (T)

Cardiac Lifestyle Knowledge Questionnaire

1. All heart patients should change their diets significantly.   (F)

2. It does not help to quit smoking after many years because one's health is   (F)
   already damaged.

3. If one stops smoking but gains weight as a result, one's health is not   (F)
   benefited.

4. The risk to one's health from cigarette smoking depends on how long one   (T)
   has smoked.

5. After a typical heart infarction physical training may lead to the same   (T)
   physical fitness as before the heart attack, or better.

6. After a typical heart infarction the patient must always avoid physical   (F)
   exertion.

7. Almost everyone can resume their sexual activities after a typical heart   (T)
   infarction.

Please rate the risk for heart infarction in:

8. Overweight   (2, 3, 4)
9. Heavy physical work   (1, 2)
10. Excessive alcohol consumption   (1, 2, 3)
11. Cigarette smoking   (4, 5)
12. High cholesterol blood level   (3, 4)
13. Heavy coffee consumption   (1, 2)
14. Sedentary occupation   (1, 2, 3)
15. High blood pressure   (3, 4)

1: very low risk for heart infarction
2: low risk
3: some risk
4: high risk
5: very high risk

Cardiac Misconceptions Questionnaire

1. Physical training after a typical heart infarction is dangerous and should   (F)
   only be performed under medical supervision.

2. A heart infarction will result in a weak area in the heart wall that can   (F)

easily rupture.

3. After a typical heart infarction the patient will be physically impaired permanently. (F)

4. After a typical heart infarction the damage to the heart is repaired within the first two to three months. (T)

5. After a typical heart infarction the patient must remain physically inactive for the first 6 weeks. (F)

6. After a typical heart infarction the risk of recurrences will be high indefinitely. (F)

7. After a typical heart infarction the patient should start gradual physical exercise within a few days after hospital discharge. (T)

8. Air travel may be dangerous after a typical heart infarction. (F)

9. People can resume their normal activities usually two to three months after a typical heart infarction. (T)

10. Three out of ten patients return to work after a typical heart infarction. (F)

From: Maeland, J. G., & Havik, O. E. (1987). Measuring cardiac knowledge. *Scandinavian Journal of Caring Sciences, 1,* 23–31. Used with permission of Blackwell Science Ltd.

40. Heart Failure Patient Learning Needs Inventory*

Developed by Dianne Wehby and Phyllis Brenner

INSTRUMENT DESCRIPTION, ADMINISTRATION, AND SCORING GUIDELINES

Heart Failure Patient Learning Needs Inventory (HFPLNI), originally developed as Cardiac Patients Learning Needs Inventory (CPLNI), has evolved into a cluster of instruments, each used to assess patients' learning needs related to cardiac conditions. It has been altered to be specific to coronary artery bypass graft (CABG) patient learning needs and in some versions includes both a rating of how important it is to learn and how realistic the patient thinks it is to learn (Moranville-Hunziker, Sagehorn, Conn, & Hagenoff, 1993), coronary artery disease (Czar & Engler, 1997), and a percutaneous transluminal coronary angioplasty (PTCALNI) for angina patients (Brezynskie, Pendon, Lindsay, & Adam, 1998). Heart Failure PLNI has been used in several studies (Hagenoff, Feutz, Conn, Sagehorn, & Moranville-Hunziker, 1999; Fratini, Lindsay, Kerr, & Park, 1998) again revised by Wehby and Brenner (1999).

Item scores are summed and frequency means obtained for content clusters. Norms are available in most of the citations. Some authors reported time to complete at 30 minutes (Czar & Engler, 1997).

PSYCHOMETRIC CHARACTERISTICS

Expert review supported content validity (Gerard & Peterson, 1984; Moranville-Hunziker, Sagehorn, Conn, & Hagenoff, 1993) and PLNI instruments modified for particular disease entities generally followed the same procedure (Hagenoff, Feutz, Conn, Sagehorn, & Moranville-Hunziker, 1994).

Internal consistency reliability for the total CPLNI was .91 and for the various informational categories: introduction to coronary care unit .68, anatomy and physiology .96, psychological concerns .69, risk factors .86, medications .89, dietary information .89, physical activity .81, and miscellaneous information .84, and in a replication study .95 total test and .77–.85 for the informational categories (Karlik & Yarcheski, 1987). In the CABG PLNI, alpha levels ranged from .77–.95 for importance to learn and .90–.96 for realistic to learn (Moranville-Hunziker, Sagehorn, Conn, & Hagenoff, 1993). Versions adapted for other populations may change these clusters and points on the rating scales. PTCALNI alpha was .94 and for individual categories of items .75–.91 (Brezynskie, Pendon, Lindsay, & Adam, 1998). Internal consistency reliability for the CHFPLNI was .94, .81–.95 for the seven categories (Frattini, Lindsay, Kerr, & Park, 1998).

---

*Originally Cardiac Patient Learning Needs Inventory (CPLNI) developed by Peggy S. Gerard.

In some studies, patients had difficulty understanding whether importance had to do with their preference or with how important it was to have the content discussed with them (Czar & Engler, 1997).

CRITIQUE AND SUMMARY

CPLNI was originally used to compare nurses' and patients' perceptions of learning needs or patients' intentions to comply with the medical regimen (Gerard & Peterson, 1984; Karlik & Yarchesi, 1987; Karlik, Yarchesi, Braun, & Wu, 1990) and has been consistently used that way. It was used in studies with small sample sizes and generated very little data about validity of the instrument or its sensitivity to interventions. While sometimes referred to as subscales, evidence of statistical testing of the clusters of items by topic could not be located. Recent use of CPLNI could not be located; recent use has involved PLNIs modified for use with particular diagnostic groups especially congestive heart failure. A check of currentness of content would be important as treatment approaches change.

REFERENCES

Brezynskie, H., Pendon, E., Lindsay, P., & Adam, M. (1998). Identification of the perceived learning needs of balloon angioplasty patients. *Canadian Journal of Cardiovascular Nursing, 9*(2), 8–14.

Czar, M. L., & Engler, M. M. (1997). Perceived learning needs of patients with coronary artery disease using a questionnaire assessment tool. *Heart & Lung, 26,* 109.

Fratinni, E., Lindsay, P., Kerr, E., & Park, Y. J. (1998). Learning needs of congestive heart failure patients. *Progress in Cardiovascular Nursing, 13*(2), 11–16, 33.

Gerard, P. S., & Peterson, L. M. (1984). Learning needs of cardiac patients. *Cardiovascular Nursing, 20*(2), 7–11.

Hagenoff, B. D., Feutz, C., Conn, V. S., Sagehorn, K. K., & Moranville-Hunziker, M. B. (1994). Patient education needs as reported by congestive heart failure patients and their nurses. *Journal of Advanced Nursing, 19,* 685–690.

Karlik, B. A., & Yarcheski, A. (1987). Learning needs of cardiac patients: A partial replication study. *Heart & Lung, 16,* 544–551.

Karlik, B. A., Yarcheski, A., Braun, J., & Wu, M. (1990). Learning needs of patients with angina: An extension study. *Journal of Cardiovascular Nursing, 4*(2), 70–82.

Moranville-Hunziker, M. B., Sagehorn, K. K., Conn, V., & Hagenoff, B. (1993). Patients' perceptions of learning needs during the first phase of cardiac rehabilitation following coronary artery bypass graft surgery. *Rehabilitation Nursing Research, 10,* 73–80.

Wehby, D., & Brenner, P. S. (1999). Perceived learning needs of patients with heart failure. *Heart & Lung, 28,* 31–40.

HEART FAILURE PATIENT LEARNING NEEDS INVENTORY

Part I—Patient Version

For each of the following statements, please check how **important** you feel the information is for you to know.

Topic	Not important	Somewhat important	Important	Moderately important	Very important
I need to know ...					
1. ... why I am short of breath.					
2. ... what the heart looks like and how it works.					
3. ... what causes heart failure.					
4. ... what happens when someone has heart failure.					
5. ... can the heart's function improve.					
6. ... if any other tests will be done after I leave the hospital.					
7. ... the reason for further testing after I go home.					
8. ... where my family can go to learn CPR.					
9. ... the normal emotional response to having a chronic illness.					
10. ... the importance of talking to someone about my fears, feelings, and thoughts.					
11. ... what effect stress has on my heart.					
12. ... what I can do to reduce stress while in the hospital.					
13. ... what I can do to reduce stress when I go home.					
14. ... what support groups are available.					
15. ... which factors may have contributed to the onset of my heart disease.					
16. ... how these factors affect the heart.					
17. ... what I can do to improve my heart function.					

Topic	Not important	Somewhat important	Important	Moderately important	Very important
18. . . . general rules about taking medications.					
19. . . . why I am taking each medication.					
20. . . . what the side-effects of each medication are.					
21. . . . what to do if I have problems with medications.					
22. . . . how to adapt to taking medications every day.					
23. . . . general rules about eating.					
24. . . . how diet affects my heart disease.					
25. . . . what the words sodium, salt, and NaCl mean.					

For each of the following statements, check how **important** you feel the information is for a patient with heart failure to know.

I need to know . . .	Not important	Somewhat important	Important	Moderately important	Very important
26. . . . what my diet restrictions are, if any.					
27. . . . how to adapt the recommended diet to my lifestyle.					
28. . . . what fluid restriction means.					
29. . . . how to adapt the recommended fluid restriction to my lifestyle.					
30. . . . why daily weights are needed.					
31. . . . how to adapt daily weights to my lifestyle.					
32. . . . how alcohol affects the heart.					
33. . . . why I may not be able to do as much physically as I could before developing heart failure.					

(continued)

I need to know . . .	Not important	Somewhat important	Important	Moderately important	Very important
34. . . . general guidelines for physical activity.					
35. . . . what my physical activity restrictions are, if any.					
36. . . . how to tell if I can increase my activity.					
37. . . . when I can engage in sexual activity.					
38. . . . how significant my heart failure is.					
39. . . . what advanced directives are.					
40. . . . what is my long-term life expectancy.					
41. . . . what can happen if I do not follow my doctor's recommendations.					
42. . . . what my quality of life is expected to be.					
43. . . . what advice should be given to my family in the event of a sudden death outside the hospital.					
44. . . . what symptoms are caused by heart failure.					
45. . . . what are the signs and symptoms of worsening heart failure.					
46. . . . what I should do if symptoms worsen.					
47. . . . when to call the doctor.					
48. . . . the signs and symptoms of other heart problems.					
49. Please write in the space below any additional item that you think is important for the patient to learn that was not on this list and rate this item using the scale to the right.					

Part II—Patient Version

As you continue the survey, you will notice that you have read each of the following items in the first half of the survey. Now, please check how **realistic** you feel it is to learn this information during hospitalization.

Topic	Not realistic	Somewhat realistic	Realistic	Moderately realistic	Very realistic
During my stay in the hospital, it is realistic to learn . . .					
50. . . . why I am short of breath.					
51. . . . what the heart looks like and how it works.					
52. . . . what causes heart failure.					
53. . . . what happens when someone has heart failure.					
54. . . . can the heart's function improve.					
55. . . . if any other tests will be done after I leave the hospital.					
56. . . . the reason for further testing after I go home.					
57. . . . where my family can go to learn CPR.					
58. . . . the normal emotional response to having a chronic illness.					
59. . . . the importance of talking to someone about my fears, feelings, and thoughts.					
60. . . . what effect stress has on my heart.					
61. . . . what I can do to reduce stress while in the hospital.					
62. . . . what I can do to reduce stress when I go home.					
63. . . . what support groups are available.					
64. . . . which factors may have contributed to the onset of my heart disease.					
65. . . . how these factors affect the heart.					
66. . . . what I can do to improve my heart function.					
67. . . . general rules about taking medications.					

(continued)

Topic	Not realistic	Somewhat realistic	Realistic	Moderately realistic	Very realistic
68. ... why I am taking each medication.					
69. ... what the side-effects of each medication are.					
70. ... what to do if I have problems with medications.					
71. ... how to adapt to taking medications every day.					
72. ... general rules about eating.					
73. ... how diet affects my heart disease.					
74. ... what the words sodium, salt, and NaCl mean.					

For each of the following statements, check how **realistic** you feel the information is for a patient with heart failure to know.

During my stay in the hospital, it is realistic to learn ...	Not realistic	Somewhat realistic	Realistic	Moderately realistic	Very realistic
75. ... what my diet restrictions are, if any.					
76. ... how to adapt the recommended diet to my lifestyle.					
77. ... what fluid restriction means.					
78. ... how to adapt the recommended fluid restriction to my lifestyle.					
79. ... why daily weights are needed.					
80. ... how to adapt daily weights to my lifestyle.					
81. ... how alcohol affects the heart.					
82. ... why I may not be able to do as much physically as I could before developing heart failure.					
83. ... general guidelines for physical activity.					

During my stay in the hospital, it is realistic to learn . . .	Not realistic	Somewhat realistic	Realistic	Moderately realistic	Very realistic
84. . . . what my physical activity restrictions are, if any.					
85. . . . how to tell if I can increase my activity.					
86. . . . when I can engage in sexual activity.					
87. . . . how significant my heart failure is.					
88. . . . what advanced directives are.					
89. . . . what is my long-term life expectancy.					
90. . . . what can happen if I do not follow my doctor's recommendations.					
91. . . . what my quality of life is expected to be.					
92. . . . what advice should be given to my family in the event of a sudden death outside the hospital.					
93. . . . what symptoms are caused by heart failure.					
94. . . . what are the signs and symptoms of worsening heart failure.					
95. . . . what I should do if symptoms worsen.					
96. . . . when to call the doctor.					
97. . . . the signs and symptoms of other heart problems.					
98. Please write in the space below any additional item that you think is realistic that was not on this list and rate this item using the scale to the right.					

HEART FAILURE PATIENT LEARNING NEEDS INVENTORY

Part I—Nurse Version

For each of the following statements, please check how **important** you feel the information is for a patient with heart failure to know.

The heart failure patient needs to know . . .	Not important	Somewhat important	Important	Moderately important	Very important
1. . . . why they are short of breath.					
2. . . . what the heart looks like and how it works.					
3. . . . what causes heart failure.					
4. . . . what happens when someone has heart failure.					
5. . . . can the heart's function improve.					
6. . . . if any other tests will be done after leaving the hospital.					
7. . . . the reason for further testing after going home.					
8. . . . where their family can go to learn CPR.					
9. . . . the normal emotional response to having a chronic illness.					
10. . . . the importance of talking to someone about their fears, feelings, and thoughts.					
11. . . . what effect stress has on the heart.					
12. . . . what they can do to reduce stress while in the hospital.					
13. . . . what they can do to reduce stress when they go home.					
14. . . . what support groups are available.					
15. . . . which factors may have contributed to the onset of their heart disease.					
16. . . . how these factors affect the heart.					

The heart failure patient needs to know . . .	Not important	Somewhat important	Important	Moderately important	Very important
17. . . . what they can do to improve the heart function.					
18. . . . general rules about taking medications.					
19. . . . why they are taking each medication.					
20. . . . what the side-effects of each medication are.					
21. . . . what to do if they have problems with medications.					
22. . . . how to adapt to taking medications every day.					
23. . . . general rules about eating.					
24. . . . how diet affects heart disease.					
25. . . . what the words sodium, salt, and NaCl mean.					
26. . . . what their diet restrictions are, if any.					
27. . . . how to adapt the recommended diet to their lifestyle.					
28. . . . what fluid restriction means.					
29. . . . how to adapt the recommended fluid restriction to their lifestyle.					
30. . . . why daily weights are needed.					
31. . . . how to adapt daily weights to their lifestyle.					
32. . . . how alcohol affects the heart.					
33. . . . why they may not be able to do as much physically as before developing heart failure.					
34. . . . general guidelines for physical activity.					

(continued)

The heart failure patient needs to know . . .	Not important	Somewhat important	Important	Moderately important	Very important
35. . . . what their physical activity restrictions are, if any.					
36. . . . how to tell if they can increase their activity.					
37. . . . when they can engage in sexual activity.					
38. . . . how significant their heart failure is.					
39. . . . what are advanced directives.					
40. . . . what is their long-term life expectancy.					
41. . . . what can happen if they do not follow their doctor's recommendations.					
42. . . . what their quality of life is expected to be.					
43. . . . what advice should be given to their family in the event of a sudden death outside the hospital.					
44. . . . what symptoms are caused by heart failure.					
45. . . . what are the signs and symptoms of worsening heart failure.					
46. . . . what they should do if symptoms worsen.					
47. . . . when to call the doctor.					
48. . . . the signs and symptoms of other heart problems.					
49. Please write in the space below any additional item that you think is important for the patient to learn that was not on this list and rate this item using the scale to the right.					

Part II—Nurse Version

As you continue the survey, you will notice that you have read each of the following items in the first half of the survey. Now, please check how **realistic** you feel it is for a heart failure patient to learn this information during hospitalization.

Topic	Not realistic	Somewhat realistic	Realistic	Moderately realistic	Very realistic
50. . . . why they are short of breath.					
51. . . . what the heart looks like and how it works.					
52. . . . what causes heart failure.					
53. . . . what happens when someone has heart failure.					
54. . . . can the heart's function improve.					
55. . . . if any other tests will be done after leaving the hospital.					
56. . . . the reason for further testing after going home.					
57. . . . where their family can go to learn CPR.					
58. . . . the normal emotional response to having a chronic illness.					
59. . . . the importance of talking to someone about their fears, feelings, and thoughts.					
60. . . . what effect stress has on their heart.					
61. . . . what they can do to reduce stress while in the hospital.					
62. . . . what they can do to reduce stress when they go home.					
63. . . . what support groups are available.					
64. . . . which factors may have contributed to the onset of their heart disease.					
65. . . . how these factors affect their heart.					

(continued)

Topic	Not realistic	Somewhat realistic	Realistic	Moderately realistic	Very realistic
66. ... what they can do to improve their heart function.					
67. ... general rules about taking medications.					
68. ... why they are taking each medication.					
69. ... what the side-effects of each medication are.					
70. ... what to do if they have problems with medications.					
71. ... how to adapt to taking medications every day.					
72. ... general rules about eating.					
73. ... how diet affects heart disease.					

For each of the following statements, check how **realistic** you feel the information is for a patient with heart failure to know.

During their stay in the hospital, it is realistic to learn ...	Not realistic	Somewhat realistic	Realistic	Moderately realistic	Very realistic
74. ... what the words sodium, salt, and NaCl mean.					
75. ... what their diet restrictions are, if any.					
76. ... how to adapt the recommended diet to their lifestyle.					
77. ... what fluid restriction means.					
78. ... how to adapt the recommended fluid restriction to their lifestyle.					
79. ... why daily weights are needed.					
80. ... how to adapt daily weights to their lifestyle.					
81. ... how alcohol affects the heart.					
82. ... why they may not be able to do as much physically as they could before developing heart failure.					

During their stay in the hospital, it is realistic to learn . . .	Not realistic	Somewhat realistic	Realistic	Moderately realistic	Very realistic
83. . . . general guidelines for physical activity.					
84. . . . what their physical activity restrictions are, if any.					
85. . . . how to tell if they can increase their activity.					
86. . . . when they can engage in sexual activity.					
87. . . . how significant their heart failure is.					
88. . . . what advanced directives are.					
89. . . . what is their long-term life expectancy.					
90. . . . what can happen if they do not follow their doctor's recommendations.					
91. . . . what their quality of life is expected to be.					
92. . . . what advice should be given to their family in the event of a sudden death outside the hospital.					
93. . . . what symptoms are caused by heart failure.					
94. . . . what are the signs and symptoms of worsening heart failure.					
95. . . . what they should do if symptoms worsen.					
96. . . . when to call the doctor.					
97. . . . the signs and symptoms of other heart problems.					
98. Please write in the space below any additional item that you think is realistic that was not on this list and rate this item using the scale to the right.					

41. Cardiac Surgical Patient Teaching Satisfaction Inventory

Developed by Susan Barnason and Lani Zimmerman

INSTRUMENT DESCRIPTION, ADMINISTRATION, AND SCORING GUIDELINES

Coronary artery disease education is used to equip patients with skills to manage both recovery from surgery and the lifestyle modifications necessary to decrease coronary disease risk factors. The purpose of the Cardiac Surgical Patient Teaching Satisfaction Inventory (CSPTSI) is to assess patient satisfaction with this essential teaching. The score is the mean of the summed item scores, with higher scores indicating more satisfaction (Barnason & Zimmerman, 1995).

PSYCHOMETRIC CHARACTERISTICS

Content validity of the CSPTSI was established through nurse specialist review. Ninety patients admitted for elective CABG surgery completed the instrument. Cronbach's alpha was .96. Although the authors indicate six subscales: disease knowledge, psychological adjustment, medication management, dietary management, exercise activity modification, and self-care management, these were not substantiated by statistical means. Patients who had five or more vessels bypassed and longer hospital stays had less satisfaction with the teaching they had received for post hospitalization self-care management. This finding would be predicted by teaching/learning theory that more complex skills are harder to learn and sicker patients harder to teach.

CRITIQUE AND SUMMARY

Very beginning work has been accomplished in studying the performance of CSPTSI. It is included in this collection in part because measures of patient satisfaction with teaching are rare. Increasing expectations that patient education programs be evaluated by measurement of functional health status, clinical outcomes, satisfaction and cost (Barnason & Zimmerman, 1995) make development and refinement of instruments such as CSPTSI important.

REFERENCE

Barnason, S., & Zimmerman, L. (1995). A comparison of patient teaching outcomes among postoperative coronary bypass graft (CABG) patients. *Progress in Cardiovascular Nursing, 10*(4), 11–20.

CARDIAC SURGICAL PATIENT TEACHING SATISFACTION INVENTORY (CSPTSI)

Directions: Please rate how "satisfied" you are with the information you received on each topic. Darken circle in the column for each question based on the following scale:

0 = I **DID NOT RECEIVE** any information on this topic
1 = I was **DISSATISFIED** with the information I received
2 = I was **SLIGHTLY DISSATISFIED** with the information I received
3 = I was **SATISFIED** with the information I received
4 = I was **VERY SATISFIED** with the information I received

Rate the teaching information you have received:	0	1	2	3	4
1. Why I have chest pain	O	O	O	O	O
2. What my heart looks like and how it works	O	O	O	O	O
3. What causes a heart attack	O	O	O	O	O
4. What happens when someone has a heart attack	O	O	O	O	O
5. How the heart heals	O	O	O	O	O
6. Why my heartbeat may be irregular or I may have "skipped beats"	O	O	O	O	O
7. How people feel when finding out they have a serious illness	O	O	O	O	O
8. The importance of talking to someone about my fears, feelings, and thoughts	O	O	O	O	O
9. How stress affects my heart	O	O	O	O	O
10. What I can do to reduce stress while in the hospital	O	O	O	O	O
11. What I can do to reduce stress when I go home	O	O	O	O	O
12. What the term "risk factor" means	O	O	O	O	O
13. Which risk factors may have contributed to my heart disease	O	O	O	O	O
14. What I can do to decrease my chances of having a heart attack, or of having another heart attack	O	O	O	O	O
15. How these risk factors affect my heart	O	O	O	O	O
16. General rules about taking medications	O	O	O	O	O
17. Why I am taking each of my medications	O	O	O	O	O
18. What the side effects of each medication are	O	O	O	O	O
19. What to do if I have problems with my medications	O	O	O	O	O

(continued)

Rate the teaching information you have received:	0	1	2	3	4
20. General rules about eating	O	O	O	O	O
21. How diet affects my heart disease	O	O	O	O	O
22. What the words "cholesterol" and "triglycerides" mean	O	O	O	O	O
23. What foods contain cholesterol and triglycerides	O	O	O	O	O
24. What my diet restrictions are, if any	O	O	O	O	O
25. How to include the recommended foods into my daily diet	O	O	O	O	O
26. What my physical activity restrictions are, if any	O	O	O	O	O
27. Why I am not able to do as much physically as I was before I had my bypass surgery	O	O	O	O	O
28. How to tell if I can increase my activity	O	O	O	O	O
29. When I can engage in sexual activity	O	O	O	O	O
30. How to care for my incisions	O	O	O	O	O
31. How to take my pulse	O	O	O	O	O
32. The signs and symptoms of angina and a heart attack	O	O	O	O	O
33. The signs and symptoms of congestive heart failure	O	O	O	O	O
34. When to call the doctor	O	O	O	O	O
35. If any other tests will be done after I go home	O	O	O	O	O
36. The reason for further testing after I go home	O	O	O	O	O
37. Where my family can go to learn CPR	O	O	O	O	O

Used with permission of Susan Barnason.

42. Needs Inventory for Patients Who Wait

Developed by Patrice Lindsay, Heather Sherrard, Lorna Bickerton, Patricia Doucette, Carol Harkness, and Joanne Morin

INSTRUMENT DESCRIPTION, ADMINISTRATION, AND SCORING GUIDELINES

In some areas of Canada, waiting periods for cardiac surgery have been 2–6 months. During this time, patients and families have concerns and educational needs. Specifically, new research has shown clinical depression and anxiety to be common during this time, as well as concerns about success of the operation, early postoperative recovery, complications, and lifestyle changes that would be required afterward. Family members frequently have similar reactions and concerns. Preoperative education traditionally has been given 1–2 weeks prior to surgery. The Needs Inventory for Patients Who Wait (NIPW) was designed to measure the importance of specific educational topics (10 items) and areas of concern (26 items). Patients and family members are asked to rate the importance of each statement on a 4-point scale (Lindsay et al., 1997).

PSYCHOMETRIC CHARACTERISTICS

Items were based on clinical practice and findings previously reported in the literature and evaluated for face and content validity by a panel of cardiovascular clinical nurse experts. Cronbach's alpha was .95 for the total scale, .89 for the Desired Information subscale, and .95 for the Areas of Concern subscale (Lindsay et al., 1997).

CRITIQUE AND SUMMARY

Very beginning work on NIPW has been accomplished. Further validity and sensitivity to intervention work remains to be addressed. This and other instruments will be important tools in research about how best to manage what can be a lengthy presurgical waiting period.

REFERENCE

Lindsay, P., Sherrard, H., Bickerton, L., Doucette, P., Harkness, C., & Morin, J. (1997). Educational and support needs of patients and their families awaiting cardiac surgery. *Heart & Lung, 26,* 458–465.

NEEDS INVENTORY FOR PATIENTS WHO WAIT

Desired Information Subscale

Information Item	Not Very Important			Very Important
	1	2	3	4
Activity after the operation				
Time to resume normal lifestyle				
Convalescence				
Changes to make after surgery				
Diet after the operation				
The surgical procedure				
Expectations during hospital stay				
Admission procedures for the Heart Institute				
Visiting guidelines				
When return to work				

Areas of Concern Subscale

Maintaining present state of health
Surviving the surgery
Surgical date
Becoming critically ill
Surviving until surgery
The effect on family (the patient)
Being treated as an individual
Losing independence
Loss of control
Feelings of anxiety
Feeling stressed
Meeting family responsibilities
Feeling fatigued
Feeling irritable
Receiving pain medication
Number of people involved in care

From: Lindsay, P., Sherrard, H., Bickerton, L., Doucette, P., Harkness, C., & Morin, J. (1997). Educational and support needs of patients and their families awaiting cardiac surgery. *Heart and Lung, 26,* 458–465. Used with permission.

43.   Stroke Care Information Test

Developed by Ron L. Evans, Sue Pomeroy, Tad vander Weele, and Margaret Hammond

INSTRUMENT DESCRIPTION, ADMINISTRATION, AND SCORING GUIDELINES

Information about the consequences of a stroke is essential for family members providing home care. Physical loss, cognitive and perceptual disorders, language impairment, and effects on sexuality are domains of knowledge thought to be needed (Evans, Pomeroy, vanderWeele, & Hammond, 1985).

Possible range of scores is 0–36 with higher scores indicating greater knowledge. Completion time is ten minutes.

PSYCHOMETRIC CHARACTERISTICS

Family members of stroke patients who had at least three months posthospital home care were the source of content for SCIT.

Split-half reliability coefficient was .78 (Evans, Pomeroy, vander Weele, & Hammond, 1985). Stroke Care Information Test (SCIT) was shown to differentiate participants in stroke education from nonparticipants, and an educational intervention including mutual problem solving did yield changes in SCIT sustained at one year, showing sensitivity of the instrument (Evans, Matlock, Bishop, Stranahan, & Pederson, 1988). So also, SCIT has been demonstrated sensitive to a rehabilitation program which includes an educational component (Clark & Smith, 1998a). Patients at risk for less than optimal home care had caregivers who were below average about knowledge in stroke care (Evans, Bishop, & Haselkorn, 1991).

CRITIQUE AND SUMMARY

Prior research indicates that informed, supportive families are essential to recovery from stroke (Evans, Bishop, & Haselkorn, 1991). Additional research has shown that core knowledge of stroke among patients and their families is poor (Clark & Smith, 1998a). SCIT is one of a battery of instruments that could be used to predict which patients are at risk for suboptimal home care poststroke and to evaluate interventions with a goal of optimal family functioning. It can be used to document the level of knowledge of stroke in communities and in patients and families; this knowledge is frequently very low despite stroke being a major cause of disability (Clark & Smith, 1998b).

REFERENCES

Clark, M. S., & Smith, D. S. (1998a). Knowledge of stroke in rehabilitation and community samples. *Disability & Rehabilitation, 20,* 90–96.

Clark, M. S., & Smith, D. S. (1998b). Factors contributing to patient satisfaction with rehabilitation following stroke. *International Journal of Rehabilitation Research, 21,* 143–154.

Evans, R. L., Bishop, D. S., & Haselkorn, J. K. (1991). Factors predicting satisfactory home care after stroke. *Archives Physical Medicine & Rehabilitation, 72,* 144–147.

Evans, R. L., Matlock, A., Bishop, D. S., Stranahan, S., & Pederson, C. (1988). Family intervention after stroke: Does counseling or education help? *Stroke, 19,* 1243–1249.

Evans, R. L., Pomeroy, S., vander Weele, T., & Hammond, M. C. (1985). Reliability of a stroke care information test for family caretakers. *International Journal of Rehabilitation Research, 8,* 199–201.

STROKE CARE INFORMATION TEST

Name:

Age:

Circle the letter of the most correct answer

1. Depression after stroke is usually due to:
   a. Reaction to losses
   b. Medication
   c. Family problems
   d. Brain damage

2. The #1 risk factor leading to stroke is:
   a. Age
   b. High blood pressure
   c. Stress
   d. Being overweight

3. The likelihood of a second stroke is:
   a. Slightly less than before
   b. Over 75
   c. Cannot be determined
   d. Reduced with good health care

4. Predicting stroke recovery can best be done by:
   a. Observing walking
   b. Waiting several weeks
   c. Observing initial improvement
   d. Knowing condition prior to the stroke

5. Most people who have a stroke will feel depressed:
   a. For several weeks
   b. As they realize their limitations
   c. For several years
   d. About being in thc hospital

6. Stroke patients with a severe language disorder:
   a. Understand normal conversation
   b. Remember what they read
   c. Rarely lose all language
   d. Cannot recognize familiar objects

7. Information on sexual ability after stroke is:
   a. Available from informed hospital staff
   b. Scarce
   c. Unnecessary
   d. Too sensitive for discussion

8. After the initial phase of stroke recovery, desire for sex:
   a. Is reduced

(continued)

    b.   Can be replaced by exercises

    c.   Returns to normal

    d.   Cannot be satisfied

9. After a stroke, sexual functioning:
   a. Is usually impaired
   b. Returns to normal
   c. Is rarely possible
   d. Should be avoided

10. Most patients who cannot understand language:
    a. Do not understand demonstration either
    b. Still enjoy reading
    c. Understand their native tongue
    d. Benefit from demonstration

11. A person recovering from memory loss:
    a. Will benefit from reminders
    b. May hallucinate past events
    c. Will remember recent events first
    d. Should not go out of the house alone

12. Decreased motivation in stroke patients is due to:
    a. Poor attention span
    b. Inability to initiate activity
    c. Loss of energy
    d. Their diet

13. Sexual performance after stroke is usually:
    a. Altered
    b. Not advisable
    c. Not a problem
    d. Absent

14. Recovery from paralysis caused by stroke usually begins:
    a. In the hip
    b. In the lower leg
    c. In the shoulder
    d. By strengthening the unaffected side

15. Proper positioning in bed can prevent:
    a. A second stroke
    b. Contractures
    c. Headaches
    d. Bladder incontinence

16. Which of the following is not a learning impairment:
    a. Paralysis
    b. Distractibility
    c. Short attention span
    d. Memory loss

17. A person who has lost the sense of touch:
    a. Cannot feel pain

b. Will forget more easily
c. Should eat alone
d. Might do dangerous things

18. A person who has lost the sense of touch should:
    a. Not be reminded of this deficit
    b. Be taught safety precautions
    c. Help out in the kitchen
    d. Smoke moderately

19. Which of the following is a physical loss:
    a. Forgetting
    b. Poor concentration
    c. Falling
    d. Paralysis

20. If a person is paralyzed on one side of the body, you should:
    a. Assist walking by supporting the affected side
    b. Not mention the problem
    c. Eliminate noise
    d. Sit close to the patient

21. Passive range of motion exercises mean that:
    a. Patient sits while exercising
    b. The limb is moved by a force other than itself
    c. Someone must assist
    d. Limbs remain motionless

22. Hemiplegia means:
    a. Poor blood clotting
    b. Weakness in both legs
    c. Paralysis on one side of the body
    d. Inability to speak

23. Family members should encourage the patient to get dressed:
    a. Without frustration
    b. With help from one person
    c. As often as possible
    d. With as little assistance as needed

24. A patient who is weak may benefit from:
    a. Hand rails on stairs
    b. Scatter rugs
    c. Shirt buttons
    d. Reclining chair

25. After initial recovery from stroke, interest in sex is:
    a. More than before
    b. Less than before
    c. Same as before
    d. Unknown

(continued)

26. Emotional lability means that a person:
    a. Has difficulty controlling emotions
    b. Is emotionless
    c. Is depressed
    d. Feels no emotion

27. A person who is labile may not:
    a. Recognize friends
    b. Detect other's moods
    c. Benefit from encouragement
    d. Express actual feelings reliably

28. Aphasia means that a person:
    a. Is unable to learn
    b. Has difficulty communicating
    c. Chokes when eating
    d. Loses balance easily

29. Stroke patients may sound emotionless because they:
    a. Cannot feel emotion
    b. Express emotions unreliably
    c. Tire easily
    d. Cannot remember emotions

30. Demonstrating instructions to stroke patients may be necessary because of:
    a. Hearing loss
    b. Personality changes
    c. Slowness
    d. Language problems

31. A stroke on the left side of the brain usually results in:
    a. Language impairment
    b. Confusion
    c. Visual loss
    d. Left sided paralysis

32. A person who perseverates:
    a. Dwells on details
    b. Cannot concentrate
    c. Should not read
    d. Cannot stop performing

33. Memory loss is most easily detected by:
    a. Old learning
    b. Performance of old habits
    c. New learning
    d. Driving ability

34. Perceptual error may lead to inability to:
    a. Recall colors
    b. Use familiar objects
    c. Experience pain
    d. Remember faces

35. The most common result of stroke is:
    a. Diabetes
    b. Loss of appetite
    c. Learning impairment
    d. Poor bladder control

36. A stroke on the right side of the brain usually means the person will be:
    a. Unable to speak
    b. Impulsive
    c. Paralyzed on the right side
    d. Incontinent

Key:

1. d
2. b
3. d
4. c
5. b
6. c
7. a
8. a
9. a
10. d
11. a
12. b
13. a
14. a
15. b
16. a
17. d
18. b
20. a
21. b
22. c
23. d
24. a
25. c
26. a
27. d
28. b
29. b
30. d
31. a
32. d
33. c
34. b
35. c
36. b

Used with permission of Ron L. Evans.

44. Knowledge Inventory: A Measure of Knowledge of Important Factors in Cardiac Rehabilitation

Developed by Pamela McHugh Schuster, Cynthia Wright, and Patricia Tomich

INSTRUMENT DESCRIPTION, ADMINISTRATION, AND SCORING GUIDELINES

Patients in need of cardiac rehabilitation may elect to participate in structured programs (20%) or more likely be given information on home rehabilitation programs that can be performed independently on discharge. Patients are also given reading materials and exercise instructions. It is well known that knowledge is one of the several elements necessary for successfully accomplishing self-care and lifestyle behavioral changes necessary for rehabilitation. The Knowledge Inventory was used in a study comparing the outcomes of structured and home rehabilitation programs. It assesses the patient's knowledge of heart disease, bypass surgery, diagnostic tests, exercise guidelines, smoking, nutrition, medications, and stress. Scores range from 0 to 50 with 50 indicating greatest knowledge (Schuster, Wright, & Tomich, 1995).

PSYCHOMETRIC PROPERTIES

Sixty-four patients who had coronary bypass surgery at a single Ohio medical center were studied. All but one were White. The test was reviewed for clarity, content, and face validity by 10 cardiac rehabilitation professionals (nurses and exercise physiologists) and administered to 10 rehabilitation patients to establish its clarity, adequacy, and freedom from bias. It was pilot tested on 54 hospitalized and outpatient cardiac patients before being used in the study. Internal consistency measured at .84. Findings of the study showed that males but not females in structured cardiac rehabilitation programs showed increased knowledge. Mean scores for males and females in home and in structured rehabilitation programs ranged from 28 to 39 as long as 6 months postprogram; further breakdown in scores may be found in Schuster and colleagues (1995). The authors describe the Knowledge Inventory as a criterion-referenced mastery test, which means that each learner should attain a certain score level to be successful.

CRITIQUE AND SUMMARY

Further details or an independent assessment of content validity are needed. Although the domains indicated are those commonly included in cardiac rehabilitation programs, it is not clear whether judges, including patients, explicitly concurred that the items adequately represent these domains and whether other domains are important. Testing on a larger and more diverse population of patients is necessary, as is further evidence of sensitivity of the inventory to instruction. Because adequate cardiac rehabilitation is the desired outcome goal, the ability of the inventory and other measures, such as self-efficacy and self-care practices to predict rehabilitation is an essential step. It is particularly essential in selecting the criterion score on the Knowledge Inventory that should be reached with or without instruction. No such score could be located in the report of development and use of this instrument.

REFERENCE

Schuster, P. M., Wright, C., & Tomich, P. (1995). Gender differences in the outcomes of participants in home programs compared to those in structured cardiac rehabilitation programs. *Rehabilitation Nursing, 20,* 93–101.

KNOWLEDGE INVENTORY

1.   The function of the coronary arteries is to

    Ⓐ.   supply the heart muscle with blood and oxygen.
    B.   connect the heart to the lungs.
    C.   maintain an even rate of the heart.
    D.   circulate blood to the rest of the body.
    E.   Don't know

2.   Atherosclerosis is

    A.   chest pain not relieved by medication.
    B.   a clot in the coronary artery.
    Ⓒ.   a build-up of cholesterol and other materials inside the arteries.
    D.   an inflammation around the sac covering the heart.
    E.   Don't know

3.   A heart attack means the heart

    A.   has a hole in it.
    Ⓑ.   has been damaged.
    C.   has been enlarged.
    D.   stops beating.
    E.   Don't know

4.   Angina or chest pain is caused by

    A.   a muscle spasm of the chest.
    B.   a blood clot in the lungs.
    C.   leaking of blood around the heart.
    Ⓓ.   lack of oxygen to the heart muscle.
    E.   Don't know

5.   A heart attack usually begins with

    A.   nausea.
    Ⓑ.   chest discomfort.
    C.   palpitations.
    D.   dizziness.
    E.   Don't know

6.   If the incision (in your chest) from cardiac surgery is draining a yellowish, thick, foul-smelling substance you should

    A.   cover it with a clean bandage and change it every day.
    B.   wash it with soap and water and place alcohol around the edge.
    Ⓒ.   contact your physician and follow his instructions.

D. leave it open to the air so it can heal faster.

E. Don't know

7. Which of the following situations will indicate the need to call your doctor

A. weight gain of 1 1/2 pounds in one week.

B. feeling of breathlessness when you run up the stairs.

Ⓒ. weight gain of 3–4 pounds overnight.

D. increase of 15 beats of your resting heart rate during your exercise program.

E. Don't know

8. The purpose of coronary artery bypass surgery is to

A. clean and open up the arteries in the heart.

B. remove an artery from the leg.

Ⓒ. increase the amount of blood to the heart muscle.

D. prevent blockages from developing in the heart's arteries.

E. Don't know

9. The healing of the breast bone (sternum) after cardiac surgery usually takes

A. 2 weeks.

Ⓑ. 4–6 weeks.

C. 3 months.

D. 1 year.

E. Don't know

10. Which statement is TRUE about smoking?

A. Cigarettes with filters and low tar are safe.

B. Smoking decreases the heart rate.

Ⓒ. Smoking decreases the amount of oxygen to the heart.

D. Men's hearts are more affected by smoking than women's hearts.

E. Don't know

11. Which statement about nicotine in cigarettes is TRUE?

A. It is non-addictive.

B. It lowers blood pressure.

Ⓒ. It raises heart rate.

D. It lowers pulse rate.

E. Don't know

12. Once you stop smoking, how long before your risk of smoking is reduced to that of a non-smoker?

A. 1 year

B. 5 years

Ⓒ. 10 years

D. Never

E. Don't know

(continued)

13. The amount of salt intake is directly related to INCREASED

    A. appetite.
    B. chest pain.
    C. heart rate.
    (D). water retention.
    E. Don't know

14. An increase of which food items is strongly recommended after a heart attack?

    A. Citrus fruits.
    B. Red meats.
    C. Yellow vegetables.
    (D). High fiber foods.
    E. Don't know

15. Which sandwich has the highest amount of cholesterol?

    A. A hot dog sandwich.
    (B). An egg sandwich.
    C. A sardine sandwich.
    D. A peanut butter sandwich.
    E. Don't know

16. The appropriate selection of an entree at a restaurant would be

    (A). broiled fish.
    B. fried chicken.
    C. steamed liver.
    D. a western omelet.
    E. Don't know

17. Which practice would be useful to lower blood cholesterol?

    A. Increase fiber in food.
    (B). Reduce saturated fat intake.
    C. Weight reduction.
    D. Decrease salt intake.
    E. Don't know

18. How many calories must be eliminated to loose one pound?

    A. 500
    B. 1,000
    C. 1,500
    (D). 3,500
    E. Don't know

19. The medication commonly prescribed for the relief of chest pain (angina) is

    A. lasix.
    B. lanoxin.
    (C). nitroglycerin.
    D. quinidine.
    E. Don't know

20. If you are experiencing chest pain (angina) and have a prescription for nitroglycerine, the total number of tablets you may take before going to the hospital is

    A.   one.
    B.   two.
    Ⓒ.   three.
    D.   four.
    E.   Don't know

21. You took three nitroglycerin tablets as prescribed. The chest pain is NOT relieved. You should

    Ⓐ.   go to the emergency room.
    B.   take two tablets at once and wait 20 minutes.
    C.   lay down for the rest of the day.
    D.   take an antacid.
    E.   Don't know

22. You take a heart medication every eight hours at 8 am, 4 pm, and 12 midnight. This morning it is 10:30 am and you remember your 8 am dosage of medication. The best thing to do is

    A.   skip the 8 am dose and double the 4 pm dosage.
    B.   take half the dose at the time you remembered it and take the full dose at 4 pm and 12 midnight.
    Ⓒ.   take this dose and delay the 4 pm dose about an hour and resume the normal schedule at 12 midnight.
    D.   skip the 8 am dose and just take the 4 pm and 12 midnight dose for that day.
    E.   Don't know

23. The process of emotionally adjusting to heart disease in most people usually takes

    Ⓐ.   1–6 months.
    B.   7–12 months.
    C.   2 years.
    D.   5 years.
    E.   Don't know

24. You are in a traffic jam, and will probably be late for work. You would

    A.   find another route, and try to get there as soon as you can.
    B.   blow your horn, shout and try to get the traffic moving.
    C.   leave your car and find a ride to work.
    Ⓓ.   realize that you will probably be late and practice some relaxation.
    E.   Don't know

25. A recommended method of relaxation for the person with heart disease is to

    A.   tighten the muscle of your extremities for 15 seconds and relax them for 5 seconds.
    B.   breathe shallow and rapidly for 30 seconds.
    C.   take a deep breath and hold it for 10 seconds.

(continued)

      Ⓓ.   inhale slowly through your nose and exhale slowly through your mouth.
      E.   Don't know

26.   Continued prolonged stress on the body may result in

      A.   reduced blood pressure.
      B.   high energy levels.
      C.   increased exercise endurance.
      Ⓓ.   high blood pressure.
      E.   Don't know

27.   In order to develop and maintain fitness, what is the minimum number of days per week exercise should be done?

      A.   One.
      B.   Two.
      Ⓒ.   Three.
      D.   Four.
      E.   Don't know

28.   Which of these factors is LEAST important to an exercise prescription?

      A.   Current fitness level.
      B.   Intensity and duration of exercise.
      C.   Frequency and type of exercise.
      Ⓓ.   Body composition.
      E.   Don't know

29.   In general, as the intensity of exercise INCREASES

      A.   blood pressure decreases.
      B.   breathing rate decreases.
      Ⓒ.   heart rate increases.
      D.   pulse rate decreases.
      E.   Don't know

30.   In order to maintain fitness, the length of each exercise session (not counting warm-up and cool-down periods)

      A.   should be 5–10 minutes each session.
      Ⓑ.   should be 15–60 minutes each session.
      C.   should be 65–70 minutes each session.
      D.   should be 75–80 minutes each session.
      E.   Don't know

31.   Warm-up before exercise is important because it

      Ⓐ.   prevents injury to muscles.
      B.   extends the exercise time period.
      C.   reduces body fat.
      D.   builds muscle strength.
      E.   Don't know

32. The cool-down phase

    A. increases blood pressure.
    Ⓑ. decreases heart rate gradually.
    C. increases the chance of skipped heart beats.
    D. decreases the chance of having a heart attack.
    E. Don't know

33. What action should be taken when symptoms occur during exercise (chest discomfort, shortness of breath)?

    A. Heart rate should be kept in the heart rate range.
    B. The heart rate can be exceeded.
    Ⓒ. The exercise should be gradually discontinued.
    D. Exercise can be done even if symptoms occur.
    E. Don't know

34. All of the following symptoms indicate that the intensity of exercise should be decreased except

    A. Chest discomfort.
    B. Skipped heart beats.
    Ⓒ. Flushed skin color.
    D. Shortness of breath.
    E. Don't know

35. You have just finished your exercise program. You are beginning to cool down and your heart rate is 15 beats above your resting heart rate. You should

    Ⓐ. complete your cool-down exercises and stretches and recheck your pulse.
    B. skip cool-down activities and relax the rest of the day.
    C. reduce the time of cool down to two minutes.
    D. resume your exercise program.
    E. Don't know

36. After your exercise program it is acceptable to feel

    Ⓐ. pleasantly tired.
    B. chest tightness and heaviness.
    C. your heart racing.
    D. dizzy and sweating.
    E. Don't know

37. The temperature outside is "0" F, and there is a heavy wind. The doctor has instructed you to walk 30 minutes per day. You should

    A. cancel the walk for that day.
    B. walk only half the recommended distance.
    Ⓒ. walk indoors.
    D. call the doctor for instructions.
    E. Don't know

(continued)

38. After a heart attack, sexual intercourse with your usual partner generally can be safely resumed how long after discharge from the hospital?

A.   Immediately.
B.   2–4 weeks.
C.   3 months.
D.   Never again.
E.   Don't know

39. After bypass surgery, sexual intercourse with your usual partner generally can be safely resumed how long after discharge from the hospital?

A.   Immediately.
B.   2–4 weeks.
C.   3 months.
D.   Never again.
E.   Don't know

40. When should the pulse rate be counted?

A.   Before and after each activity.
B.   Before and during each activity.
C.   During and after each activity.
D.   Before, during, and after each activity.
E.   Don't know

41. Which of the following is the BEST way to check the pulse during exercise?

A.   Count the pulse for 10 seconds and multiply the number by 6.
B.   Count the pulse for 60 seconds.
C.   There is no need to count the pulse because the pulse rate does not have to be checked during exercise.
D.   Count the pulse for 15 seconds and multiply the number by 4.
E.   Don't know

42. What are the three major risk factors associated with the development of coronary artery disease that can be controlled?

A.   Smoking, high blood pressure, cholesterol
B.   High blood pressure, age, stress
C.   Heredity, cholesterol, stress
D.   Obesity, diabetes, sex
E.   Don't know

43. A heart catheterization is a diagnostic test that

A.   measures the size of the heart.
B.   records the electrical activity of the heart.
C.   visualizes the blood vessels and chambers of the heart.
D.   calculates the strength of the heart.
E.   Don't know

44. An electrocardiogram (EKG) is a test that

    A.   looks the same for everyone.
    Ⓑ.   records the electrical impulses generated by the heart.
    C.   is rarely done since new tests have become available.
    D.   uses sound waves to outline the chambers of the heart.
    E.   Don't know

45. Which statement is true about a stress test (exercise test)?

    A.   It determines the extent of blockage of the coronary arteries.
    B.   It measures the size of the chest.
    C.   It provides very little information about the heart.
    Ⓓ.   It determines how much work the heart can safely do.
    E.   Don't know

Correct answer circled.

46. What are the risk factors that you believe influenced your development of heart disease? Circle those that apply to you.

    don't know
    high blood pressure   lack of exercise   smoking
    high cholesterol   stress   heredity
    overweight   diabetes   age

47. What is the highest heart rate (maximum heart rate) that you should not go above WHILE EXERCISING?

    _____ beats per minute

    _____ don't know

48. What is the lowest heart rate (minimum heart rate) that you should not go below WHILE EXERCISING?

    _____ beats per minute

    _____ don't know

49. What is your (average) resting heart rate?

    _____ beats per minute

    _____ don't know

50. List your medications and what they are for.

(continued)

1. example: Nitroglycerine for chest discomfort

_____

2. _____

3. _____

4. _____

5. _____

Answers are individualized, based on patient paramenters.

45. Beliefs About Medication Compliance Scale and Beliefs About Dietary Compliance Scale

Developed by Susan J. Bennett, Lesley Milgrom, Victoria Champion, and Gertrude A. Huster

INSTRUMENT DESCRIPTION, ADMINISTRATION, AND SCORING GUIDELINES

The Beliefs About Medication Compliance Scale (BMCS) and the Beliefs About Dietary Compliance Scale (BDCS) were developed specifically to measure beliefs about compliance with behaviors that affect sodium retention in persons with heart failure. The health belief model constructs of perceived benefits and barriers have been found useful in studying adherence and were used for development of this instrument. Items were built on past studies of perceived benefits and barriers in this population of patients, on previously well validated scales for mammography, and on patient focus groups.

Because persons with heart failure often report decreased attention span and concentration ability, items are short. Each scale is 12 items in length, each rated on a 5-point response (1 = strongly disagree to 5 = strongly agree). On the BMCS, six items each were designed to measure perceived benefits and barriers, with a possible score range of 6–30. On the BDCS, five items were developed to measure perceived benefits (score range 5–25) and seven items to measure perceived barriers (score range 7–35). Reading level for BMCS was grade 6 and for BDCS grade 4 (Bennett, Milgrom, Champion, & Huster, 1997). Complete scoring directions accompany the instruments.

PSYCHOMETRIC PROPERTIES

The content validity index was .81. Factor analysis confirmed the barriers and benefits scales outlined in the HBM with two patient samples of 101 and 234, the latter largely indigent. Internal consistencies of the subscales ranged from .68–.91 with BMCS having some estimates lower than .70. Test–retest reliability estimates ranged from .07–.57 (Bennett, Milgrom, Champion, & Huster, 1997; Bennett et al., 2001). Pilot work on sensitivity of the scales to educational messages tailored to their beliefs was inconclusive (Bennett, Hays, Embree, & Arnould, 2000).

CRITIQUE AND SUMMARY

The scales are misnamed—in essence they are about compliance with diuretics and low salt diets—two elements important in management of heart failure. The authors agree that the scales should be tested in more diverse populations beyond Caucasian men with Heart Association Class III heart failure, with whom they were developed. Extension of initial work on psychometric properties including improvement in reliability and definitive work on sensitivity to psychosocial intervention, is needed.

The hope is that BMCS and BDCS will provide information about each person's unique perceptions of the benefits and barriers to compliance with these elements of therapy and that this information can be used to provide targeted interventions to decrease barriers (Bennett, Milgrom, Champion, & Huster, 1997). This action presumably will increase compliance, although this presumption has apparently not yet been tested.

REFERENCES

Bennett, S. J., Hays, L. M., Embree, J. L., & Arnould, M. (2000). Heart Messages: A tailored message intervention for improving heart failure outcomes. *Journal of Cardiovascular Nursing, 14*(4), 94–105.

Bennett, S. J., Milgrom, L., Champion, V., & Huster, G. A. (1997). Beliefs about medication and dietary compliance in people with heart failure: An instrument development study. *Heart & Lung, 26,* 273–279.

Bennett, S. J., Perkins, S. M., Lane, K. A., Forthofer, M. A., Brater, D. C., & Murray, M. D. (2001). Reliability and validity of the compliance belief scales among patients with heart failure, *Heart and Lung, 30,* 177–185.

BELIEFS ABOUT DIETARY COMPLIANCE SCALE

INSTRUCTIONS: These are questions about the good and bad things about following a low sodium (low salt) diet. As I read each sentence to you, please mark the number that best describes how much you agree or disagree with the statement. Choose 1 if you strongly disagree, 2 if you disagree, 3 if you are undecided, 4 if you agree, and 5 if you strongly agree with the sentences. Here we go.

1 = Strongly Disagree
2 = Disagree
3 = Undecided
4 = Agree
5 = Strongly Agree

	SD	D	U	A	SA
1. Eating a low salt diet will keep me healthy.	1	2	3	4	5
2. Salty food is not good for me.	1	2	3	4	5
3. Eating a low salt diet will keep my heart healthy.	1	2	3	4	5
4. Eating a low salt diet will keep my swelling down.	1	2	3	4	5
5. Eating a low salt diet will keep fluid from building up in my body.	1	2	3	4	5
6. Eating a low salt diet makes it hard to go to restaurants.	1	2	3	4	5
7. Food does not taste good on the low salt diet.	1	2	3	4	5
8. Following a low salt diet costs too much money.	1	2	3	4	5
9. Following a low salt diet takes too much time.	1	2	3	4	5
10. Following a low salt diet is too hard to understand.	1	2	3	4	5
11. When I follow my low salt diet, I feel better.	1	2	3	4	5
12. Eating a low salt diet will help me breathe easier.	1	2	3	4	5

BELIEFS ABOUT DIET

Benefits and Barriers Coding Sheet

Benefit	1.	Eating a low salt diet will keep me healthy.
Benefit*	2.	Salty food is not good for me.
Benefit	3.	Eating a low salt diet will keep my heart healthy.
Benefit	4.	Eating a low salt diet will keep my swelling down.
Benefit	5.	Eating a low salt diet will keep fluid from building up in my body.
Barrier	6.	Eating a low salt diet makes it hard to go to restaurants.
Barrier	7.	Food does not taste good on the low salt diet.
Barrier	8.	Following a low salt diet costs too much money.
Barrier	9.	Following a low salt diet takes too much time.
Barrier	10.	Following a low salt diet is too hard to understand.
Benefit	11.	When I follow my low salt diet, I feel better.
Benefit	12.	Eating a low salt diet will help me breathe easier.

*Recode when scoring.

Copyright © 1998 Susan J. Bennett, DNS, RN. Used with permission.

BELIEFS ABOUT MEDICATION COMPLIANCE SCALE

INSTRUCTIONS: These are questions about the good and bad things about taking your medicines. As I read each sentence to you, please mark the number that best describes how much you agree or disagree with the statement. Choose 1 if you strongly disagree, 2 if you disagree, 3 if you are undecided, 4 if you agree, and 5 if you strongly agree with the sentences. Here we go.

1 = Strongly Disagree
2 = Disagree
3 = Undecided
4 = Agree
5 = Strongly Agree

	SD	D	U	A	SA
1. When I take my water pills, I do not worry as much about my heart disease.	1	2	3	4	5
2. If I take my water pills, I will lower my chance of being in the hospital.	1	2	3	4	5

	SD	D	U	A	SA
3. Taking water pills is hard to remember.	1	2	3	4	5
4. Taking water pills is unpleasant.	1	2	3	4	5
5. I have to take too many water pills each day.	1	2	3	4	5
6. Taking water pills makes it hard to go away from home.	1	2	3	4	5
7. Taking my water pills lessens my swelling.	1	2	3	4	5
8. I forget to take my water pills.	1	2	3	4	5
9. Taking water pills makes me worry about my heart disease.	1	2	3	4	5
10. Taking my water pills helps me breathe better.	1	2	3	4	5
11. Taking my medicine improves my quality of life.	1	2	3	4	5
12. Taking water pills makes me wake up at night to go to the bathroom.	1	2	3	4	5

BELIEFS ABOUT MEDICATION

Benefits and Barriers Coding Sheet

Benefit	1.	When I take my water pills, I do not worry as much about my heart disease.
Benefit	2.	If I take my water pills, I will lower my chance of being in the hospital.
Barrier	3.	Taking water pills is hard to remember.
Barrier	4.	Taking water pills is unpleasant.
Barrier	5.	I have to take too many water pills each day.
Barrier	6.	Taking water pills makes it hard to go away from home.
Benefit	7.	Taking my water pills lessens my swelling.
Barrier	8.	I forget to take my water pills.
Benefit*	9.	Taking water pills makes me worry about my heart disease.
Benefit	10.	Taking my water pills helps me breathe better.
Benefit	11.	Taking my medicine improves my quality of life.
Barrier	12.	Taking water pills makes me wake up at night to go to the bathroom.

*Recode 9 when scoring.

Instructions for Scoring the Beliefs About Compliance Scales
Susan J. Bennett, DNS, RN

Each Belief Scale has two scores: A Benefits Score and a Barriers Score. Scores are obtained as follows:

1. Score all individual items as:
    1 = "Strongly Disagree"
    2 = "Disagree"
    3 = "Undecided"
    4 = "Agree"
    5 = "Strongly Agree"
2. Reverse code item 9 on the Belief About Medication Scale.
3. Reverse code item 2 on the Beliefs About Diet Scale.
4. Compute a Benefits Score and a Barriers Score for each instrument by summing individual items of each subscale.

Section F

Cancer

There appear to be a smaller group of instruments for cancer although they reflect the range of assessment, self-efficacy, and knowledge tests.

---

46. Toronto Informational Needs Questionnaire–Breast Cancer

Developed by Susan Galloway, Jane Graydon, Dianne Harrison, Sherrol Palmer-Wickham, Stephanie Burlein-Hall, Louanne Rich-van der Bij, Pamela West, and Barbara Evans-Boyden

INSTRUMENT DESCRIPTION, ADMINISTRATION, AND SCORING GUIDELINES

The Toronto Informational Needs Questionnaire–Breast Cancer (TINQ-BC) is designed to elicit women's perceptions of their informational needs related to their experience of breast cancer. Its development was guided by Lazarus and Folkman's theory of stress and coping, suggesting that people want information to clarify elements of a new experience, determine implications for their well-being, and help manage and control their emotions.

The instrument can be completed in about 20 minutes (Galloway et al., 1997). Each item begins with the stem: "To help me with my illness it is important for me to know" and rates each item on a scale of 1 (not important) to 5 (extremely important). The questionnaire yields a total score with a minimum of 51 and a maximum of 255. Higher scores represent higher information needs. Individual subscales may be calculated using percentages as there are unequal numbers of items in the subscales (Galloway et al., n.d.).

PSYCHOMETRIC PROPERTIES

Items were generated from findings in the literature and 11 oncology nurse experts. Each expert independently placed each item on one subscale, yielding an interrater reliability of item assignment to category of .91. Thirty-four women, including those with and without breast cancer, lay people, and health care providers, assessed the questionnaire for clarity in the wording of items. The TINQ-BC was administered to 114 women with a recent diagnosis of breast cancer during chemotherapy ($n = 39$), radiation therapy ($n = 40$), or surgery ($n = 35$). Items important to the majority of women were retained with interitem correlations between .20 and .80. The five subscales may be seen in Table 46.1. Intercorrelations of the subscale scores were .38–.73 (Galloway et al., 1997). Informational needs of the women were high with mean scores over 200 and the greatest needs in the areas of diagnosis or treatment. Findings are congruent with the theory on which it is based (Galloway, 1993).

There is beginning evidence of construct validity. Women newly diagnosed with breast cancer report high informational needs as measured by the TINQ-BC, and women experiencing a recurrence of breast cancer also place high importance on having information. These findings are congruent with the theoretical perspective of Lazarus and Folkman (1984) that people in threatening situations will seek information to understand what is happening, and with results of previous studies. Younger women reported a greater need for information than did older women. Scores on the TINQ-BC have shown variability in women's responses. The instrument has shown internal consistency reliabilities between .85 and .90 for the subscales and .94 for the total questionnaire (Galloway et al., n.d.).

In a second study of 20 female breast cancer patients after excisional biopsy and axillary node dissection, 20 completed TINQ-BC in the first week of radiation therapy, and 20 did so in the first clinic visit after completion of radiation therapy. Although all women had informational needs on all TINQ scales, treatment was the highest area of informational need, with the physical subscale being second. These findings were common with both groups and at both times in the treatment cycle. In general, patient informational needs were high (Harrison-Woermke & Graydon, 1993).

More recently, Graydon and colleagues (1997) studied seventy women with breast cancer and found that those treated by surgery, chemotherapy, or radiation therapy showed no

TABLE 46.1 Subscale Definitions of the TINQ-BC

Subscale	Definition and item nos.
Disease	Assess need for information about the nature of the disease, its process, and prognosis. (Items: 2, 7, 10, 12, 14, 18, 37, 42, 50)
Investigative tests	Assess need for information about procedures used to assess extent of disease, how and why they are done, and sensations that may be experienced. (Items: 1, 15, 16, 19, 33, 47, 48, 51)
Treatments	Assess need for information regarding various cancer treatments, how they work, how they are performed, sensations that may be experienced, and possible side effects. (Items: 3, 5, 6, 9, 13, 17, 27, 28, 29, 30, 32, 35, 40, 41, 45, 46)
Physical	Assess need for information regarding the preventive, restorative, and maintenance care which the body requires as a result of the disease. (Items: 4, 21, 23, 24, 31, 36, 38, 39, 43, 44, 52)
Psychosocial	Assess the need for information about how to handle the patient's or their family's feelings and concerns. (Items: 8, 11, 20, 22, 25, 26, 34, 49)

differences in information needs although younger women had more information needs. Scores for these groups may be found in Graydon and colleagues (1997), with all having high information needs. Harrison and colleagues (1999) also found high informational needs among women receiving a course of radiation therapy for breast cancer. In this study, two items specific to radiation therapy were added to TINQ-BC. Cronbach's alpha was .97 for the total scale and .75–.97 for the subscales.

CRITIQUE AND SUMMARY

This instrument demonstrates good content validity, high internal consistency reliability and beginning construct validity. It requires further evaluation of construct validity by factor analysis and longitudinal studies to determine how informational needs alter over time to determine the best timing and methods for delivering information and whether TINQ-BC is sensitive enough to detect these changes. Almost all testing has been done on well-educated Canadian women (Galloway, 1993).

TINQ-BC can be used in needs assessment for individuals or groups of women, so that teaching interventions can be targeted. Availability of the information patients need should contribute to realistic expectations, to self-care, to a sense of control, and to trust in providers. Sensitivity of TINQ-BC to instruction and its ability to predict these important outcomes should be established including with patients who cope best by avoidance of information.

This tool should also be useful as one of several measures to evaluate the quality of communication in a care program for persons with breast cancer to see that most patients get the information they need and want, and to feel secure with their care. Perception of inadequate information can occur because patients cannot absorb what is being given to them or feel that no one has a sustained interest in and commitment to their care and symptoms. Sometimes it is not information that patients desire but rather intensified support of their hopes, concern for their person, and confirmation of the validity of what they think they know (Cassileth, Volckmar, & Goodman, 1980).

REFERENCES

Cassileth, B. R., Volckmar, D., & Goodman, R. L. (1980). The effect of experience on radiation therapy patients' desire for information. *International Journal Radiation Oncology Biophysics, 6,* 493–496.

Galloway, S. (1993). Informational needs questionnaire for women with breast cancer. *Oncology Nursing Forum, 20,* 336.

Galloway, S., Graydon, J., Harrison, D., Evans-Boyden, B., Palmer-Wickham, S., Burlein-Hall, S., Rich-van der Bij, L., West, P., & Blair, A. (1997). Informational needs of women with a recent diagnosis of breast cancer: Development and initial testing of a tool. *Journal of Advanced Nursing, 25,* 1175–1183.

Galloway, S., Graydon, J., Harrison, D., Palmer-Wickham, S., Evans-Boyden, B., Burlein-Hall, S., Rich-van der Bij, L., & West, P. (n.d.). *Toronto Informational Needs Questionnaire–Breast Cancer.* University of Toronto, Ontario, Canada.

Graydon, J., Galloway, S., Palmer-Wickham, S., Harrison, D., Rich-Van der Bij, L., West, P., Burlein-Hall, S., & Evans-Boyden, B. (1997). Information needs of women during early treatment for breast cancer. *Journal of Advanced Nursing, 26,* 59–64.

Harrison, D. E., Galloway, S., Graydon, J. E., Palmer-Wickham, S., & Rich-van der Bij, L. (1999). Information needs and preferences for information of women with breast cancer over a first course of radiation therapy. *Patient Education & Counseling, 38,* 217–225.

Harrison-Woermke, D. E., & Graydon, J. E. (1993). Perceived informational needs of breast cancer patients receiving radiation therapy after excisional biopsy and axillary node dissection. *Cancer Nursing, 16,* 449–455.

Lazarus, R., & Folkman, S. (1984). *Stress, appraisal and coping.* New York: Springer Publishing Co.

TORONTO INFORMATIONAL NEEDS QUESTIONNAIRE—BREAST CANCER

We are interested in knowing the types of information women with breast cancer need. Please read each of the following statements and circle the number that best describes how important it is for you to have this information.

1 = not important
2 = slightly important
3 = moderately important
4 = very important
5 = extremely important

It is important for me to know:

1.	How I will feel during the tests (e.g., x-ray, bone scans).	1	2	3	4	5
2.	If the breast cancer will come back.	1	2	3	4	5
3.	How to prepare for my treatment.	1	2	3	4	5
4.	When to examine my breasts.	1	2	3	4	5
5.	How I will feel after my treatment.	1	2	3	4	5
6.	Who I should call if I have questions while I am still getting treatment.	1	2	3	4	5
7.	How breast cancer acts in the body.	1	2	3	4	5
8.	If there are groups where I can talk with other people with cancer.	1	2	3	4	5
9.	If there are ways to prevent treatment side effects.	1	2	3	4	5
10.	How the illness may affect my life over the next few months.	1	2	3	4	5
11.	If there will be changes in the usual things I can do with and for my family.	1	2	3	4	5
12.	If there is cancer anywhere else in my body.	1	2	3	4	5
13.	Who I should call if I have questions after all the treatments are over.	1	2	3	4	5
14.	If it is known what causes breast cancer.	1	2	3	4	5
15.	How the tests (e.g., x-rays, bone scans) are done.	1	2	3	4	5
16.	Why they need to test my blood.	1	2	3	4	5
17.	Who to talk with if I hear about treatments other than surgery, radiation, or chemotherapy.	1	2	3	4	5
18.	How the illness may affect my life in the future.	1	2	3	4	5

(continued)

1 = not important
2 = slightly important
3 = moderately important
4 = very important
5 = extremely important

It is important for me to know:

19.	What the results of my blood tests mean.	1	2	3	4	5
20.	Where my family can go if they need help dealing with my illness.	1	2	3	4	5
21.	How to care for my wound or incision.	1	2	3	4	5
22.	What to do if I become concerned about dying.	1	2	3	4	5
23.	If I can continue my usual hobbies and sports.	1	2	3	4	5
24.	If I can wear a brassiere.	1	2	3	4	5
25.	Where I can get help to deal with my feelings about my illness.	1	2	3	4	5
26.	How to talk to family/friends about my illness.	1	2	3	4	5
27.	If I have side effects, how to deal with them.	1	2	3	4	5
28.	The possible side effects of my treatment.	1	2	3	4	5
29.	What side effects I should report to the doctor/nurse.	1	2	3	4	5
30.	If I am prone to infection because of my treatment.	1	2	3	4	5
31.	How long my wound/incision will take to heal.	1	2	3	4	5
32.	How long I will be receiving treatment.	1	2	3	4	5
33.	How I will feel after the tests (e.g., x-rays, bone scans).	1	2	3	4	5
34.	Where I can get help if I have problems feeling as attractive as I did before.	1	2	3	4	5
35.	How the treatment works against the cancer.	1	2	3	4	5
36.	If there are special arm exercises to do.	1	2	3	4	5
37.	The medical name for my type of breast cancer.	1	2	3	4	5
38.	If there are any physical things I should not do.	1	2	3	4	5
39.	If I'm going to need help taking care of myself.	1	2	3	4	5
40.	How my treatment is done.	1	2	3	4	5
41.	If the treatment will alter the way that I look.	1	2	3	4	5
42.	How to tell if the cancer has come back.	1	2	3	4	5
43.	Which foods I can or cannot eat.	1	2	3	4	5

1 = not important
2 = slightly important
3 = moderately important
4 = very important
5 = extremely important

It is important for me to know:

44.	If I can take a bath or shower.	1	2	3	4	5
45.	What types of treatment are available.	1	2	3	4	5
46.	Why the doctor suggested this treatment plan for me.	1	2	3	4	5
47.	The reasons my doctor suggests certain tests (e.g., x-rays, bone scans).	1	2	3	4	5
48.	How to prepare for the tests (e.g., x-rays, bone scans).	1	2	3	4	5
49.	What to do if I feel uncomfortable in social situations.	1	2	3	4	5
50.	If my illness is hereditary.	1	2	3	4	5
51.	When to have a mammogram.	1	2	3	4	5
52.	If I can continue my usual social activities.	1	2	3	4	5

47. English/Spanish Self-Efficacy Scale for Breast Self-Examination

Developed by Judith T. Gonzalez-Calvo and Virginia M. Gonzalez

INSTRUMENT DESCRIPTION, ADMINISTRATION, AND SCORING GUIDELINES

Women of color and from lower socioeconomic groups have higher rates of breast cancer deaths, a greater percentage of which are considered preventable by early detection. Prior study has shown that among low-income Mexican-American women, self-efficacy was the most significant predictor of breast self-examination (BSE). Study of this population is important because self-efficacy may include not only skills specific to a particular task but also related behaviors, such as communication with the health care provider or educator, to learn the complex performance of BSE and ability or motivation to break down barriers of access to health care (Gonzalez & Gonzalez, 1990).

Scores are obtained by adding the Likert scores of the original items. Items are available in both English and Spanish. Rating scales are adjectives describing degrees of intensity, found to work better with this group than did a 100-point visual analog scale used in other measures of self-efficacy (Gonzalez & Gonzalez, 1990).

PSYCHOMETRIC PROPERTIES

The scale was initially tested on a convenience sample of 106 low-income, primarily Spanish-speaking Mexican American women attending a clinic in Tucson. Average years of schooling was 8.7. Although 62% reported having had a breast examination by a physician in the past year, and 39% reported they examined their own breasts at least once a month, few possessed adequate knowledge of correct procedure (Gonzalez & Gonzalez, 1990). Alpha coefficient was .79. Factor analysis showed three subdimensions of self-efficacy: BSE skill related items (items 1 to 3), communication skill related (items 4 to 7), and ability to surmount barrier to health care (items 8 to 11). Self-efficacy was significantly correlated with actual skill measures for BSE (although with low interrater reliability), English language proficiency, and reported frequency of BSE, providing some evidence of validity. The mean self-efficacy score for this group was 48, *SD* 8.7, and median 4.8 (Gonzalez & Gonzalez, 1990).

A more recent study (Mishra et al., 1998) with a similar population found Cronbach's alphas .70 at pretest and .80 and .73 at posttest. More than half of the women were either undecided or somewhat uncertain about their ability to effectively interact with their health providers, overcome environmental barriers to care, and skillfully perform BSE. The English/Spanish Self Efficacy Scale was sensitive to a theoretically potent intervention in a quasi-experimental study.

CRITIQUE AND SUMMARY

Little research has been conducted among Mexican Americans relating self-efficacy to health outcomes; further use of this scale can provide more evidence. The author notes the possibility that responses to the scale and the reported skill in performing BSE are indicative of a tendency others have noted of Mexican Americans to give socially desirable responses. Traditional views of the human body in Mexico consider touching of the breasts as a breach of decency. Test–retest reliability was not assessed. This measure should also be compared with other methods of assessing self-efficacy to reevaluate construct validity. It should also be tested in other settings, with Mexican American females who do not receive regular medical care, and in research testing the amount of change in self-efficacy related to training interventions (Gonzalez & Gonzalez, 1990).

Although in an early stage of development, this scale is important in part because it addresses cross-cultural issues. Not only is it important to develop scales in appropriate language and response modes, it is also important to incorporate self-efficacy beliefs related to the central skill of BSE (communication and overcoming barriers), and essential to carrying out the appropriate health action. While breast cancer is the most commonly diagnosed cancer among Latinas in the United States, this group is less likely to practice breast cancer screening examinations.

REFERENCES

Gonzalez, J. T., & Gonzalez, V. M. (1990). Initial validation of a scale measuring self-efficacy of breast self-examination among low-income Mexican American women. *Hispanic Journal of Behavioral Sciences, 12,* 277–291.

Mishra, S. I., Chavez, L. R., Magana, J. R., Nava, P., Valdez, R. B., & Hubbell, F. A. (1998). Improving breast cancer control among Latinas: Evaluation of a theory-based educational program. *Health Education & Behavior, 25,* 653–670.

ENGLISH/SPANISH SELF-EFFICACY SCALE
FOR BREAST SELF-EXAMINATION

English Response Choices

(1)   uncertain
(2)   somewhat uncertain
(3)   neither certain nor uncertain
(4)   somewhat certain
(5)   certain

Spanish Response Choices

(1)   muy insegura
(2)   algo insegura
(3)   ni segura, ni insegura
(4)   algo segura
(5)   segura

1.   How certain are you that you can do a breast self-examination without anyone's help?
     ¿Hasta qué punto se siente segura de que puede hacerse la auto-examinación de los senos sin la ayuda de otra persona?

2.   How certain are you that you can find a lump on your breast when you do the breast self-examination without help?
     ¿Hasta qué punto se siente segura de que puede encontrar un bulto en el seno al hacerse la auto-examinación sin la ayuda de nadie?

3.   How certain are you that you can teach another woman how to examine her breasts?
     ¿Qué tan segura se siente de que puede enseñarle a otra mujer como examinarse los senos?

4.   How certain are you that you can ask the doctor the necessary questions to get the information that you need about your health condition?
     ¿Qué tan segura se siente de que puede hacerle al médico las preguntas necesarias para obtener la información que Ud. necesita respecto a su condición física?

5.   How certain are you that you can understand the doctor's explanation about your health condition?
     ¿Qué tan segura se siente de que puede comprender la explicación que le da el médico respecto a su condición física?

6.   How certain are you that you can understand what the doctor is doing when he/she examines you?
     ¿Hasta qué punto se siente segura de que puede comprender lo que está haciendo el médico cuando la examina?

English Response Choices

(1) uncertain
(2) somewhat uncertain
(3) neither certain nor uncertain
(4) somewhat certain
(5) certain

Spanish Response Choices

(1) muy insegura
(2) algo insegura
(3) ni segura, ni insegura
(4) algo segura
(5) segura

7. Sometimes it is necessary to explain to our friends and family the results of pap smear. How certain are you that you can explain the results to another person?
   A veces es necesario explicarle a sus amigas y familia los resultados del examen de la cervix (Pap smear). ¿Hasta qué punto se siente segura de que puede explicarle los resultados a otra persona?

8. If needed, how certain are you that you can get someone to help you with child care so that you can get to the doctor?
   Si fuera necesario, ¿qué tan segura se siente de que puede conseguir a alguien que le ayude con el cuidado de los niños para que Ud. pueda ir con el doctor?

9. How certain are you that you can keep your next appointment with the doctor?
   ¿Qué tan segura se siente Ud. de que pudrá ir a su siguiente cita con el médico?

10. How certain are you that you can do what the doctor recommends for required follow-up care?
    ¿Qué tan segura se siente que Ud. puede hacer lo que recomienda el doctor/la doctora en cuanto el cuidado necesario después de su consulta?

11. If needed, how certain are you that you can get a friend or family member to give you a ride to the clinic?
    Si fuera necesario, ¿qué tan segura se siente de que puede conseguir que una amiga o un familiar la lleve a la clinica?

48. Breast Cancer and Hereditary Knowledge Scale

Developed by Nancy Ondrusek, Ellen Warner, and Vivek Goel

INSTRUMENT DESCRIPTION, ADMINISTRATION, AND SCORING GUIDELINES

Breast cancer is the most common cancer among North American women, who currently face a 1 in 9 lifetime risk of the disease. Although women with very strong family histories are frequently referred to specialized familial breast cancer clinics with extensive counseling, whether women with less striking family histories are getting and understanding the information they need about risk is not known. BCHK is a brief self-administered knowledge scale about breast cancer and heredity specifically for women at low to moderate risk for hereditary breast cancer (HBC).

Correct response to a statement of "strongly agree" or "strongly disagree" is assigned a value of 2, "agree" or "disagree" a 1, unsure 0, with incorrect responses given a negative value. Scores are summed. Reading level is grade 8.2. The scale can be completed in less than five minutes (Ondrusek, Warner, & Goel, 1999).

PSYCHOMETRIC CHARACTERISTICS

Content for BCHK was developed from focus groups of women as well as from relevant professionals. Knowledge about genetics and HBC was generally poor, supporting the need for the instrument. The Breast Cancer and Hereditary Knowledge Scale (BCHK) examines knowledge in four breast cancer subject areas: incidence and etiology (3 items); screening, disease presentation, and treatment (4 items); and genetics (4 items).

Test–retest reliability at 2–4 weeks was .76. Construct validity and sensitivity to change is currently being examined (Ondrusek, Warner, & Goel, 1999). BCHK did show sensitivity to intervention with a decision aid (form of instruction meant to facilitate patient decision making) (Warner et al., 1999).

CRITIQUE AND SUMMARY

BCHK addresses an important need. The authors caution that until more is known about its psychometric characteristics, BCHK use should be limited to well-defined research studies (Ondrusek, Warner, & Goel, 1999).

REFERENCES

Ondrusek, N., Warner, E., & Goel, V. (1999). Development of a knowledge scale about breast cancer and heredity (BCHK). *Breast Cancer Research & Treatment, 53,* 69–75.

Warner, E., Goel, V., Ondrusek, N., Thiel, E. C., Lickley, L. A., Chart, P. L., Meschino, W. S., Doan, B. D., Carroll, J. C., & Taylor, K. M. (1999). Pilot study of an information aid for women with a family history of breast cancer. *Health Expectations, 2,* 118–128.

BREAST CANCER HEREDITARY
KNOWLEDGE SCALE

A. Genetics domain:

Testing for breast cancer gene mutations will tell a woman if she has breast cancer.   (F)

Men cannot inherit breast cancer gene mutations.   (F)

A woman whose mother was diagnosed with breast cancer at age 69 is considered to be at high risk for breast cancer.   (F)

Ovarian cancer and breast cancer in the same family can be a sign of hereditary breast cancer.   (T)

B. Incidence domain:

Out of every 100 women who are diagnosed with breast cancer, 75 are alive and well after 10 years.   (T)

Stress has been proven to increase the risk of breast cancer.   (F)

Women who are over 50 years of age are more likely to get breast cancer than are younger women.   (T)

Over a lifetime, 1 out of 9 women will develop breast cancer.   (T)

C. Disease presentation and treatment domain:

Swelling or enlargement of one breast is a possible sign of breast cancer.   (T)

Chemotherapy is always used in the treatment of breast cancer.   (F)

Women over age 50 should have mammograms at least every 2 years.   (T)

From: Warner, E., Goel, V., Ondrusek, N., Thiel, E. C., Lickley, L. A., Chart, P. L., Meschino, W. S., Doan, B. D., Carroll, J. C., & Taylor, K. M. (1999). Pilot study of an information aid for women with a family history of breast cancer. *Health Expectations, 2,* 118–128. Used with permission.

49. Colorectal Cancer Knowledge Questionnaire

Developed by Sally P. Weinrich, Martin C. Weinrich, Marilyn D. Boyd, Edna Johnson, and Marilyn Frank-Stromberg

INSTRUMENT DESCRIPTION, ADMINISTRATION, AND SCORING GUIDELINES

Colorectal cancer is the second leading cause of death in the United States; yet the survival rate for patients could be increased with screening and early detection in conjunction with appropriate management. Although not sufficient by itself to promote behavioral change, adequate levels of knowledge are prerequisite to such behavior. The possible range of scores on the questionnaire is 0 to 12, with each correct answer counting as 1 point and higher scores reflecting greater knowledge. Responses were obtained by interview for those who had difficulty reading and writing, with each interview lasting 12 minutes (Weinrich, Weinrich, Boyd, Johnson, & Frank-Stromberg, 1992).

PSYCHOMETRIC PROPERTIES

Only one study using the questionnaire could be located. Participants were socioeconomically disadvantaged adults with an average age of 72 years, contacted in 12 Southern congregate meal sites sponsored by the Council on Aging (Weinrich et al., 1992). A socioeconomically disadvantaged population has been shown to be least likely to participate in screening and also most likely to die from colorectal cancer, and studies have documented inadequate knowledge of cancer among this group. Half of the participants in the present study were Black and half White.

The Colorectal Cancer Knowledge Questionnaire (CCKQ) was adapted for the study population from the American Cancer Society's Colorectal Health Check Questionnaire. The CCKQ was administered before and after a program using four different educational methods to which participants were randomly assigned: peer education, educational modification to accommodate normal aging changes including increased time for learning and decrease in short-term memory, a combination of these approaches, and the traditional method. Pretest scores ranged from 2 to 12, with an overall mean of 8 and *SD* of 2.6; posttest scores administered 6 days later had a range of 1 to 12, mean of 8.7, and *SD* of 2.5, a significant change in scores. Cronbach's alpha was 0.69, with a test–retest reliability of 0.65 for a subset of 19 people from the sample.

Fewer subjects in this sample had undergone screening for colorectal cancer than the national average, although having been screened was not significantly associated with cancer knowledge. Score on the CCKQ was a predictor of participation in fecal occult blood testing made available at the time of education. Powe (1995) found a significant negative relationship between scores on CCKQ and a measure of cancer fatalism, again supportive of validity.

An intervention study using a culturally sensitive video and an educational audio, showed improvements in scores on the CCKQ. In this sample, Cronbach's alpha ranged from .66 to .77 (Powe & Weinrich, 1999).

CRITIQUE AND SUMMARY

Little information about validity of the CCKQ, including content validity, was made available. Particularly with a knowledge test, explicit definition of the domains from which items were generated and then chosen is expected. Relationship between CCKQ scores and additional target behaviors such as diet would also be helpful. Reliability is modest. In addition, the questionnaire has been tested with only one sociodemographically homogeneous set of participants. Because more educated persons could be anticipated to have greater knowledge of cancer, it is not clear whether ceiling effects might occur when such persons were tested with the CCKQ. This is a particular problem when testing sensitivity to teaching interventions.

REFERENCES

Powe, B. D., & Weinrich, S. (1999). An intervention to decrease cancer fatalism among rural elders. *Oncology Nursing Forum, 26,* 583–588.

Powe, B. D. (1995). Perceptions of cancer fatalism among African Americans: The influence of education, income and cancer knowledge. *Journal of the National Black Nurses' Association, 7*(2), 41–48.

Weinrich, S. P., Weinrich, M. C., Boyd, M. D., Johnson, E., & Frank-Stromborg, M. (1992). Knowledge of colorectal cancer among older persons. *Cancer Nursing, 15,* 322–330.

KNOWLEDGE OF COLORECTAL CANCER QUESTIONNAIRE

Tell me if you think these questions are true, false, or don't know.

Do you think or believe that:	Yes (true)	No (false)	Don't know
1. Men get cancer of the bowel more often than women.	T	F	DK
2. Bowel cancer is always a deadly disease.	T	F	DK
3. To check for blood in your bowel movement, you need to have a bowel movement blood test.	T	F	DK
4. You think you would always have pain if you had cancer of the bowel.	T	F	DK
5. You think your chances of getting cancer of the bowel are greater if you have a family member who had cancer of the bowel.	T	F	DK
6. Blood in your bowel movement means you have cancer for sure.	T	F	DK
7. You need to check your bowel movement for blood even if your bowel habits are normal.	T	F	DK
8. You think testing bowel movements for hidden blood would be very painful.	T	F	DK
9. Almost all the people who get bowel cancer are 50 years old or older.	T	F	DK
10. Most people who get cancer of the bowel could be saved if it were found and treated at an early stage.	T	F	DK
11. A diet with a lot of roughage, like fruits, vegetables, and grains, may reduce your chances of getting cancer of the bowel.	T	F	DK
12. You should have your bowel movement tested for hidden blood every year if you are 50 years or older.	T	F	DK

Correct answers: 1, 2, 4, 6, and 8 are false; 3, 5, 7, 9, 10, 11, and 12 are true.

From Weinrich, S. P., Weinrich, M. C., Boyd, M. D., Johnson, E., & Frank-Stromberg, M. (1992). Knowledge of colorectal cancer among older persons. *Cancer Nursing, 15*(5), 322–330.

50.   Family Inventory of Needs

Developed by Linda J. Kristjanson, Jan Atwood, and Lesley F. Degner

INSTRUMENT DESCRIPTION, ADMINISTRATION, AND SCORING GUIDELINES

The Family Inventory of Needs (FIN) is designed to measure the importance of care needs of families of advanced cancer patients (FIN-Importance of Needs Subscale) and the extent to which families perceive their care needs have been met (FIN-Fulfillment of Needs Subscale). FIN was designed to be used with individual family members whose needs may be different, not with the family as a unit. This kind of care is known to be important to family satisfaction and functioning and to recovery from grieving. FIN is based on fulfillment theory which hypothesizes that the greater degree to which needs are fulfilled, the higher a family's satisfaction with care (Kristjanson, Sloan, Dudgeon, & Adaskin, 1996).

The two subscales are scored separately. A score of 0 on FIN-Importance of Care Needs means the item is not important at all; if it is, respondent scores it 1–10 with 10 being a very important need. A simple count of the number of items scored indicates the number of needs a family member identifies (range 0–20) with the raw score as total score (0–200). FIN-Need Fulfillment Subscale is scored by assigning a "met" response as 1 and "not met" as 0, yielding a raw score of 0–20. Comparison with the Importance of Care Needs Scale shows the number of needs met. FIN is brief, which is important for highly stressed populations (Kristjanson, Atwood, & Degner, 1995).

Kilpatrick, Kristjanson, Tataryn, and Fraser (1998) and Kilpatrick, Kristjanson, and Tataryn (1998) have developed FIN-Husbands (FIN-H), tested on those whose wives have recently undergone surgery for breast cancer. This instrument incorporates some items from FIN and added others. It is not reproduced here but can be obtained from its developer.

PSYCHOMETRIC CHARACTERISTICS

Content validity was addressed using a panel of family members of advanced cancer patients. Each subscale was found to be unidimensional, supporting construct validity. FIN-Fulfillment subscale correlated .77–.79 with an independent care satisfaction scale, supporting criterion validity and providing some support for construct validity. Internal consistency of FIN-Importance of Needs subscale was .83 and of FIN-Fulfillment of Care Needs .91–.95, with a test–retest reliability of .91. FIN-H also met content validity standards and had an alpha coefficient of .91 and test–retest reliability of .82 and .76 (Kristjanson, Atwood, & Degner, 1995).

CRITIQUE AND SUMMARY

Many of the needs included in FIN are oriented to information and expectations and so could be met by educational programs, although no sensitivity data could be located. The authors suggest further testing of the tool in more racially mixed populations in other countries to determine how culturally robust it is (Kristjanson, Atwood, & Degner, 1995).

REFERENCES

Kilpatrick, M. G., Kristjanson, L. J., & Tataryn, D. J. (1998). Measuring the information needs of husbands of women with breast cancer: Validity of the Family Inventory of Needs-Husbands. *Oncology Nursing Forum, 25,* 1347–1351.

Kilpatrick, M. G., Kristjanson, L. J., Tataryn, D. J., & Fraser, V. H. (1998). Information needs of husbands of women with breast cancer. *Oncology Nursing Forum, 25,* 1595–1601.

Kristjanson, L. J., Atwood, J., & Degner, L. F. (1995). Validity and reliability of the Family Inventory of Needs (FIN): Measuring the care needs of families of advanced cancer patients. *Journal of Nursing Measurement, 3,* 109–126.

Kristjanson, L. J., Sloan, J. A., Dudgeon, D., & Adaskin, E. (1996). Family members' perceptions of palliative cancer care: Predictors of family functioning and family members' health. *Journal of Palliative Care, 12*(4), 10–20.

FAMILY INVENTORY OF NEEDS (FIN)

Below is a list of needs identified by some family members of cancer patients. Please rate how important each item is from 0–10 as it relates to your present situation. If an item is not at all important to you, give it a 0. If it is very important to you give it a 10. If it is somewhere in between, give it a score between 0 and 10 which reflects how important it is for you. Then check whether each need is currently met or unmet.

	If you rate an item higher than 0, check if met or unmet		
RATINGS FORM			
I Need to:	0–10	Met	Unmet
1. have my questions answered honestly	_____	_____	_____
2. know specific facts concerning the patients' prognosis	_____	_____	_____
3. feel that the professionals care about the patients	_____	_____	_____
4. be informed of changes in the patient's condition	_____	_____	_____
5. know exactly what is being done to the patient	_____	_____	_____
6. know what treatment the patient is receiving	_____	_____	_____
7. have explanations given in terms that are understandable	_____	_____	_____
8. be told about changes in treatment plans while they are being made	_____	_____	_____
9. feel there is hope	_____	_____	_____
10. be assured that the best possible care is being given to the patient	_____	_____	_____
11. know what symptoms the treatment or disease can cause	_____	_____	_____
12. know when to expect symptoms to occur	_____	_____	_____
13. know the probable outcome of the patient's illness	_____	_____	_____
14. know why things are done for the patient	_____	_____	_____
15. know the names of health professionals involved in the patient's care	_____	_____	_____
16. have information about what to do for the patient at home	_____	_____	_____
17. feel accepted by the health professionals	_____	_____	_____
18. help with the patient's care	_____	_____	_____
19. have someone be concerned with my health	_____	_____	_____
20. be told about people who could help with problems	_____	_____	_____

From: Kristjanson, L. J., Atwood, J., & Degner, L. F. (1995). Validity and reliability of the Family Inventory of Needs (FIN): Measuring the care of families of advanced cancer patients. *Journal of Nursing Measurement, 3,* 109–126. Used with permission.

Section G

Pregnancy, Childbirth, and Parenting

This field has historically had a rich array of instruments including a number of self-efficacy scales covering a range of behaviors.

---

51.   Pregnancy Anxiety Scale

Developed by Jeffrey S. Levin

INSTRUMENT DESCRIPTION, ADMINISTRATION, AND SCORING GUIDELINES

Many studies have identified an association of higher anxiety and deleterious pregnancy outcomes. The Pregnancy Anxiety Scale (PAS) is a 10-item scale of maternal anxiety during pregnancy. It is intended to be useful as a diagnostic tool related to the pregnancy experience and more useful than general anxiety inventories would be. Its authors see it as useful in research. It is not yet known if it has specific clinical applications with cutoff points that would indicate a need for further assessment and intervention. The 10 items are scored 0 = no, 1 = yes, and summed (Levin, 1991).

PSYCHOMETRIC PROPERTIES

The 13-item PAS was tested on 266 postpartum mothers, largely African-American and Hispanic, and showed reliability of .63. Factor analysis shows three factors: anxiety about being pregnant (items 1 to 3), anxiety about childbirth (items 4 to 7), and anxiety about hospitalization (items 8 to 10). Based on these measurement characteristics three items were removed, leaving 10. A full and detailed description of the psychometric analysis may be found in Levin (1991). More recently, PAS was used in a small study of stress in pregnancy showing that PAS scores were not significantly correlated with pregnancy outcome and had a low correlation with the State-Trait Anxiety Inventory, indicating little overlap in the constructs assessed by these measures (Milad, Klock, Moses, & Chatterton, 1998).

SUMMARY AND CRITIQUE

The scale's latent structure has not yet been confirmed separately with African-American and Hispanic mothers, or with other groups like Anglo Whites.

It is reasonable to expect education to be one means of lowering excess anxiety, through teaching anxiety reduction strategies or changing misconceptions that produce anxiety. The PAS requires additional developmental work including exploration of the use of expanded response categories and its structure after prospective use during pregnancy (Levin, 1991).

REFERENCES

Levin, J. S. (1991). The factor structure of the Pregnancy Anxiety Scale. *Journal of Health and Social Behavior, 21,* 368–381.

Milad, M. P., Klock, S. C., Moses, S., & Chatterton, R. (1998). Stress and anxiety do not result in pregnancy wastage. *Human Reproduction, 13,* 2296–2300.

PREGNANCY ANXIETY

Anxiety about Being Pregnant   Yes   No

Did any one frighten you about having a baby?
Did you read anything that frightened you about having a baby?
Did you fear that you would fall and hurt your baby?

Anxiety about Childbirth

Were you afraid the pain of childbirth would be bad?
Did you ask for pain medicine before childbirth?
Did you have any fear about being torn or cut when the baby was born?
Were you afraid your baby would not be normal?

Anxiety about Hospitalization

Were you afraid you would be alone in the hospital?
Were you worried that the doctors might not be friendly?
Were you worried that the nurses might not be friendly?

From Levin, J. S. (1991) The Factor Structure of the Pregnancy Anxiety Scale. *Journal of Health and Social Behavior,* *32* (Dec.), 368–381. Reprinted Table 1, "Pregnancy Anxiety Indicators by Dimensions" with permission.

52. Maternal Serum Screening Knowledge Questionnaire

Developed by Vivek Goel, Richard Glazier, Stephen Holzapfel, Patricia Pugh, and Anne Summers

INSTRUMENT DESCRIPTION, ADMINISTRATION, AND SCORING GUIDELINES

Maternal serum screening (MSS) is used to estimate risk for fetal birth defects. Potentially serious problems may arise including raised levels of anxiety among women with false-positive tests, false reassurance among women with negative test results, lack of timely follow up of positive tests, and in certain populations and locations, problems with access to follow-up services. For these reasons and because there is currently limited understanding of how comprehensible this test is, the Maternal Serum Screening Knowledge Questionnaire (MSSKQ) is expected to be a useful measure of patient knowledge of MSS and its implications.

Questions were designed to assess four knowledge domains a fully informed woman should have prior to testing: test characteristics, timing and indications for MSS, role of ancillary tests and perceived risk of these tests, and target conditions and knowledge of risk factors for the conditions. Items were given a value of 2 if the correct response was given with a "strongly agree" or "disagree," a value of 1 for a correct response with "agree" or "disagree." Incorrect responses were assigned a value of −2 or −1, whereas 0 was assigned for a "not sure" response. A score of 0 reflects guessing or complete lack of information, scores of −2 to 0 are most likely due to incorrect understanding of the information, 0–.5 a low level of knowledge, .5–1.0 a moderate level, and more than 1.0 a high level of knowledge. Reading level was grade 8; the instrument can be completed in a few minutes (Goel, Glazier, Holzapfel, Pugh, & Summers, 1996).

PSYCHOMETRIC CHARACTERISTICS

Items were selected based on a review of educational materials, the literature, and expert opinion. They were pretested for comprehensibility and ambiguity in a convenience sample, and administered to 1084 women attending a maternal registration clinic. Content validity was supported by the fact that question content adhered closely to consumer MSS information pamphlets distributed to health care providers in Ontario.

Chronbach's alpha was .74, test–retest reliability .76. Mean MSSKQ scores were significantly higher among those reporting having an opportunity to discuss maternal serum screening with their health care provider and receiving written material about it. A study by Glazier and others (1997) showed MSSKQ to be sensitive to an educational pamphlet in comparison with a group receiving a control pamphlet.

CRITIQUE AND SUMMARY

The authors suggest MSSKQ should be valuable in assessing knowledge and level of informed consent in women receiving maternal serum screening and in evaluating implementation of MSS programs.

So far, MSSKQ has been used with highly educated women, and its reading level of grade 8 could be expected to be problematic for many populations. Scores obtained by this group may be found in Goel, Glazier, Holzapfel, Pugh, and Summers (1996). The fact that these women showed important information gaps raises questions about the degree to which women in this setting are giving informed consent when they have MSS.

REFERENCES

Goel, V., Glazier, R., Holzapfel, S., Pugh, P., & Summers, A. (1996). Evaluating patients' knowledge of maternal serum screening. *Prenatal Diagnosis, 16,* 425–430.

Glazier, R., Goel, V., Holzapfel, S., Summers, A., Pugh, P., & Yeung, M. (1997). Written patient information about triple-marker screening: A randomized controlled trial. *Obstetrics & Gynecology, 90,* 769–774.

MATERNAL SERUM SCREENING
KNOWLEDGE QUESTIONNAIRE (MSSKQ)

	Strongly Agree	Agree	Disagree	Strongly Disagree	Not Sure

Domain: test characteristics

If maternal serum screening is abnormal, further tests are needed to tell if anything is wrong (A)

Maternal serum screening (also called alpha plus or triple test) detects only Down syndrome (D)

If maternal serum screening is abnormal, something is usually wrong with the baby (D)

Women who have normal maternal serum screening can be sure that they will have a normal baby (D)

Domain: indications and timing

Maternal serum screening is not accurate when done at the wrong time during the pregnancy (A)

Having maternal serum screening is routine for all pregnant women (A)

Domain: ancillary tests

Ultrasound can be used to detect every kind of birth defect (D)

Amniocentesis can cause miscarriage in about 1 out of 200 women (A)

Amniocentesis is a test of the mother's blood which can detect Down syndrome (D)

Domain: target conditions

The chance of having a baby with Down syndrome is higher the older the mother (A)

Open neural tube defects include spina bifida (an opening in the bones around the spinal cord) and anencephaly (missing much of the skull and brain) (A)

	Strongly Agree	Agree	Disagree	Strongly Disagree	Not Sure
All children born with Down syndrome have severe physical and mental disabilities which require life-long care in an institution (D)					
If amniocentesis shows Down syndrome, the only options are to have a baby with Down syndrome or to end the pregnancy (A)					
The chance of having an open neural tube defect is higher the older the mother (D)					

From: Goel, V., Glazier, R., Holzapfel, S., Pugh, P., & Summers, A. (1996). Evaluating patients' knowledge of maternal serum screening. *Prenatal Diagnosis, 16,* 425–430. © John Wiley & Sons. Reproduced with permission.

Correct answers are indicated at the end of each item.

53. Labour Agentry Scale: A Measure of a Woman's Sense of Control Over the Childbirth Experience

Developed by Ellen Hodnett

INSTRUMENT DESCRIPTION, ADMINISTRATION, AND SCORING GUIDELINES

The Labour Agentry Scale (LAS) measures perceived control during childbirth, that is, a woman's sense of mastery over internal and environmental forces. This control has been linked to improved learning and functioning on various tasks and decreased need for analgesia and anesthesia during childbirth, and is considered to be a key component of birth satisfaction (Hodnett & Abel, 1986). The LAS has been translated into and validated in French, Spanish, Swedish, Danish, and Hebrew. It can be used to measure either expectations or experiences of control, depending on timing of administration (antepartum or postpartum). Scores are obtained from summing item scores, with a possible range from 29 (very low control) to 203. Low scores indicate low expectancies of experiences of control over oneself and one's environment during labor; high scores indicate high expectancies/experiences. The LAS takes 10 minutes to complete.

PSYCHOMETRIC PROPERTIES

Most subjects asked open-ended questions about what contributed to a positive birth experience indicated that aspects of personal control were important to them during labor. In psychometric and field studies, alpha reliability coefficients for the LAS have ranged from .91 to .98 (Hodnett & Abel, 1986). Subjects who experienced the highest levels of control over self and environment during labor by ambulating, foregoing analgesia and anesthesia, and having spontaneous births had the highest LAS scores, evidence supporting concurrent validity. There was also a significant inverse relationship between use of pharmacological pain-relief measures and LAS scores, a significant positive relationship between levels of perceived human support during childbirth and LAS scores. Experienced control was distinct from, but related to, maternal childbirth satisfaction. Antepartum mean scores ranged from 156.5 to 162.38, and postpartum scores from 152.19 to 156.89. LAS scores remained stable at 2 weeks, 1 month, and 3 months postpartum. Factor analysis and dual scaling yielded evidence of a unifactorial scale (Hodnett & Simmons-Tropea, 1987).

In one study (Hodnett & Abel, 1986), the 80 women with home births had a significantly higher mean (174.7; $SD = 24.43$) LAS score than did the 80 with hospital births (mean score = 150.9; $SD = 25.38$). Multigravidas had significantly higher mean LAS scores than did primigravidas. Such findings are congruent with perceived environmental control. Hodnett and Osborn (1989) found greater increases in LAS scores and significantly less analgesia and anesthesia when continuous support (emotional, informational, physical, and advocacy) from montrices was provided during labor than under conditions of usual nursing care. Thus, the LAS showed sensitivity to intervention.

More recently, LAS has been used in three studies of various approaches to managing labor. In a study with more than 5000 women carried out in six countries, Cronbach's alpha reliability was greater than .85 in each language version of LAS. Women who had a previous cesarean delivery and those who were smokers had lower levels of control, whereas multiparity was associated with an increase of 6.5 points in LAS scores (Hodnett et al., 1998).

In a group of women making slow progress in the active phase of labor and with intact membranes, Blanch, Lavender, Walkinshaw, and Alfirevic (1998) found those who received interventions of oxytocin and/or amniotomy had a higher sense of control than did those who received only expectant management, perhaps because of a feeling that "something is being done to shorten labor." Among women suffering from low back pain during labor, Labrecque, Nouwen, Bergeron, and Rancourt (1999) found no significant difference in LAS scores among those randomly assigned to receive intracutaneous sterile water injections, TENS, or standard care.

LAS is being actively used to study outcomes of various interventions to better manage labor.

CRITIQUE AND SUMMARY

Although several thousands of patients have been tested with LAS, the level of score that constitutes control relevant to women is uncertain (Blanch et al., 1998).

Expected control has been inversely related to prenatal anxiety and education can decrease this problem. One of the key elements of professional care during labor is information and instruction. Thus, the LAS would seem to be a useful tool for patient assessment and tailoring of interventions, and for research on the influence of expectations in both physiological and psychological outcomes of pregnancy and birth. LAS has also been used in studies addressing environmental conditions for birth and support during labor (Hodnett & Simmons-Tropea, 1987).

REFERENCES

Blanch, G., Lavender, T., Walkinshaw, S., & Alfirevic, Z. (1998). Dysfunctional labour: A randomized trial. *British Journal of Obstetrics and Gynaecology, 105*, 117–120.

Hodnett, E. D., & Abel, S. M. (1986). Person-environment interaction as a determinant of labor length variables. *Health Care for Women International, 7*, 341–356.

Hodnett, E. D., & Osborn, R. W. (1989). Effect of continuous intrapartum professional support on childbirth outcomes. *Research in Nursing and Health, 12*, 289–297.

Hodnett, E. D., & Simmons-Tropea, D. A. (1987). The Labour Agentry Scale: Psychometric properties of an instrument measuring control during childbirth. *Research in Nursing and Health, 10*, 301–310.

Hodnett, E. D., Hannah, M. E., Weston, J. A., Ohlsson, A., Myhr, T. L., Wang, E. E. I., Hewson, S. A., Willan, A. R., & Farine, D., for the TermPROM Study Group. (1998). Women's evaluations of induction of labor versus expectant management for prelabor rupture of the membranes at term. *Birth, 24,* 117–120.

Labrecque, M., Nouwen, A., Bergeron, M., & Rancourt, J. (1999). A randomized controlled trial of nonpharmacologic approaches for relief of low back pain during labor. *Journal of Family Practice, 48,* 259–263.

LABOUR AGENTRY SCALE

6–8 Weeks Postpartum

Section J: Your Childbirth Experience

PART 1: Your Feelings About Your Childbirth Experience

Just as no two women are exactly alike, no two women have exactly the same experiences during childbirth. Please try to recall your labor and your baby's birth as vividly as you can. Think about your feelings during labor and birth. Of course, you probably had many different feelings, but try to remember what it was generally like for you during this time.

INSTRUCTIONS ON HOW TO USE THIS SCALE:

This question is used as an example.

I felt confident	Almost always	○ ○ ○ ○ ○ ○ ○	Rarely
		1 2 3 4 5 6 7	
If you felt confident <u>almost all of the time</u> *mark this position*	Almost always	● ○ ○ ○ ○ ○ ○ 1 2 3 4 5 6 7	Rarely
If you felt confident <u>a lot but not always</u> *mark this position*	Almost always	○ ● ○ ○ ○ ○ ○ 1 2 3 4 5 6 7	Rarely
If you felt confident <u>a little more than half the time</u> *mark this position*	Almost always	○ ○ ● ○ ○ ○ ○ 1 2 3 4 5 6 7	Rarely
If you felt confident <u>about half the time</u> *mark this position*	Almost always	○ ○ ○ ● ○ ○ ○ 1 2 3 4 5 6 7	Rarely
If you felt confident <u>slightly less than half</u> the time *mark this position*	Almost always	○ ○ ○ ○ ● ○ ○ 1 2 3 4 5 6 7	Rarely
If you <u>sometimes</u> felt confident *mark this position*	Almost always	○ ○ ○ ○ ○ ● ○ 1 2 3 4 5 6 7	Rarely
If you <u>never or almost never</u> felt confident *mark this position*	Almost always	○ ○ ○ ○ ○ ○ ● 1 2 3 4 5 6 7	Rarely

Please try to rate each statement on its own. Do not consider the other statements. The position of the boxes in relation to "almost always" and "rarely" is what is important, not the numbers under the boxes.

Fill in bubbles like this: ●   Not like this: ⊗ Ⓞ̸

Section J: Your Childbirth Experience

PART 1: Your Feelings About Your Childbirth Experience

Please see the previous page for instructions on completing this scale.

J1.	I felt tense	Almost Always	○ ○ ○ ○ ○ ○ ○ Rarely 1 2 3 4 5 6 7
J2.	I felt important	Almost Always	○ ○ ○ ○ ○ ○ ○ Rarely 1 2 3 4 5 6 7
J3.	I felt confident	Almost Always	○ ○ ○ ○ ○ ○ ○ Rarely 1 2 3 4 5 6 7
J4.	I felt in control	Almost Always	○ ○ ○ ○ ○ ○ ○ Rarely 1 2 3 4 5 6 7
J5.	I felt fearful	Almost Always	○ ○ ○ ○ ○ ○ ○ Rarely 1 2 3 4 5 6 7
J6.	I felt relaxed	Almost Always	○ ○ ○ ○ ○ ○ ○ Rarely 1 2 3 4 5 6 7
J7.	I felt good about my behavior	Almost Always	○ ○ ○ ○ ○ ○ ○ Rarely 1 2 3 4 5 6 7
J8.	I felt helpless (powerless)	Almost Always	○ ○ ○ ○ ○ ○ ○ Rarely 1 2 3 4 5 6 7
J9.	I felt I was with people who care about me	Almost Always	○ ○ ○ ○ ○ ○ ○ Rarely 1 2 3 4 5 6 7
J10.	I felt like a failure	Almost Always	○ ○ ○ ○ ○ ○ ○ Rarely 1 2 3 4 5 6 7

Scoring the 10-item version:

Reverse the item scores for the *positively-worded* items, e.g., Items #2, 3, 4, 6, 7, and 9, then sum the item scores. The higher the score, the higher the level of experienced control.

54. Childbirth Self-Efficacy Inventory

Developed by Nancy K. Lowe

INSTRUMENT DESCRIPTION, ADMINISTRATION, AND SCORING GUIDELINES

Self-efficacy (SE) involves an individual's evaluation of her capabilities to cope with stressful situations and perform required behaviors, certainly of concern during labor. Perceptions of self-efficacy developed before an event predict whether an individual will even try to cope with the situation and how long the effort will be sustained.

Confidence in the ability to cope with labor can be considered a motivational or conceptual factor affecting a woman's interpretation of painful labor stimuli. The importance of confidence to the perception of pain during labor is supported by data from clinical studies, which indicate that more than one half of the variance in early labor pain and about one third of the variance in active labor pain may be explained by the single variable of maternal confidence in the ability to cope. Women who express greater confidence in their ability to cope with labor report having less pain during labor. Those with the highest levels of SE will anticipate being able to execute coping behaviors during the most stressful times of labor including absence of a significant other, complications of labor, and concerns for fetal well-being. Confidence can be significantly increased by childbirth education including observation of others performing successfully during labor (Lowe, 1991).

The Childbirth Self-Efficacy Inventory (CBSEI) measures both outcome expectancies (belief that a given behavior will lead to a given outcome) and self-efficacy expectancies (conviction that one can successfully perform required behaviors in a given situation) for coping with an approaching childbirth. An individual may believe that a certain behavior could help someone cope with the potentially aversive event but feel incapable of personally performing the behavior in the particular situation (Lowe, 1993).

Reading level of the scale has been measured at grade 7 or 8. Scale scores are the sum of responses (1 to 10) to each item. In each part, the first half of the items measures outcome expectation and the second half measure self-efficacy expectations. Thus, active labor outcome and self-efficacy scores may range from 15 to 150, whereas the parallel second-stage scores have a potential range of 16 to 160 each. Total CBSEI outcome and self-efficacy expectancy scores are the sum of the corresponding scores from active and second stage labor and may range from 31 to 310 (Lowe, 1993).

PSYCHOMETRIC PROPERTIES

Fifty-six items were generated for the CBSEI through content analysis of postpartum interviews with 23 primiparous and 25 multiparous women who had experienced the uncomplicated vaginal birth of a normal term infant within the preceding 48 hours. The interview guide elicited each subject's perceptions of the specific behaviors she used to cope with labor, the adequacy of her individual strategies, and the perceived deficiencies in her ability to cope. Fifty percent of the sample had attended childbirth preparation classes. Rating of the items by an expert panel of university professors and nurse specialists in the care of childbearing women, or self-efficacy theory and removal of redundancies reduced the item pool to 20 items.

Pilot data from 96 healthy pregnant women led to further revision including separation of items into two phases of labor: when contractions are 5 or fewer minutes apart (active labor) and when pushing the baby out to give birth; change of the response scale; and addition of outcome expectancy scales. The CBSEI was then administered to 351 women attending community-based childbirth classes in the third trimester of pregnancy. The range of scores indicated that the CBSEI was sensitive to various levels of outcome and self-efficacy expectancies for childbirth and in differentiating outcome from self-efficacy expectancies (Lowe, 1993).

Internal consistency estimates ranged from .86 to .95, and item-total correlations were greater than .30 for all items on each scale. Correlations of test–retest scores over a 2-week period ranged from .46 to .76. Validity of the CBSEI was supported by significant positive correlations with measures of generalized self-efficacy, self-esteem, and internal locus of control, and by significant negative correlations with external health locus of control and learned helplessness. Validity was also supported by significantly higher self-efficacy scores for multiparous compared with nulliparous pregnant women. Factor analysis suggested that each CBSEI scale is unidimensional. Mean scores were 128 for outcome expectancy during active labor, 103 for SE during active labor, 130 for outcome expectancy during birth, 107 for SE during birth, 258 total outcome expectancy score, and 210 total SE score (Lowe, 1993).

A pilot study found that women choosing elective repeat cesarean delivery (rather than vaginal birth after cesarean section) had lower scores of CBSEI than did primagravidas or multigravidas who elected a vaginal birth after previous section. This finding would be predicted by SE theory undergirding CBSEI. It raises the question of whether childbirth classes specifically designed to build SE in women who have had a previous cesarean birth would be successful and whether the instrument would be sensitive to these interventions (Dilks & Beal, 1997).

Drummond and Rickwood (1997) studied psychometric characteristics of CBSEI in a sample of 100 pregnant Australian women. Consistent with U.S. data, the measure was shown to have high internal consistency (above .90) on all four subscales. Consistent with self-efficacy theory, having a prior good birth experience and knowledge about childbirth had significant effects on childbirth SE, supporting validity of the CBSEI. Other variables which might also be predicted by theory to relate to SE (parity, social support, and anxiety) were not significantly related to CBSEI scores. These findings support CBSEI validity.

Factor analysis showed a distinction between outcome and SE expectancies but not between active labor and birth as originally found by Lowe (1993). The authors suggest that the factor structure needs to be confirmed in other samples.

Sinclair and O'Boyle (1999) studied the performance of CBSEI in a Northern Ireland convenience sample of 126 women. This study confirmed earlier findings including reliability estimates of .91–.95 for the four subscales and outcome and SE as different constructs. Factor analysis was not done.

SUMMARY AND CRITIQUE

Self-efficacy has been shown to have a considerable effect on a woman's childbirth experience, affecting not only how well she copes physically, but also how she thinks and feels about the experience (Drummond & Rickwood, 1997). An obvious direction for research is to investigate the effectiveness of particular strategies used in childbirth preparation to enhance women's confidence in coping with labor. It is important to understand how to tailor this education to individual variations in personality and skills that a woman may bring to her pregnancy experience including previous experience with childbirth, or stressful and painful medical events. Most of the participants on whom the instrument has been tested were White, married, highly educated, nulliparous, and recruited from childbirth education classes. The instrument must be tested in more diverse demographic samples and in women unexposed to childbirth education. In addition, prospective study using the CBSEI during pregnancy and outcome measures during labor and birth will provide additional evidence for its validity. Because outcome expectancies are not conceptually well developed in the SE theory literature, their distinctiveness from SE in relation to coping with experiences such as childbirth should be further studied (Lowe, 1991).

The CBSEI was developed through a well-planned and conceptualized series of studies.

REFERENCES

Dilks, F. M., & Beal, J. A. (1997). Role of self-efficacy in birth choice. *Journal of Perinatal and Neonatal Nursing, 11*(1), 1–9.

Drummond, F. M., & Rickwood, D. (1997). Childbirth confidence: Validating the childbirth self-efficacy inventory (CBSEI) in an Australian sample. *Journal of Advanced Nursing, 26,* 613–622.

Lowe, N. K. (1991). Maternal confidence in coping with labor: A self-efficacy concept. *JOGN Nursing, 20,* 457–463.

Lowe, N. K. (1993). Maternal confidence for labor: Development of the Childbirth Self-Efficacy Inventory. *Research in Nursing and Health, 16,* 141–149.

Sinclair, M., & O'Boyle, C. (1999). The Childbirth Self-Efficacy Inventory: A replication study. *Journal of Advanced Nursing, 30,* 1416–1423.

CHILDBIRTH SELF-EFFICACY INVENTORY (CBSEI)

CBSEI: Part I (Labor)

Think about how you imagine labor will be and feel when you are having contractions 5 minutes apart or less. For each of the following behaviors, indicate how helpful you feel the behavior could be in helping you cope with this part of labor by circling a number between 1, *not at all helpful*, and 10, *very helpful*.

		Not at All Helpful									Very Helpful
1.	Relax my body.	1	2	3	4	5	6	7	8	9	10
2.	Get ready for each contraction.	1	2	3	4	5	6	7	8	9	10
3.	Use breathing during labor contractions.	1	2	3	4	5	6	7	8	9	10
4.	Keep myself in control.	1	2	3	4	5	6	7	8	9	10
5.	Think about relaxing.	1	2	3	4	5	6	7	8	9	10
6.	Concentrate on an object in the room to distract myself.	1	2	3	4	5	6	7	8	9	10
7.	Keep myself calm.	1	2	3	4	5	6	7	8	9	10
8.	Concentrate on thinking about the baby.	1	2	3	4	5	6	7	8	9	10
9.	Stay on top of each contraction.	1	2	3	4	5	6	7	8	9	10
10.	Think positively.	1	2	3	4	5	6	7	8	9	10
11.	Not think about the pain.	1	2	3	4	5	6	7	8	9	10
12.	Tell myself that I can do it.	1	2	3	4	5	6	7	8	9	10
13.	Think about others in my family.	1	2	3	4	5	6	7	8	9	10
14.	Concentrate on getting through one contraction at a time.	1	2	3	4	5	6	7	8	9	10
15.	Listen to encouragement from the person helping me.	1	2	3	4	5	6	7	8	9	10

Part I Continued

Continue to think about how you imagine labor will be and feel when you are having contractions 5 minutes apart or less. For each behavior, indicate how certain you are of your ability to use the behavior to help you cope with this part of labor by circling a number between 1, *not at all sure*, and 10, *completely sure*.

		Not at All Sure									Completely Sure
16.	Relax my body.	1	2	3	4	5	6	7	8	9	10
17.	Get ready for each contraction.	1	2	3	4	5	6	7	8	9	10
18.	Use breathing during labor contractions.	1	2	3	4	5	6	7	8	9	10
19.	Keep myself in control.	1	2	3	4	5	6	7	8	9	10
20.	Think about relaxing.	1	2	3	4	5	6	7	8	9	10
21.	Concentrate on an object in the room to distract myself.	1	2	3	4	5	6	7	8	9	10
22.	Keep myself calm.	1	2	3	4	5	6	7	8	9	10
23.	Concentrate on thinking about the baby.	1	2	3	4	5	6	7	8	9	10
24.	Stay on top of each contraction.	1	2	3	4	5	6	7	8	9	10
25.	Think positively.	1	2	3	4	5	6	7	8	9	10
26.	Not think about the pain.	1	2	3	4	5	6	7	8	9	10
27.	Tell myself that I can do it.	1	2	3	4	5	6	7	8	9	10
28.	Think about others in my family.	1	2	3	4	5	6	7	8	9	10
29.	Concentrate on getting through one contraction at a time.	1	2	3	4	5	6	7	8	9	10
30.	Listen to encouragement from the person helping me.	1	2	3	4	5	6	7	8	9	10

(continued)

CBSEI: Part II (Birth)

Think about how you imagine labor will be and feel when you are pushing your baby out to give birth. For each of the following behaviors, indicate how helpful you feel the behavior could be in helping you cope with this part of labor by circling a number between 1, *not at all helpful*, and 10, *very helpful*.

		Not at All Helpful									Very Helpful
31.	Relax my body.	1	2	3	4	5	6	7	8	9	10
32.	Get ready for each contraction.	1	2	3	4	5	6	7	8	9	10
33.	Use breathing during labor contractions.	1	2	3	4	5	6	7	8	9	10
34.	Keep myself in control.	1	2	3	4	5	6	7	8	9	10
35.	Think about relaxing.	1	2	3	4	5	6	7	8	9	10
36.	Concentrate on an object in the room to distract myself.	1	2	3	4	5	6	7	8	9	10
37.	Keep myself calm.	1	2	3	4	5	6	7	8	9	10
38.	Concentrate on thinking about the baby.	1	2	3	4	5	6	7	8	9	10
39.	Stay on top of each contraction.	1	2	3	4	5	6	7	8	9	10
40.	Think positively.	1	2	3	4	5	6	7	8	9	10
41.	Not think about the pain.	1	2	3	4	5	6	7	8	9	10
42.	Tell myself that I can do it.	1	2	3	4	5	6	7	8	9	10
43.	Think about others in my family.	1	2	3	4	5	6	7	8	9	10
44.	Concentrate on getting through one contraction at a time.	1	2	3	4	5	6	7	8	9	10
45.	Focus on the person helping me in labor.	1	2	3	4	5	6	7	8	9	10
46.	Listen to encouragement from the person helping me.	1	2	3	4	5	6	7	8	9	10

Part II Continued

Continue to think about how you imagine labor will be and feel when you are pushing your baby out to give birth. For each behavior, indicate how certain you are of your ability to use the behavior to help you cope with this part of labor by circling a number between 1, *not at all sure*, and 10, *completely sure*.

		Not at All Sure									Completely Sure
47.	Relax my body.	1	2	3	4	5	6	7	8	9	10
48.	Get ready for each contraction.	1	2	3	4	5	6	7	8	9	10
49.	Use breathing during labor contractions.	1	2	3	4	5	6	7	8	9	10
50.	Keep myself in control.	1	2	3	4	5	6	7	8	9	10
51.	Think about relaxing.	1	2	3	4	5	6	7	8	9	10
52.	Concentrate on an object in the room to distract myself.	1	2	3	4	5	6	7	8	9	10
53.	Keep myself calm.	1	2	3	4	5	6	7	8	9	10
54.	Concentrate on thinking about the baby.	1	2	3	4	5	6	7	8	9	10
55.	Stay on top of each contraction.	1	2	3	4	5	6	7	8	9	10
56.	Think positively.	1	2	3	4	5	6	7	8	9	10
57.	Not think about the pain.	1	2	3	4	5	6	7	8	9	10
58.	Tell myself that I can do it.	1	2	3	4	5	6	7	8	9	10
59.	Think about others in my family.	1	2	3	4	5	6	7	8	9	10
60.	Concentrate on getting through one contraction at a time.	1	2	3	4	5	6	7	8	9	10
61.	Focus on the person helping me in labor.	1	2	3	4	5	6	7	8	9	10
62.	Listen to encouragement from the person helping me.	1	2	3	4	5	6	7	8	9	10

Scoring Instructions. The CBSEI is a self-report measure of outcome expectancy and self-efficacy expectancy for labor and birth. In the framework of self-efficacy theory (Bandura, 1982), *outcome expectancy* for labor and birth is defined as the belief that a given behavior will enhance coping with labor, while *self-efficacy expectancy* is a personal conviction that one can successfully perform specific behaviors during labor. This distinction is important because a woman may believe that a certain behavior could help a woman cope with labor, but feel incapable of personally performing the behavior during her own labor.

Part I of the CBSEI measures outcome expectancy and self-efficacy expectancy for active labor, while Part II measures the same constructs for second stage or birth. Scale scores are computed by summing the item responses as follows:

Outcome Expectancy Active Labor (Outcome-AL) : items 1 through 15

Self-Efficacy Expectancy Active Labor (Efficacy-AL) : items 16 through 30

Outcome Expectancy Second Stage (Outcome-SS) : items 31 through 46

Self-Efficacy Expectancy Second Stage (Efficacy-SS) : items 47 through 62

A Total Childbirth Outcome Expectancy Score (Outcome-Total) is computed by summing the Outcome-AL and Outcome-SS scale scores. A Total Self-Efficacy Expectancy Score (Efficacy-Total) is computed by summing the Efficacy-AL and Efficacy-SS scale scores.

55. Knowledge of Maternal Phenylketonuria Test

Developed by Shoshana Shiloh, Paula St. James, and Susan Waisbren

INSTRUMENT DESCRIPTION, ADMINISTRATION, AND SCORING GUIDELINES

Routine newborn screening for phenylketonuria (PKU), which identifies affected infants early enough for dietary treatment to be effective, has essentially eliminated mental retardation as a consequence of PKU in developed parts of the world. Many girls treated early with PKU are now reaching childbearing age. These women are at high risk for bearing children who have mental retardation, microcephaly, congenital heart disease, and low birth weight as a consequence of the maternal disorder, which can occur regardless of whether the child does or does not have PKU Dietary treatment during pregnancy offers at least partial protection to the developing fetus if initiated before conception. Because most young women with PKU returned to a normal diet during middle childhood, prevention of the effects of maternal PKU requires reinstitution of the difficult low-phenylalanine diet, along with careful planning of pregnancies so that the diet begins before conception (Shiloh, St. James, & Waisbren, 1990). The results of some tracking efforts indicate that women with PKU usually seek treatment after they are pregnant rather than before (Waisbren, Shiloh, St. James, & Levy, 1991).

Educational and counseling programs aimed at this problem have been conducted at several centers including Children's Hospital in Boston. In this program, group meetings include a review of PKU and definition of the maternal PKU syndrome and risk figures, and planning about reproductive health care. The Knowledge of Maternal Phenylketonuria instrument was developed to assess patients' knowledge and identify misconceptions, and to evaluate and compare educational programs. One point for each correct score is summed for a total score, with a potential range of 0 to 10. The test is written at a lower than 6th-grade reading level and can usually be completed in 5 minutes. Knowledge is reasonably presumed to be necessary but insufficient for the implicit goal of adherence to the regimen described previously (Shiloh, St. James, & Waisbren, 1990).

PSYCHOMETRIC PROPERTIES

Development and initial testing of the instrument was accomplished with 49 young hyperphenylalanimemic female patients in New England, with a mean education of 12 years. The test was developed to cover content areas of risk of maternal PKU, pregnancy planning, and dietary treatment. Initial questions from an earlier version that were answered correctly by all who took the test were excluded, and unclear questions were rephrased. Cronbach's alpha was .62, affected by the length of test, which restricts the validity upper limit. As evidence of validity, the authors show a moderate but statistically significant (.40) correlation with IQ scores. In addition, scores on the instrument were significantly different between patients who participated in educational sessions and those who did not. Mean test score was 7.1, with a standard deviation of 2.11. Scores for individual items may be found in Shiloh, St. James, and Waisbren (1990).

Other studies that have compared behaviors of young women with PKU, those with diabetes (who also have childbearing risks and needs for medical intervention prior and during pregnancy), and a comparison group showed that knowledge of maternal PKU was not significantly related to frequency of contraceptive use (Waisbren, Shiloh, St. James, & Levy, 1991; Waisbren, Hamilton, St. James, Shiloh, & Levy, 1995). A comparison study with Israeli women with PKU found that although the American group was more knowledge-able about both contraception and maternal PKU, it also had more unplanned pregnancies (Shiloh, Waisbren, Cohen, St. James, & Levy, 1993).

More recently, Antisdel and Chrisler (2000) used this instrument to study eating attitudes and behaviors of campers and staff in a camp specializing in care of young women with diabetes and PKU and found that knowledge did not differentiate those with and without aberrant eating behavior.

CRITIQUE AND SUMMARY

The Knowledge of Maternal PKU test is one of a battery of tests being used to study this clinical problem including tests of knowledge about family planning, social support for family planning, and attitudes and beliefs about contraception, sex, and childbearing (Wais-bren, Shiloh, St. James, & Levy, 1991). From a theoretical viewpoint, it is unlikely that a test of this kind will, by itself, show a strong relationship to contraceptive use. Intervention programs aimed at conscious reproductive planning would likely be peer oriented and include social support in facing issues of sexuality and contraception (Waisbren, Hamilton, St. James, Shiloh, & Levy, 1995). More explicit domain validation would be helpful to establish that the domains and items contained in the test represent those most likely to be important to what should be an explicit goal of informed patient decision making. This goal is more justifiable than is compliance with a medical regimen.

REFERENCES

Antisdel, J. E., & Chrisler, J. C. (2000). Comparison of eating attitudes and behaviors among adolescent and young women with type 1 diabetes and phenylketonuria. *Developmental & Behavioral Pediatrics, 21,* 81–86.

Shiloh, S., St. James, P., & Waisbren, S. (1990). The development of a patient knowledge test on maternal phenylketonuria. *Patient Education and Counseling, 16,* 139–146.

Shiloh, S., Waisbren, S. E., Cohen, B. E., St. James, P., & Levy, H. L. (1993). Cross-cultural perspectives on coping with the risks of maternal phenylketonuria. *Psychology and Health, 8,* 435–446.

Waisbren, S. E., Hamilton, B. D., St. James, P. J., Shiloh, S., & Levy, H. L. (1995). Psychosocial factors in maternal phenylketonuria: Women's adherence to medical recom-mendations. *American Journal of Public Health, 85,* 1636–1641.

Waisbren, S. E., Shiloh, S., St. James, P., & Levy, H. L. (1991). Psychosocial factors in maternal phenylketonuria: Prevention of unplanned pregnancies. *American Journal of Public Health, 81,* 299–304.

KNOWLEDGE OF MATERNAL PKU®

Please circle the best answer.

1.   PKU is _____.

     A.   a blood disease
     Ⓑ.   an enzyme deficiency
     C.   a kidney disorder
     D.   a protein deficiency
     E.   an iron deficiency

2.   Mental retardation in babies born to mothers with PKU is most likely caused by _____.

     A.   an enzyme deficiency in the baby
     B.   PKU in the baby
     Ⓒ.   high blood phenylalanine in the mother during pregnancy
     D.   the father carrying a gene for PKU
     E.   too little protein in the mother's diet during pregnancy

3.   The best known treatment for maternal PKU to prevent damage to the baby is _____.

     A.   following a well-balanced diet
     B.   following a vegetarian diet
     C.   following a high-protein diet during pregnancy
     D.   following a low-phenylalanine diet after a positive pregnancy test
     Ⓔ.   following a low-phenylalanine diet before conception and throughout pregnancy

4.   In addition to mental retardation, other problems that have been seen in babies born to mothers with PKU include _____.

     A.   low birth weight
     B.   heart problems
     C.   small head size
     Ⓓ.   all of the above
     E.   none of the above

5.   Twenty mg/dl is considered a high blood phenylalanine level. On a low phenylalanine diet during pregnancy, blood phenylalanine levels should be controlled to what level?

     A.   less than 1 mg/dl
     Ⓑ.   2–6 mg/dl
     C.   6–8 mg/dl
     D.   10–15 mg/dl
     E.   16–20 mg/dl

6.   Which of the following snacks has the least amount of phenylalanine?

     A.   chocolate chip cookies

(B). apple
C.   hamburger
D.   potato chips
E.   bagel with jelly

7. Children born to mothers with PKU _____.

   A.   never have PKU
   B.   have a 1 in 1,000 chance of having PKU
   C.   have a 1 in 100 chance of having PKU if the father carries the gene for PKU
   (D). have a 50–50 chance of having PKU if the father carries the gene for PKU
   E.   will always have PKU

8. The problems that have been seen in babies born from untreated pregnancies in mothers with PKU _____.

   A.   are entirely reversible
   B.   can all be corrected with surgery
   C.   can be corrected by treating the baby with a low phenylalanine diet
   (D). generally result in the child having mental retardation, learning difficulties, birth defects, and the need for special services
   E.   go away as the child grows older

9. After a child is born to a mother with PKU it is important _____.
   A.   to place the child on a high-protein diet
   (B). to perform newborn screening for PKU with special care and consideration so that if the child has PKU, he or she can begin dietary treatment
   C.   to hold off on newborn screening for PKU for a month since the baby has had enough stress
   D.   for the mother to be on a high-protein diet
   E.   to immediately place the child on a low-protein diet

10. The best advice to give a young woman with PKU who thinks she might be pregnant is to _____.

    A.   wait and see if it's true
    B.   wait but stop eating meat in the meantime
    C.   wait but start birth control
    (D). immediately contact the PKU Clinic for guidance
    E.   contact her friends for guidance

The score is the total number of correct responses (circled). Range of scores is 0 to 10.

Reprinted from Shiloh, S., St. James, P., & Waisbren, W. *The Development of a Patient Knowledge Test on Maternal Phenylketonuria,* Volume 16, 1990, pp. 139–146. With kind permission to reproduce Appendix I: Knowledge of Maternal PKU® from Elsevier Science Ireland Ltd, Bay 15K, Shannon Industrial Estate, Co. Clare, Ireland.

56. Parent Expectations Survey

Developed by Susan McClennan Reece

INSTRUMENT DESCRIPTION, ADMINISTRATION, AND SCORING GUIDELINES

Reece (1992) describes preliminary development of the Parent Expectations Survey (PES) to measure self-efficacy in early parenting. Self-efficacy (SE) in parenting is defined as the confidence a new mother has in her ability to meet the demands and responsibilities of parenthood. For the new mother, perceptions of SE in parenting stem from her own past experiences in caring for infants; her observations of other new mothers viewed as similar to herself; encouragement from others; and environmental feedback, such as that received from the baby or family. With these sources of information, the mother develops her own judgments as to whether she is capable of carrying out a certain level of performance in the care of her infant. Clinical usefulness of the PES is believed to be in identification of those women at risk for increased stress in the role of new parent because of a low level of SE (Reece, 1992).

The PES takes about 10 minutes to complete and is scored by summing individual items and dividing by the total number of items (20) to determine the mean PES score (Reece, 1992).

PSYCHOMETRIC PROPERTIES

Items were generated from the literature and clinical experience of the author and colleagues. Seven nurse and other experts in the field of SE and instrument development judged content validity. Appropriateness of the items for measuring tasks of mothering were validated by requesting feedback on the scale from four pediatric/family nurse practitioners.

The PES was then completed by 82 first-time mothers between the ages of 35 and 42 years. Most were college educated and had attended graduate school and were recruited from childbirth education programs; 45% had a cesarean section (Reece, 1992). PES scores at 1 and 3 months postpartum showed moderate correlations with the Self-Evaluation subscale of the "What Being the Parent of a Baby is Like" questionnaire (.40 to .75). Self-efficacy at 1 month ($r = .28$) and at 3 months ($r = .40$) postpartum was associated with greater maternal confidence in parenting 1 year after delivery. PES scores at 3 months postpartum had a negative association ($r = .28$) with perceived stress at 1 year. These results imply that women with higher self-efficacy early in the transition to parenthood have increased confidence in parenting and less stress 1 year after delivery. All of these results are supportive of validity.

The alpha coefficient for the PES administered at 1 month postpartum was .91 and at 3 months .86. Because of the theoretical expectation that self-efficacy in parenting would change over time, test–retest reliability was not calculated (Reece, 1992). Scores on the PES from as yet unpublished research were: mean = 7.83 and $SD = 1.08$ for mothers in the last trimester; mean = 7.63 and *SD* = .97 for fathers in the last trimester; mean = 8.77 and *SD* = .71 for mothers 4 months after delivery; and mean = 8.06 and *SD* = 1.01 for fathers 4 months after delivery (S. M. Reece, personal communication, 1996). A more recent study (Roberts, Paynter, & McEwen, 2000) found interventions of conventional cuddling and kangaroo mother care were associated with high PES scores. In addition, they found that the neonatal intensive care unit experience was not related to PES scores.

CRITIQUE AND SUMMARY

The PES is in preliminary stages of development and has only been tested with a group of mothers with a limited range of demographic characteristics. Correspondence with the author indicates that the PES is undergoing active revision to include interactive behaviors of the parent and infant, and affective tasks of early parenthood. PES might be used by clinicians during the perinatal period to ascertain a mother's early perceptions of self-efficacy in parenting. For those found to be low, a number of self-efficacy developing interventions could reasonably be expected to be effective including use of parenting support groups, verbal persuasion, and others (Reece, 1992). Content validity for the PES might be checked with parents as well as with practitioners. Additional studies of validity will be necessary.

REFERENCES

Reece, S. M. (1992). The Parent Expectations Survey. *Clinical Nursing Research, 1,* 336–346.

Roberts, K. L., Paynter, C., & McEwan, B. (2000). A comparison of kangaroo mother care and conventional cuddling care. *Neonatal Network, 19*(4), 31–35.

PARENT EXPECTATIONS SURVEY

The following statements describe what some parents-to-be believe about their abilities to take care of their infants. After reading each statement, please circle which number that *you* feel most closely describes how you feel about *yourself* in relation to parenting. Because these are statements about beliefs, there are no right or wrong answers. Please answer each of the 25 questions below.

1. I will be able to manage the feeding of my baby.

Cannot Do   Moderately Certain Can Do   Certain Can Do
0   1   2   3   4   5   6   7   8   9   10

2. I will be able to manage the responsibility of my baby.

Cannot Do   Moderately Certain Can Do   Certain Can Do
0   1   2   3   4   5   6   7   8   9   10

3. I will always be able to tell when my baby is hungry.

Cannot Do   Moderately Certain Can Do   Certain Can Do
0   1   2   3   4   5   6   7   8   9   10

4. I will be able to deal effectively with the baby when h/she cries for "no reason."

Cannot Do   Moderately Certain Can Do   Certain Can Do
0   1   2   3   4   5   6   7   8   9   10

5. I will be able to tell when my baby is sick.

Cannot Do   Moderately Certain Can Do   Certain Can Do
0   1   2   3   4   5   6   7   8   9   10

6. I will be able to tell when to add different food items to my baby's diet.

Cannot Do   Moderately Certain Can Do   Certain Can Do
0   1   2   3   4   5   6   7   8   9   10

7. I will be able to manage my household as well as before, meanwhile caring for the baby.

Cannot Do   Moderately Certain Can Do   Certain Can Do
0   1   2   3   4   5   6   7   8   9   10

8. When I think the baby is sick, I will be able to take his/her temperature accurately.

Cannot Do   Moderately Certain Can Do   Certain Can Do
0   1   2   3   4   5   6   7   8   9   10

9. I will be able to give my baby a bath without him/her getting cold or upset.

Cannot Do   Moderately Certain Can Do   Certain Can Do
0   1   2   3   4   5   6   7   8   9   10

10. I will work out my concerns about working or not working once the baby arrives.

Cannot Do				Moderately Certain Can Do					Certain Can Do	
0	1	2	3	4	5	6	7	8	9	10

11. I will be able to keep my baby from crying.

Cannot Do				Moderately Certain Can Do					Certain Can Do	
0	1	2	3	4	5	6	7	8	9	10

12. I will be able to maintain my relationship with my partner during this next year.

Cannot Do				Moderately Certain Can Do					Certain Can Do	
0	1	2	3	4	5	6	7	8	9	10

13. I will be able to meet all the demands placed on me once the baby is here.

Cannot Do				Moderately Certain Can Do					Certain Can Do	
0	1	2	3	4	5	6	7	8	9	10

14. I will easily be able to get the baby and myself out for a doctor appointment.

Cannot Do				Moderately Certain Can Do					Certain Can Do	
0	1	2	3	4	5	6	7	8	9	10

15. I have good judgment in deciding how to care for the baby.

Cannot Do				Moderately Certain Can Do					Certain Can Do	
0	1	2	3	4	5	6	7	8	9	10

16. I can make the right decisions for my baby.

Cannot Do				Moderately Certain Can Do					Certain Can Do	
0	1	2	3	4	5	6	7	8	9	10

17. I will be able to get the baby on a good nighttime routine.

Cannot Do				Moderately Certain Can Do					Certain Can Do	
0	1	2	3	4	5	6	7	8	9	10

18. I will be able to give the baby the attention h/she needs.

Cannot Do				Moderately Certain Can Do					Certain Can Do	
0	1	2	3	4	5	6	7	8	9	10

19. I will be able to hire a babysitter when I need one.

Cannot Do				Moderately Certain Can Do					Certain Can Do	
0	1	2	3	4	5	6	7	8	9	10

20. I will be able to tell what my baby likes and dislikes.

Cannot Do				Moderately Certain Can Do					Certain Can Do	
0	1	2	3	4	5	6	7	8	9	10

(continued)

21.   I will be able to sense my baby's moods.

Cannot Do				Moderately Certain Can Do					Certain Can Do	
0	1	2	3	4	5	6	7	8	9	10

22.   I will be able to show my love for my baby.

Cannot Do				Moderately Certain Can Do					Certain Can Do	
0	1	2	3	4	5	6	7	8	9	10

23.   I will be able to calm my baby when h/she is upset.

Cannot Do				Moderately Certain Can Do					Certain Can Do	
0	1	2	3	4	5	6	7	8	9	10

24.   I will be able to support my baby during stressful times such as at the doctor's office.

Cannot Do				Moderately Certain Can Do					Certain Can Do	
0	1	2	3	4	5	6	7	8	9	10

25.   I will be able to stimulate my baby by playing with him/her.

Cannot Do				Moderately Certain Can Do					Certain Can Do	
0	1	2	3	4	5	6	7	8	9	10

POSTPARTUM PARENTAL EXPECTATIONS SURVEY

The following statements describe what some new parents believe about their abilities to take care of their infants. After reading each statement, please circle which number that *you* feel most closely describes how you feel about *yourself* in relation to parenting. Because these are statements about beliefs, there are no right or wrong answers. Please answer each of the 25 questions below.

1. I can manage the feeding of my baby.

Cannot Do   Moderately Certain Can Do   Certain Can Do
0   1   2   3   4   5   6   7   8   9   10

2. I can manage the responsibility of my baby.

Cannot Do   Moderately Certain Can Do   Certain Can Do
0   1   2   3   4   5   6   7   8   9   10

3. I can tell when my baby is hungry.

Cannot Do   Moderately Certain Can Do   Certain Can Do
0   1   2   3   4   5   6   7   8   9   10

4. I can deal effectively with the baby when h/she cries for "no reason."

Cannot Do   Moderately Certain Can Do   Certain Can Do
0   1   2   3   4   5   6   7   8   9   10

5. I can tell when my baby is sick.

Cannot Do   Moderately Certain Can Do   Certain Can Do
0   1   2   3   4   5   6   7   8   9   10

6. I can tell when to add different food items to my baby's diet.

Cannot Do   Moderately Certain Can Do   Certain Can Do
0   1   2   3   4   5   6   7   8   9   10

7. I can manage my household as well as before, meanwhile caring for the baby.

Cannot Do   Moderately Certain Can Do   Certain Can Do
0   1   2   3   4   5   6   7   8   9   10

8. When I think the baby is sick, I can take his/her temperature accurately.

Cannot Do   Moderately Certain Can Do   Certain Can Do
0   1   2   3   4   5   6   7   8   9   10

9. I can give my baby a bath without him/her getting cold or upset.

Cannot Do   Moderately Certain Can Do   Certain Can Do
0   1   2   3   4   5   6   7   8   9   10

(continued)

10. I can work out my concerns about working or not working once the baby arrives.

Cannot Do   Moderately Certain Can Do   Certain Can Do
0   1   2   3   4   5   6   7   8   9   10

11. I can keep my baby from crying.

Cannot Do   Moderately Certain Can Do   Certain Can Do
0   1   2   3   4   5   6   7   8   9   10

12. I can maintain my relationship with my partner during this next year.

Cannot Do   Moderately Certain Can Do   Certain Can Do
0   1   2   3   4   5   6   7   8   9   10

13. I can meet all the demands placed on me now that the baby is here.

Cannot Do   Moderately Certain Can Do   Certain Can Do
0   1   2   3   4   5   6   7   8   9   10

14. I can easily get the baby and myself out for a doctor's visit.

Cannot Do   Moderately Certain Can Do   Certain Can Do
0   1   2   3   4   5   6   7   8   9   10

15. I have good judgment in deciding how to care for the baby.

Cannot Do   Moderately Certain Can Do   Certain Can Do
0   1   2   3   4   5   6   7   8   9   10

16. I can make the right decisions for my baby.

Cannot Do   Moderately Certain Can Do   Certain Can Do
0   1   2   3   4   5   6   7   8   9   10

17. I can get the baby on a good nighttime routine.

Cannot Do   Moderately Certain Can Do   Certain Can Do
0   1   2   3   4   5   6   7   8   9   10

18. I can give the baby the attention h/she needs.

Cannot Do   Moderately Certain Can Do   Certain Can Do
0   1   2   3   4   5   6   7   8   9   10

19. I can hire a babysitter when I need one.

Cannot Do   Moderately Certain Can Do   Certain Can Do
0   1   2   3   4   5   6   7   8   9   10

20. I can tell what my baby likes and dislikes.

Cannot Do   Moderately Certain Can Do   Certain Can Do
0   1   2   3   4   5   6   7   8   9   10

21. I can sense my baby's moods.

Cannot Do				Moderately Certain Can Do					Certain Can Do	
0	1	2	3	4	5	6	7	8	9	10

22. I can show my love for my baby.

Cannot Do				Moderately Certain Can Do					Certain Can Do	
0	1	2	3	4	5	6	7	8	9	10

23. I can calm my baby when h/she is upset.

Cannot Do				Moderately Certain Can Do					Certain Can Do	
0	1	2	3	4	5	6	7	8	9	10

24. I can support my baby during stressful times such as at the doctor's office.

Cannot Do				Moderately Certain Can Do					Certain Can Do	
0	1	2	3	4	5	6	7	8	9	10

25. I can stimulate my baby by playing with him/her.

Cannot Do				Moderately Certain Can Do					Certain Can Do	
0	1	2	3	4	5	6	7	8	9	10

57.   Infant Care Survey

Developed by Robin D. Froman and Steven V. Owen

INSTRUMENT DESCRIPTION, ADMINISTRATION, AND SCORING GUIDELINES

The Infant Care Survey (ICS) was developed to assess mothers' self-efficacy in caring for babies under 1 year of age. Social learning theory forms the framework for this work, with self-efficacy defined as a person's belief that he can successfully accomplish some particular behavior. A new mother may understand a behavior, but not attempt it because she has little confidence in her ability or expects failure. Responses on the ICS from A (very little confidence = 1) to E (quite a lot of confidence = 5) are summed into an average total score, with ranges from 1 to 5 (Froman & Owen, 1989).

PSYCHOMETRIC PROPERTIES

An initial pool of 48 statements that represent usual and important infant care behaviors was written and reviewed by nursing faculty members, visiting nurses, and hospital-based maternity nurses to assess relevance of each task to infant care, adequacy of domain sampling, and readability of the items. Items were grouped into those requiring knowledge or skill to foster feelings of efficacy and partitioned into content subgroups of health, diet, and safety behaviors. Data were collected in hospital regular and high-risk obstetrical units, home visits to new mothers, clinical nursing sites, and college classrooms among White, Hispanic, and Black groups, to provide response variation ($N = 142$) (Froman & Owen, 1989).

Alpha internal consistency estimate for the total scale was .98, and for the subgroups of knowledge and skill items .94 and .96, respectively. In a more recent study, alpha reliability was .92 for the knowledge subscale, .91 for the skills subscale, and .96 for the total scale (Ruchala & James, 1997), and .95 for both mothers and fathers (Hudson, Elek, & Fleck, 2001). Factor analysis showed a single major construct: infant care self-efficacy with modest empirical support for the groupings of items into logical subdomains. Construct validity was supported by findings that would be predicted by self-efficacy theory—behaviors commonly performed successfully or observed showed the highest means, such as holding a baby (average score = 4.46), changing diapers (average score = 4.40), and those behaviors difficult to master showed the lowest, such as relieving gas pains (average score = 2.82) or treating diarrhea (average score = 2.92). The fact that being female, and age and number of children, was predictive of ICS scores also is congruent with self-efficacy theory because these groups have more opportunity to perform infant care success-fully (Froman & Owen, 1989).

A second study of a convenience sample of 200 new mothers and the nurses caring for them addressed not only variables related to mothers' sense of infant care self-efficacy as indicated by scores on the ICS, but also differences between the mothers' reports and nurses' ratings of mothers' skills at those tasks. Factor analysis and measure of internal consistency were consistent with the first study as was the relationship with number of children and age. Other more specific relationships between demographic variables and self-efficacy for various parenting tasks measured in the ICS may be found in Froman and Owen (1990).

Trends between health of the child and self-efficacy ratings suggested that mothers of special care neonates do not share the same sense of confidence for infant care activities that mothers of healthy infants enjoy. The implication of this finding is that extra time and special effort should be spent to build these mothers' self-confidence even beyond demonstration of adequate skill in the care of these infants. In this sample, there is little evidence that nurses' estimates of mothers' proficiency explain perceptions beyond established demographic factors. This means that nurses should not base decisions about how much teaching mothers need on demonstrated skill alone (Froman & Owen, 1990).

Ruchala and James (1997) found a strong relationship between knowledge of infant development and scores on the ICS, especially for adolescents who had less information than did adult mothers. The authors believed that adolescents might need more information about infant development to increase their confidence in caring for new infants. In studying first-time mothers' and fathers' transitions to parenthood, Hudson, Elek, and Fleck (2001) found ICS scores significantly related to parenting change scores, as would be predicted by SE theory.

CRITIQUE AND SUMMARY

ICS incorporates both knowledge and confidence in the ability to perform a task, both of which are necessary for real-world performance. Teaching should focus on including the multiple ways in which self-efficacy can be developed (actual successful experience, modeling, and persuasion). Because providing such potent learning experiences may require special effort in most health care settings, the ICS can be used to evaluate how well current teaching efforts are doing to yield high self-efficacy.

The predictive worth of ICS needs to be documented (Froman & Owen, 1989), and further study is needed to show whether specific efficacy-building attempts by nurses are associated with changes in maternal self-beliefs (Froman & Owen, 1990). In response to the first study, Barnard (1989) suggests addition of a new domain called Communication Skills: talking to your baby, expressing love and affection, sensing the baby's moods, helping the baby modulate state, communicating security to the baby, recognizing distress cues, and responding contingently to the baby constitute an important part of social and emotional infant care. She also notes that future samples should include parents of preterm infants, adolescent mothers, and adoptive parents. The second study addresses the health of the infant.

Although mean self-ratings were found to be high, there was also wide variation in efficacy perceptions among mothers and across tasks. Routine use of the ICS before discharge may help to identify those mothers who seem skilled but suffer from low-efficacy expectations and offer diagnostic advice to help individualize maternity education. It may also be used to assess those at risk and those needing to be drawn into the health care system (Froman & Owen, 1990).

REFERENCES

Barnard, K. (1989). Response to "Infant care self-efficacy." *Scholarly Inquiry for Nursing Practice: An International Journal, 3,* 213–215.

Froman, R. D., & Owen, S. V. (1989). Infant care self-efficacy. *Scholarly Inquiry for Nursing Practice: An International Journal, 3,* 199–211.

Froman, R. D., & Owen, S. V. (1990). Mothers' and nurses' perceptions of infant care skills. *Research in Nursing and Health, 13,* 247–253.

Hudson, D. B., Elek, S. M., & Fleck, M. O. (2001). First-time mothers' and fathers' transition to parenthood. *Issues in Comprehensive Pediatric Nursing, 24,* 31–43.

Ruchala, P. L., & James, D. C. (1997). Social support, knowledge of infant development, and maternal confidence among adolescent and adult mothers. *Journal of Obstetrical, Gynecologic and Neonatal Nursing, 26,* 685–689.

INFANT CARE SURVEY

DIRECTIONS: Your responses are confidential and will help us to improve our services. There are no right or wrong answers. How much confidence do you have about doing each of the behaviors listed below?

A	B	C	D	E
Quite a lot	←-- -- -- -- -- -- -- -- -- -- -- -- -- -- -- -- -- -- --→			Very little
	C O N F I D E N C E			

quite a lot			very little			Health Knowledge
A	B	C	D	E	1.	Knowing immunization schedules.
A	B	C	D	E	2.	Knowing schedule for physical exam.
A	B	C	D	E	3.	Recognizing signs of an ear infection.
A	B	C	D	E	4.	Identifying diaper rash.
A	B	C	D	E	5.	Knowing when to get help from the clinic, emergency room, or doctor.
A	B	C	D	E	6.	Recognizing teething.
A	B	C	D	E	7.	Knowing regular breathing sounds of babies.
A	B	C	D	E	8.	Describing the tonic neck reflex.
A	B	C	D	E	9.	Recognizing congestion.
A	B	C	D	E	10.	Recognizing an allergic response.
A	B	C	D	E	11.	Recognizing croup.
A	B	C	D	E	12.	Knowing expected weight gain patterns for an infant.
A	B	C	D	E	13.	Recognizing constipation.
A	B	C	D	E	14.	Recognizing diarrhea.
A	B	C	D	E	15.	Recognizing gas pains.
A	B	C	D	E	16.	Knowing normal growth and development patterns.

quite a lot			very little			Diet Knowledge
A	B	C	D	E	17.	Knowing how much to feed your baby.
A	B	C	D	E	18.	Selecting the best formula.
A	B	C	D	E	19.	Selecting baby foods.
A	B	C	D	E	20.	Planning a balanced diet for your baby.
A	B	C	D	E	21.	Knowing how to use a baby bottle.

(continued)

quite a lot				very little		Safety Knowledge
A	B	C	D	E	22.	Identifying safety hazards in the house.
A	B	C	D	E	23.	Choosing safe baby toys.
A	B	C	D	E	24.	Choosing safe baby furniture.
A	B	C	D	E	25.	Choosing safe baby clothes.
A	B	C	D	E	26.	Knowing which medications are dangerous.
A	B	C	D	E	27.	Knowing safe positions for a baby after feeding.
A	B	C	D	E	28.	Knowing what articles are safe to leave with your baby in the crib or baby seat.

quite a lot				very little		Health Skills
A	B	C	D	E	29.	Treating a diaper rash.
A	B	C	D	E	30.	Burping your baby.
A	B	C	D	E	31.	Weighing your baby.
A	B	C	D	E	32.	Taking your baby's temperature.
A	B	C	D	E	33.	Changing a diaper.
A	B	C	D	E	34.	Relieving pain from teething.
A	B	C	D	E	35.	Relieving congestion.
A	B	C	D	E	36.	Giving your baby a liquid medication.
A	B	C	D	E	37.	Relieving croup.
A	B	C	D	E	38.	Treating constipation.
A	B	C	D	E	39.	Treating diarrhea.
A	B	C	D	E	40.	Relieving gas pains.
A	B	C	D	E	41.	Establishing a sensible sleeping schedule.
A	B	C	D	E	42.	Soothing your crying baby.

quite a lot				very little		Diet Skills
A	B	C	D	E	43.	Breast or bottle feeding your baby (circle whichever way your baby is fed).
A	B	C	D	E	44.	Spoon feeding your baby.

quite a lot				very little		Diet Skills
A	B	C	D	E	45.	Preparing baby food.
A	B	C	D	E	46.	Introducing new food into baby's diet.
A	B	C	D	E	47.	Establishing a sensible feeding schedule.

quite a lot				very little		Safety Skills
A	B	C	D	E	48.	Holding your baby.
A	B	C	D	E	49.	Bathing your baby.
A	B	C	D	E	50.	Using a car seat.
A	B	C	D	E	51.	Walking while holding your baby.
A	B	C	D	E	52.	Playing with your baby.

58.   Toddler Care Questionnaire

Developed by Deborah Gross and Lorraine Rocissano

INSTRUMENT DESCRIPTION, ADMINISTRATION, AND SCORING GUIDELINES

The Toddler Care Questionnaire (TCQ) is a measure of maternal confidence specifically for the developmental issues that arise in children between 12 and 36 months of age. Changing behaviors in the developing child require changing behaviors in the parent because skills learned during the first year of life are not necessarily the most relevant skills for the second year of life. Such a measure is important because maternal confidence has been correlated with indices of maternal and child competence including mothers' self-esteem, mental health, adaptation to parenthood, and perception of infant temperament (Conrad, Gross, Fogg, & Ruchala, 1992). TCQ was designed to be used as a research measure and clinical assessment tool (Gross & Tucker, 1994).

Maternal confidence is defined as a mother's perception that she can effectively manage a variety of tasks or situations related to parenting her toddler. The theoretical framework used to guide this program of research is Bandura's theory of self-efficacy. Knowing what is typical behavior for a 2-year-old is not the same as feeling confident that you can manage your 2-year-old's behavior.

The TCQ can be completed in about 5 minutes. Item responses are scored with A to E as 1 to 5; TCQ score is the sum of the items, ranging from 37 to 185, which shows greater maternal confidence. Respondents are also asked to circle those items for which they wish more information, which offers a base for working with mothers. Because completion of the tool requires 5 minutes, it is well suited for use in busy clinical settings (Gross & Rocissano, 1988).

PSYCHOMETRIC PROPERTIES

TCQ was first tested on a convenience sample of 20 and then 50 additional middle-class mothers of toddlers. TCQ has been reviewed for content validity by five experts in the fields of maternal-child nursing, child development, and psychometrics. Each item refers to a specific parenting task or situation that typically arises during toddlerhood; making the item task-specific makes the tool consistent with self-efficacy theory. Multiple estimates of alpha reliability have ranged between .91 and .96. Test–retest reliability over a 4-week interval was .87 (Gross & Rocissano, 1988; Gross, Rocissano, & Roncoli, 1989).

Multiple studies of validity have shown a negative correlation between TCQ scores and maternal depression, a negative relationship with dimensions of difficult toddler temperament, a positive relationship with other measures of maternal confidence, extent of prior childcare experience, maternal effectiveness ratings based on observations of structured mother-toddler interactions (Gross, Conrad, Fogg, Willis, & Garvey, 1993) and with maternal knowledge of child development and parenting, and with extent of prior child-care experience, as would be predicted by self-efficacy theory. Lack of difference in TCQ scores between mothers of a first- versus second-born child could not be supported by SE theory. The combined effects of maternal knowledge and confidence were related to quality of mother-toddler interactions, congruent with SE theory. Mean TCQ scores in this study were 155.5 (SD = 16.5). The TCQ has not been significantly related to scores on the Marlow-Crowne Social Desirability Scale (Conrad, Gross, Fogg, & Ruchala, 1992).

A study of 70 mothers of toddlers who had been full term and 62 whose toddlers had been preterm showed no difference in their TCQ scores, except if the mother reported the preterm child had cerebral palsy, which would present many novel, unpredictable, and stressful experiences for parents. There may be several possible reasons for the lack of difference between the groups perhaps that these preterms were relatively healthy. The TCQ does not adequately detect the issues of concern to mothers of preterms, or these mothers may have received additional support services. Future research on this question should use multiple measures and methods (Gross, Rocissano, & Roncoli, 1989).

Gross, Conrad, Fogg, and Wothke (1994) studied 126 mothers of 1-year-olds and 126 mothers of 2-year-olds three times during a year. Data analyzed with structural equation modeling supported a model whereby (a) the more depressed the mother feels, the more likely she is to rate her toddler's temperament as difficult; (b) the more difficult the child's temperament is perceived to be, the lower the mother's estimates of her parenting self-efficacy; (c) the lower the mother's self-efficacy, the greater her depression; and (d) the more depressed the mother feels at one point in time, the more likely she is to remain depressed 6 months later. The study by Gross and Tucker (1994) compares factors that appear to influence scores on TCQ for mothers and fathers, and finds them to be different.

Gross, Fogg, and Tucker (1995) found the TCQ to be sensitive to interventions, particularly for those who completed a higher portion of the intervention and in comparison with groups who did not have the intervention. The 10-week intervention program systematically taught parents who judged their 2-year-olds to be behaviorally difficult child management techniques such as how to play with and help their children learn, how to use praise and rewards effectively, how to set limits effectively, and how to manage misbehavior. Participants practiced problem solving using videotaped vignettes (vicarious learning), homework assignments (mastery experiences), and verbal persuasion and reinforcement in the group.

The training program led to significant increases in maternal SE, decreases in maternal stress, and improvements in the quality of mother-toddler interactions and perceived improvements in child behavior. Fathers participated less in the program. The authors suggest use of the intervention with a group of children more difficult to parent (Gross, Fogg, & Tucker, 1995). A more recent study (Tucker, Gross, Fogg, Delaney, & Lapporte, 1998) provides a 1-year follow-up for the efficacy of a behavioral parent training intervention for families with two-year-olds. Significant gains in maternal self-efficacy (as measured by TCQ) were maintained. Mothers who received the intervention reported a 31-point increase in mean parenting SE score from preintervention to 1-year postintervention, whereas mothers who did not receive the intervention reported a 15-point decline. This supports sensitivity of the TCQ. These findings did not hold for fathers.

CRITIQUE AND SUMMARY

Although TCQ has been studied with ethnically diverse populations (Gross, Conrad, Fogg, Willis, & Garvey, 1993), all have been middle class and most were married and from an urban health maintenance organization population; in some samples, two thirds were college educated or beyond. The authors suggest additional longitudinal research to explore continuities and discontinuities of maternal confidence across developmental periods, and to examine the consequences for the mother-child relationship (Conrad, Gross, Fogg, & Ruchala, 1992), as well as experimental research to confirm the validity of the model of the longitudinal relationship between maternal self-efficacy, depression, and difficult temperament during toddlerhood (Gross, Conrad, Fogg, & Wothke, 1994).

TCQ has undergone considerable testing. Seven hundred seventy parents have taken the TCQ through the seven studies cited subsequently. Its internal consistency levels are in the range adequate for clinical use as well as for research. Its most obvious use is to focus interventions with mothers who have low levels of confidence in parenting their toddlers.

REFERENCES

Conrad, B., Gross, D., Fogg, L., & Ruchala, P. (1992). Maternal confidence, knowledge, and quality of mother-toddler interactions: A preliminary study. *Infant Mental Health Journal, 13,* 353–361.

Gross, D., Conrad, B., Fogg, L., Willis, L., & Garvey, C. (1993). What does the NCATS measure? *Nursing Research, 42,* 260–265.

Gross, D., Conrad, B., Fogg, L., & Wothke, W. (1994). A longitudinal model of maternal self-efficacy, depression, and difficult temperament during toddlerhood. *Research in Nursing and Health, 17,* 207–215.

Gross, D., Fogg, L., & Tucker, S. (1995). The efficacy of parent training for promoting positive parent-toddler relationships. *Research in Nursing and Health, 18,* 489–499.

Gross, D., & Rocissano, L. (1988). Maternal confidence in toddlerhood: Its measurement for clinical practice and research. *Nurse Practitioner, 13*(3), 19–27.

Gross, D., Rocissano, L., & Roncoli, M. (1989). Maternal confidence during toddlerhood: Comparing preterm and full-term groups. *Research in Nursing and Health, 12,* 1–9.

Gross, D., & Tucker, S. (1994). Parenting confidence during toddlerhood. *Nurse Practitioner, 19*(10), 25–34.

Tucker, S., Gross, D., Fogg, L., Delaney, K., & Lapporte, R. (1998). The long-term efficacy of a behavioral parent training intervention for families with 2-year-olds. *Research in Nursing and Health, 21,* 199–210.

TODDLER CARE QUESTIONNAIRE

Dear Parents,

Please complete the items below. Your responses on the questionnaire are confidential and will help us to improve our services to parents of young children. Circle the appropriate letter to indicate how much confidence you have with the following:

	A	B	C	D	E
Very					Quite
Little		CONFIDENCE			a Lot

A   B   C   D   E   1.   Knowing which toys are appropriate for your child's age.

A   B   C   D   E   2.   Knowing how to encourage your child's language development.

A   B   C   D   E   3.   Knowing about common fears children have at this time.

A   B   C   D   E   4.   Knowing what to do to help your child develop hand coordination (for example, using a spoon, stacking blocks, etc.).

A   B   C   D   E   5.   Knowing how to help your child develop body coordination (for example, walking, climbing, etc.).

A   B   C   D   E   6.   Knowing how to manage toilet training.

A   B   C   D   E   7.   Knowing how feeding patterns change between 12 and 36 months.

A   B   C   D   E   8.   Knowing which situations are likely to upset your child.

A   B   C   D   E   9.   Knowing how to make your home safe for your child.

A   B   C   D   E   10.   Knowing which situations your child is likely to enjoy.

A   B   C   D   E   11.   Predicting how your child will respond to new people and places.

A   B   C   D   E   12.   Knowing your child's daily sleep schedule.

A   B   C   D   E   13.   Knowing what foods your child will and won't eat.

A   B   C   D   E   14.   Predicting whether your child will like a new toy.

A   B   C   D   E   15.   Knowing what your child's different cries mean (for example, tiredness, hunger, pain, fear, boredom, frustration, etc.).

A   B   C   D   E   16.   Knowing how to relieve your child's distress (for example, due to being tired, hungry, in pain, frightened, bored, frustrated, etc.).

A   B   C   D   E   17.   Involving your child in activities you both enjoy.

A   B   C   D   E   18.   Knowing when your child seems to want affection from you.

A   B   C   D   E   19.   Being comfortable in showing affection to your child.

A   B   C   D   E   20.   Getting your child to smile or laugh.

(continued)

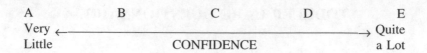

A		B	C	D		E
Very	←				→	Quite
Little			CONFIDENCE			a Lot

A B C D E   21.   Developing your child's interest in new things.

A B C D E   22.   Knowing your child's favorite toys and games.

A B C D E   23.   Knowing how to help your child play with other children.

A B C D E   24.   Helping your child adjust to new situations (for example, a new babysitter, entering daycare, vacationing, etc.).

A B C D E   25.   Setting limits on your child's destructive behaviors (for example, tearing books, breaking valuable items).

A B C D E   26.   Setting limits on your child's behavior when it looks dangerous (for example, playing with matches, electric outlets and wires, etc.).

A B C D E   27.   Knowing what types of discipline do not work with your child.

A B C D E   28.   Knowing what to do when your child has a temper tantrum.

A B C D E   29.   Getting your child to bed without a struggle.

A B C D E   30.   Keeping a consistent bedtime hour for your child.

A B C D E   31.   Knowing when rules can be "bent" or modified and when they should not be.

A B C D E   32.   Getting back to "friendly terms" with your child soon after a problem behavior has ended.

A B C D E   33.   Knowing whether your style of parenting will "spoil" your child.

A B C D E   34.   Managing your child's aggressiveness with other children (for example, hitting, biting, or pushing).

A B C D E   35.   Finding supportive services and people in your community for you and your child (for example, other parents of young children, play groups, daycare services, preschools, etc.).

A B C D E   36.   Knowing how to manage non-emergency illnesses at home (for example, fever, diarrhea, minor injuries).

A B C D E   37.   Managing separations from your child (for example, to go to the store, to go to work, to go out for the evening).

             38.   Now go back and circle the numbers of any item you would like to know more about.

Thank you.

59. Preschool Health and Safety Knowledge Assessment

Developed by Caryl Erhardt Mobley

INSTRUMENT DESCRIPTION, ADMINISTRATION, AND SCORING GUIDELINES

Injury accidents, which are the leading cause of death for children over 1 year of age, are often preventable. The Preschool Health and Safety Knowledge Assessment (PHASKA) assesses the health and safety knowledge of children 3 to 6 years of age, using a picture format so as not to be limited by the child's verbal ability.

PHASKA consists of 53 picture cards. The first three are used to establish the child's ability to point appropriately. The following 50 cards show pictures of children and adults in various situations and assess the preschooler's ability to differentiate those behaviors that promote or represent health and safety and those that do not. Cards cover safety (31 items), nutrition (6 items), general hygiene measures (5 items), and health recognition and promotion (8 items). Each card contains two or three pictures—one to set up the situation and the other two representing the choices. The preschooler is asked to point to the picture. Figure 59.1 depicts a sample item, and a manual detailing administration language and procedures has been developed. Reproduction is computerized and available in English or Spanish (Mobley, 1996).

A score is derived from the number of correct answers from the last fifty items; a mean score of 37 was obtained in the group tested. Mean scores by age may be found in Mobley and Evashevski (2000).

PSYCHOMETRIC PROPERTIES

Content was derived from a review of preschool educational materials on health and safety and from the advice of child development and early childhood education specialists. Cronbach's alpha on the last fifty items was .51, lower than acceptable for group-level comparisons, perhaps because preschool children vary in age and across categories of knowledge. Test–retest reliability in two hours was .88. Reliability across individuals administering PHKA also must be established with ninety percent or better to be considered acceptable.

Children from a variety of socioeconomic and ethnic groups have been tested, although they were from a convenience sample in one metropolitan area. Groups of older children had higher mean scores (Mobley, 1996), supportive of PHASKA's validity.

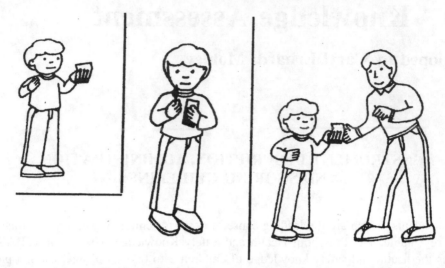

FIGURE 59.1   Sample item from the Preschool Health and Safety Knowledge Assessment.

From: Mobley, C. E., & Evashevski, J. (2000). Evaluating health and safety knowledge of preschoolers: Assessing their early start to being health smart. *Journal of Pediatric Health Care, 14,* 160–165. Used with permission.

CRITIQUE AND SUMMARY

Preschool years are an important time to incorporate health-promoting behaviors into children's lifestyles. Internal consistency reliability should continue to be studied. Since children of this age are limited in their ability to transfer knowledge from one situation to another, the relationship between PHASKA scores and health and accident risk factors should be studied.

REFERENCES

Mobley, C. E. (1996). Assessment of health knowledge in preschoolers. *Children's Health Care, 25,* 11–18.

Mobley, C. E., & Evashevski, J. (2000). Evaluating health and safety knowledge of preschoolers: Assessing their early start to being health smart. *Journal of Pediatric Health Care, 14,* 160–165.

60. Parent Report of Psychosocial Care Scale and Child Report of Psychosocial Care Scale

Developed by Joan Austin, David Dunn, Gertrude Huster, and Douglas Rose

INSTRUMENT DESCRIPTION, ADMINISTRATION, AND SCORING GUIDELINES

Each year 150,000 youths are evaluated for a new onset seizure condition. These parents and children have many fears and little knowledge and need to become competent at dealing with this new health threat. What research there is on this issue shows that parents' fears are frequently based on incomplete or inaccurate information and that negative attitudes on the part of children are related to poor self-concept. Because professionals may not understand these concerns very well, the authors suggest that psychosocial care needs be objectively assessed on a regular basis in the clinical setting (Austin, Dunn, Huster, & Rose, 1998). These scales are designed to measure: (a) satisfaction with care received, (b) perceptions of unmet needs for care, and (c) concerns and fears related to new-onset seizures.

PSYCHOMETRIC PROPERTIES

Interviews of parents in the first four months following their child's first seizure showed concerns about the effect of seizures on the brain, the child's mental health and future life, and on management of the epilepsy. The scales were reviewed by clinical nurse specialists expert in pediatric epilepsy for content validity. The child scale was used with children 8–14 years of age. Alpha reliabilities for the parent scales ranged between .83 and .94 and for the children's scales .71–.87. Construct validity was supported by correlation in the direction predicted with established instruments measuring parent stigma and mood and children's attitude toward illness (Austin, Dunn, Huster, & Rose, 1998).

CRITIQUE AND SUMMARY

In the setting in which it was tested, the Child Report showed the most unmet need to be the need for information about important aspects of managing the seizure condition (McNelis, Musick, Austin, Dunn, & Creasy, 1998). Parents were least satisfied with information about handling seizures at school. The pattern of findings in studies to date suggests that the need for information and support should be assessed at every encounter during the first six months after the child's first seizure, and that using these instruments may help identify needs that parents may be unable to verbalize on their own (Shore et al., 1998).

Evidence of the instruments' sensitivity to intervention could not be located. Beginning work on reliability and validity should be supplemented in general and in more diverse populations.

REFERENCES

Austin, J., Dunn, D., Huster, G., & Rose, D. (1998). Development of scales to measure psychosocial care needs of children with seizures and their parents. *Journal of Neuroscience Nursing, 30,* 155–160.

McNelis, A., Musick, B., Austin, J., Dunn, D., & Creasy, K. (1998). Psychosocial care needs of children with new-onset seizures. *Journal of Neuroscience Nursing, 30,* 161–165.

Shore, C., Austin, J., Musick, B., Dunn, D., McBride, A., & Creasy, K. (1998). Psychosocial care needs of parents of children with new-onset seizures. *Journal of Neuroscience Nursing, 30,* 169–174.

PARENT REPORT OF PSYCHOSOCIAL CARE

I want to remind you that your answers are confidential and stay between you and me. I will not be sharing your answers with the doctors or the nurses, so please answer honestly. I am now going to read to you a list of statements about your interactions with the doctors and nurses. Each time, I want you to pick the response that most fits your experience:

1 = Strongly Disagree
2 = Disagree
3 = Neither Agree Nor Disagree
4 = Agree
5 = Strongly Agree

Information Received

1. The doctors/nurses clearly explained the seizure condition to me.   1   2   3   4   5

2. The doctors/nurses clearly described how the medicine worked,   1   2   3   4   5
    and possible side effects of the medicine prescribed to _____.

3. The doctors/nurses described any problems from the medicine   1   2   3   4   5
    that I would need to report immediately.

4. The doctors/nurses described how to give the medicine or other   1   2   3   4   5
    treatments to _____

5. The doctors/nurses gave me the opportunity to ask questions   1   2   3   4   5
    about _____'s seizures.

6. The doctors/nurses clearly explained what to do in the event of a   1   2   3   4   5
    future seizure.

7. The doctors/nurses addressed my worries and fears   1   2   3   4   5
    about _____'s seizures.

8. The doctors/nurses explained how to handle the seizure condition   1   2   3   4   5
    at school.

Parental Worries

From our past interviews with parents, we have found parents to worry about all kinds of things, including things that almost never happen. We developed a list of these things that parents worried about, and as I read them to you, I would like for you to tell me how much each worries you now.

Please choose from the following responses:

$$
\begin{array}{rcl}
1 & = & \text{Not At All} \\
2 & = & \text{Not Often} \\
3 & = & \text{Somewhat Often} \\
4 & = & \text{Very Often} \\
5 & = & \text{All of the Time}
\end{array}
$$

9. How often do you worry that _____'s seizure condition . . .
    a. is caused by a brain tumor?   1 2 3 4 5
    b. will cause loss of intelligence?   1 2 3 4 5
    c. will cause brain damage?   1 2 3 4 5
    d. will cause death?   1 2 3 4 5
    e. medicine will cause addiction?   1 2 3 4 5

Unmet Needs for Information or Psychosocial Care

10. Although we will not be giving you information, we are interested in the areas where you desire more information about _____'s seizures, or help in handling the seizures at this time. We want to use this information to develop programs for families in the future. I am going to read some statements to you, and I want you to respond with either:

$$
\begin{array}{rcl}
1 & = & \text{No Need} \\
2 & = & \text{Some Need} \\
3 & = & \text{Strong Need}
\end{array}
$$

_____ a. Information about the seizures.
_____ b. Information about treatment.
_____ c. Information about possible causes of seizures.
_____ d. Information about handling future seizures.
_____ e. Information about any activity restrictions.
_____ f. Information about protection from injury.
_____ g. Need for encouragement and support.
_____ h. Need for help in handling responses of others (school, friends, child's peers).
_____ i. Need to discuss worries about _____'s future.
_____ j. Need to discuss fears about _____'s seizures.
_____ k. Need to discuss worries about _____'s mental health.
_____ l. Need for help with handling _____'s response to seizures.
_____ m. Need for _____ to discuss worries and fears about seizures with other children with seizures.
_____ n. Need for _____ to receive counseling about seizures.

CHILD REPORT OF PSYCHOSOCIAL CARE

I want to remind you that your answers are confidential and stay between you and me. I will not be sharing your answers with your doctors or nurses, so please answer honestly. I am now going to ask you some questions about talking with the doctors and nurses about your seizure condition.

For each question I want you to choose the best answer from this list of three answers:

> 1 = Not very much
> 2 = Some
> 3 = A lot

1. How much do the doctors and nurses explain your seizure condition to you?   1   2   3

2. How much do the doctors and nurses tell you about how your medicine works?   1   2   3

3. How much do the doctors and nurses tell you about possible problems or side effects with your medicine?   1   2   3

4. How much do the doctors and nurses tell you about things that you can and cannot do because of your seizure condition?   1   2   3

5. How much of a chance do you get to ask your doctor or nurse questions about your seizure condition?   1   2   3

6. How much do the doctors and nurses talk to you about your fears and worries about your seizure condition?   1   2   3

7. How much do the doctors and nurses tell you about how to handle your seizure condition at school?   1   2   3

Child Worries

The next set of questions ask about things that might worry you about having a seizure condition. Each time I will ask you to tell me how often you worry, using the following responses:

> 1 = Never
> 2 = Not Often
> 3 = Sometimes
> 4 = Often
> 5 = Very Often

8. How often do you worry about what causes your seizure condition?   1   2   3   4   5

9. How often do you worry about having a seizure in front of your friends?   1   2   3   4   5

(continued)

10. How often do you worry about getting hurt while having a   1   2   3   4   5
    seizure?

11. How often do you worry about your friends knowing that you   1   2   3   4   5
    have a seizure condition?

12. How often do you worry about being alone because you might   1   2   3   4   5
    have a seizure?

13. How often do you worry about being different from other kids   1   2   3   4   5
    because of the seizure condition?

14. How often do you worry that having a seizure condition might   1   2   3   4   5
    damage the way you think?

15. How often do you worry that you might get sicker?   1   2   3   4   5

16. How often do you worry that you will not be able to do some   1   2   3   4   5
    things you would like to do because of the seizure condition?

17. How often do you worry about people teasing you because of the   1   2   3   4   5
    seizure condition?

18. How often do you worry about your parents getting upset about   1   2   3   4   5
    the seizure condition?

19. How often do you worry about having to get blood tests because   1   2   3   4   5
    of your seizure condition?

20. How often do you worry about when you will have another   1   2   3   4   5
    seizure?

Need for Information or Help

Although we will not be giving you information, we are also interested in the areas where you want or need more information or more help with your seizures. Please answer each of these questions with how you feel RIGHT NOW:

$$1 = \text{Not very much}$$
$$2 = \text{Some}$$
$$3 = \text{A lot}$$

1. How much more information do you need about your seizure condition?   1   2   3

2. How much more information do you need about your medication?   1   2   3

3. How much more information do you need about possible causes of your   1   2   3
   seizure condition?

4. How much more information do you need about how to handle future   1   2   3
   seizures?

5. How much more information do you need about any things or activities   1   2   3
   you can or cannot do because of the seizure condition?

6. How much more information do you need about keeping safe during a   1   2   3
   seizure?

7. How much do you need to talk to someone about your feelings about   1   2   3
   having a seizure condition?

8. How much do you need to talk to someone about how to tell your friends about your seizure condition? 1 2 3

9. How much do you need to talk to someone about concerns or fears you have about having a seizure condition? 1 2 3

10. How much do you need to talk to someone about how your seizure condition might affect your future? 1 2 3

11. How much do you need to talk to other kids your age who also have a seizure condition? 1 2 3

12. How much do you need to talk to someone about how to handle seizures at school? 1 2 3

Scoring Instructions for Parent Report of Psychosocial Care

Subscale: Information Received
Items 1–8
Calculate mean score by dividing sum by 8.

Subscale: Parental Worries
Items 9a–9e
Calculate mean score by dividing sum by 5.

Subscale: Unmet Needs for Information
Items 10a–10f
Calculate mean score by dividing sum by 6.

Subscale: Unmet Needs for Support
Items 10g 10n
Calculate mean score by dividing sum by 8.

Scoring for Child Report of Psychosocial Care

Subscale: Information Received
Items 1–7
Calculate mean score by dividing sum by 7.

Subscale: Child Worries
Items 8–20
Calculate mean score by dividing sum by 13.

Subscale: Unmet Needs for Information
Items 1–6
Calculate mean score by dividing by 6.

Subscale: Unmet Needs for Support
Items 7–12
Calculate mean score by dividing sum by 6.

Used with permission of *Journal of Neuroscience Nursing.*

61. Contraceptive Self-Efficacy Scale

Developed by Ruth Andrea Levinson

INSTRUMENT DESCRIPTION, ADMINISTRATION, AND SCORING GUIDELINES

Contraceptive Self-Efficacy (CSE) is not only the name of this tool but also a concept believed to be important for teenagers because their sexual activity and its consequences (including sexually transmitted disease and pregnancy) are so strongly linked to their ability to control their adult lives. CSE is defined as the strength of a teenager's conviction that she should and can exercise control within sexual and contraceptive situations to achieve contraceptive protection.

Items for the CSE Scale are constructed in a hierarchy of task difficulty related to situations with increasing levels of stress. Items were based on literature that distinguishes between successful and unsuccessful contraceptive users and on the author's teaching experience with the target population.

The behavioral situations contained in the items simulate the kinds of conditions in which teenagers have been reported not to use contraceptives. They are drawn from three bodies of research literature: family planning, developmental psychology, and social psychology. They involve obtaining contraceptives, using contraceptives with a partner, talking to a partner about contraceptive use, using contraceptives despite partner or parental disapproval, interrupting an episode of unplanned sex to talk about or use a contraceptive, and preventing episodes of unprotected intercourse. It is expected that young women from different backgrounds (cultures) might feel confident in different areas. Scores on the CSE are obtained by averaging item scores, with higher numbers indicating higher CSE. Items 2, 5, 6, 8, 9, 11, 12, 14, and 15 are reverse scored. The instrument takes 10 minutes to complete (Levinson, 1986).

PSYCHOMETRIC PROPERTIES

Reliability coefficient for the CSE was .73. The CSE has been shown to be sensitive to interventions based on self-efficacy theory, with the goal of influencing teenagers to believe that they should and could influence control in sexual and contraceptive situations and to be contraceptively protected. Interventions used role-playing situations, videocassette episodes, and salient role models with persuasive communications. Several studies have found that an increase in SE contributed significantly to females' contraceptive use. Some adolescents were strongly resistant to instruction or consideration of the consequences of being sexually active (Heinrich, 1993; Levinson, 1984).

CSE has now been used with four diverse samples: suburban lower-middle to middle-class teenage girls who attended a family-planning clinic in Northern California (21%

Hispanic); in a French version with 9th- and 10th-grade male and female high school students in Montreal; in a predominantly White middle-class college sample in the United States; and inner-city, primarily poverty to middle-class African American (94%) teenage women in Chicago. Some of these samples were at high risk for pregnancy because of high frequency of unprotected intercourse and irregular use of contraceptives. Mean score for the college sample was 4.07, 3.79 for less effective user groups, and 4.26 for highly effective user groups. Item means for each of the four populations may be found in Levinson, Jaccard, Wan, and Beamer (1996), and serve as norms for other similar populations.

Although four factors emerged from factor analysis in most of the research, correlations between items have been relatively low, suggesting large amounts of unique variance in them. The factors are conscious acceptance of sexual activity (items 2, 5, 6, 12, 14, and 15); assumption of responsibility for sexual activity and contraception (items 1 and 13a to 13c); assertiveness in preventing sexual intercourse (items 4, 7, and 13d); and strong feelings of sexual arousal (items 3 and 8 to 11) (Heinrich, 1993; Levinson, 1986). At least two of the studies raised questions about which items belong to which factor and which factors are most highly predictive of contraceptive behavior.

CSE items have operated distinctly in the Chicago sample, where only item 3 was significantly correlated with contraceptive behavior. For the California sample, items 8, 10, 11, and 13c were the primary predictors of contraceptive use; for the Montreal group, items 3, 8, and 12 were the most relevant; for the college sample, items 2, 6, and 8 were most relevant. Although the CSE items as a totality were significant predictors of contraceptive behavior in all four samples, there were variations in their predictive power in different samples (Levinson et al., 1996).

CSE operated least powerfully in predicting contraceptive behavior in the Chicago sample, perhaps representing cultural differences in the issues impacting contraceptive behavior. The authors believe that although the total item set be used, the relationship between each item and contraceptive behavior should be analyzed separately because items may offer unique information about what issues are most salient to any given sample. Norms for each item for each sample described previously are available and may be used for comparison for like samples (Levinson, Jaccard, Wan, & Beamer, 1996). This work is summarized in Levinson, Wan, and Beamer (1998). The authors recommend examination of scores on each item.

Kvalem and Traeen (2000) used CSE translated into Norwegian with some rephrasing for both girls and boys in a high school. Factor analysis showed five factors (situational contraceptive communication, preventing undesired intercourse, general sexual communication, controlling passion, and public sexuality). CSE scores were related to former use of, and to some degree the intention to use, contraception, as would be predicted by SE theory. Levinson, Wan, and Beamer (1998) tested the CSE in four diverse samples to check generalizability.

CRITIQUE AND SUMMARY

Contraceptive behavior is clearly complex, and the authors are to be congratulated for testing the CSE with nearly 900 adolescents from four diverse populations to establish generalizability and to set guidelines for use of the scale (Levinson, Jaccard, Wan, & Beamer, 1996). Clearly, cultural assumptions are important in attaining a tool predictive of contraceptive behavior, and it must be understood that the outcome behavior will not be valued by everyone. More important, the issues embedded in the CSE Scale may not be the most relevant issues impacting these young women's sexual and contraceptive behavior. Reliability for the CSE is still low, and work remains to be done to obtain internally consistent factors. Most of the work on the CSE has been done with teenage girls and less with boys; yet the work already accomplished is impressive.

Because individuals who feel relatively contraceptively self-efficacious on some items might not feel so on others, it is useful to look at item scores. Yet to be established is some target score level that could be used to judge the efficacy of interventions. Theory would suggest that a teenager would need to feel relatively self-efficacious across several items.

REFERENCES

Heinrich, L. B. (1993). Contraceptive self-efficacy in college women. *Journal of Adolescent Health, 14,* 269–276.

Kvalem, I. L., & Traeen, B. (2000). Self-efficacy, scripts of love and intention to use condoms among Norwegian adolescents. *Journal of Youth & Adolescence, 29,* 337–353.

Levinson, R. A. (1984). Contraceptive self-efficacy: A primary prevention strategy. *Journal of Social Work and Human Sexuality, 3,* 1–15.

Levinson, R. A. (1986). Contraceptive self-efficacy: A perspective on teenage girls' contraceptive behavior. *Journal of Sex Research, 22,* 347–369.

Levinson, R. A., Jaccard, J., Wan, C. K., & Beamer L. A. (1996). The Contraceptive Self-Efficacy Scale: Analysis in four samples. Unpublished manuscript.

Levinson, R. A., Wan, C. K., & Beamer, L. J. (1998). The Contraceptive Self-Efficacy Scale: Analysis in four samples. *Journal of Youth & Adolescence, 27,* 773–793.

CONTRACEPTIVE SELF-EFFICACY INSTRUMENT

The items on the following page are a list of statements. Please rate each item on a 1 to 5 scale according to how true the statement is of you. Using the scale, circle one number for each question.

1 = Not at all true of me
2 = Slightly true of me
3 = Somewhat true of me
4 = Mostly true of me
5 = Completely true of me

1.   1   2   3   4   5   When I am with a boyfriend, I feel that I can always be responsible for what happens sexually with him.

2.   1   2   3   4   5   Even if a boyfriend can talk about sex, I can't tell a man how I really feel about sexual things.

3.   1   2   3   4   5   When I have sex, I can enjoy it as something that I really wanted to do.

4.   1   2   3   4   5   If my boyfriend and I are getting "turned on" sexually and I don't really want to have sexual intercourse (go all the way, get down), I can easily tell him "No" and mean it.

5.   1   2   3   4   5   If my boyfriend didn't talk about the sex that was happening between us, I couldn't either.

6.   1   2   3   4   5   When I think about what having sex means, I can't have sex so easily.

7.   1   2   3   4   5   If my boyfriend and I are getting "turned on" sexually and I don't really want to have sexual intercourse (go all the way, get down), I can easily stop things so that we don't have intercourse.

8.   1   2   3   4   5   There are times when I'd be so involved sexually or emotionally that I could easily have sexual intercourse even if I weren't protected (using a form of birth control).

9.   1   2   3   4   5   Sometimes I just go along with what my date wants to do sexually because I don't think I can take the hassle of trying to say what I want.

10.   1   2   3   4   5   If there were a man (boyfriend) to whom I was very attracted physically and emotionally, I could feel comfortable telling him that I wanted to have sex with him.

11.   1   2   3   4   5   I couldn't continue to use a birth control method if I thought that my parents might find it.

12.   1   2   3   4   5   It would be hard for me to go to the drugstore and ask for foam (Encare Ovals, a diaphragm, a pill prescription, etc.) without feeling embarrassed.

13.   If my boyfriend and I were getting really heavy into sex and moving towards intercourse and I wasn't protected . . .

(continued)

1 = Not at all true of me
2 = Slightly true of me
3 = Somewhat true of me
4 = Mostly true of me
5 = Completely true of me

(a)   1   2   3   4   5   I could easily ask him if he had protection (or tell him that I didn't).

(b)   1   2   3   4   5   I could excuse myself to put in a diaphragm or foam (if I used them for birth control).

(c)   1   2   3   4   5   I could tell him I was on the pill or had an IUD (if I used them for birth control).

(d)   1   2   3   4   5   I could stop things before intercourse, if I couldn't bring up the subject of protection.

14.   1   2   3   4   5   There are times when I should talk to my boyfriend about using contraceptives, but I can't seem to do it in the situation.

15.   1   2   3   4   5   Sometimes I end up having sex with a boyfriend because I can't find a way to stop it.

Note: The CSE scale was previously published in ''Contraceptive Self-Efficacy: A perspective on teenage girls' contraceptive behavior'' by R. A. Levinson (1986). *Journal of Sex Research, 22,* 351.

Section H

Other Clinical Topics

Measurement instruments relevant to many other topics are available, frequently one or two per disease entity. Although this is not the full range needed to do comprehensive assessments or studies, individual instruments can be helpful.

---

62. Patient/Family Pain Questionnaires

Developed by Betty R. Ferrell, Michelle Rhiner, and Lynne M. Rivera

INSTRUMENT DESCRIPTION, ADMINISTRATION, AND SCORING GUIDELINES

Ferrell, Ferrell, Rhiner, and Grant (1991) remind us that two of every three American families will have at least one member diagnosed with cancer. Family members become active caregivers whether or not they feel competent to do so, and home care is increasing as the site of cancer care, frequently for many years.

Researchers have consistently found pain to be a major concern of family caregivers including fear of drug addiction, respiratory depression, or drug tolerance. These fears may lead to undermedication of patients even though they are experiencing unrelieved pain. In addition, pain management has become increasingly complex, with use of multiple medications, adjunct drugs, and complex delivery systems, such as patient-controlled analgesia pumps, epidural catheters, or continuous parenteral infusions.

The Family Pain Questionnaire (FPQ) was developed to measure caregivers' knowledge of basic pain management. The Patient Pain Questionnaire (PPQ) and FPQ include the same items; nine are in the knowledge subscale, with a higher score indicating higher knowledge, and seven items in the experience scale, with lower scores indicating more positive experience. Scale and subscale scores are sums of item scores.

PSYCHOMETRIC PROPERTIES

The FPQ was modeled after tools that have been used extensively to measure knowledge and attitudes of health care professionals about pain but modified to be appropriate for patients and family using results of interviews and surveys of families and patients describing their pain experience. The PPQ and FPQ were first tested with 85 patients/families with cancer pain in a community hospital, a cancer center, and a home-based community hospice program. Seventy-seven percent were White. The FPQ received 90% to 100% acceptance for content validity by a panel of six cancer pain management experts. Test–retest reliability was .92 and Cronbach's alpha .81 (Ferrell, Rhiner, & Rivera, 1993).

The two subscales of knowledge and experience were defined through factor analysis. The experience subscale captures the caregivers' personal experiences, such as perceptions of the intensivity of the patient's pain, and his or her own distress regarding the patient's pain (Ferrell, Rhiner, & Rivera, 1993).

Several other studies by the authors using these instruments have been reported. Ferrell, Ferrell, Ahn, and Tran (1994) report a study of an educational intervention for pain management delivered during home visits to 80 patients 60 years and older and their family caregivers. Topics included assessment of pain, use of pain-rating scales, the use of pharmacological and nonpharmacological agents, and the need to relieve pain to promote overall comfort and quality of life. Mean of the knowledge subscale was 54 and the experience subscale 52 before the intervention. Areas of lowest scores for knowledge and attitudes included fear of respiratory depression (mean score = 43), pain distress (mean score = 38), and need to take low doses of medicines (mean score = 38).

Significant improvement was verified in eight of the experience subscales before and after the educational treatment, providing support for sensitivity of the instrument. Scores of 50 family caregivers of these patients on the FPQ before the educational intervention are reported in Ferrell, Grant, Chan, Ahn, and Ferrell (1995). Mean score on the knowledge subscale was 53 and on the experience subscale 39. Caregivers showed lowest knowledge about the inevitability of addiction, a perception that patients were often overmedicated, and the relationship between medication and respiratory distress. Again, 10 of the 14 items showed significant improvement after the educational intervention, as did the two subscale scores. Overall, patients showed more positive responses than did family members.

A study of the family experience of cancer pain management in children used the FPQ. Participants were families of patients in a pediatric cancer hospital and a community hospice. Scores on individual items of the FPQ may be seen in a report of that research. Again, low scores were found in knowledge of the danger (mean item score = 56), dose (mean item score = 44), and constancy of pain medications (mean item score = 56) (Ferrell, Rhiner, Shapiro, & Strause, 1994).

CRITIQUE AND SUMMARY

Ferrell, Ferrell, Ahn, and Tran (1994) believe that structured pain education should be provided to all patients with cancer who experience this symptom, just as it is expected that diabetes education will be provided to all who have diabetes. Indeed, the studies cited previously indicate that patients and family caregivers have important educational needs in areas related to routine dosing, pain assessment, addiction, and respiratory depression.

They also show the effectiveness of an educational intervention (Ferrell, Grant, Chan, Ahn, & Ferrell, 1995), although the most optimally effective intervention has still not been adequately investigated. Meanings that might be attached to different levels of scores are not immediately clear. Studies of the predictive validity of the scores and patient/family pain management behavior would be useful.

The PPQ was recently used to evaluate a structured pain education intervention. No new psychometric data were reported (Ferrell, Borneman, & Juarez, 1998).

REFERENCES

Ferrell, B. R., Borneman, T., & Juarez, G. (1998). Integration of pain education in home care. *Journal of Palliative Care, 14*(3), 62–68.

Ferrell, B. R., Ferrell, B. A., Ahn, C., & Tran, K. (1994). Pain management for elderly patients with cancer at home. *Cancer, 74,* 2139–2146.

Ferrell, B. R., Ferrell, B. A., Rhiner, M., & Grant, M. (1991). Family factors influencing cancer pain. *Post Graduate Medical Journal, 67*(Suppl. 2), S64–S69.

Ferrell, B. R., Grant, M., Chan, J., Ahn, C., & Ferrell, B. A. (1995). The impact of cancer pain education on family caregivers of elderly patients. *Oncology Nursing Forum, 22,* 1211–1218.

Ferrell, B., Rhiner, M., & Rivera, L. M. (1993). Development and evaluation of the Family Pain Questionnaire. *Journal of Psychosocial Oncology, 10*(4), 21–35.

Ferrell, B. R., Rhiner, M., Shapiro, B., & Strause, L. (1994). The family experience of cancer pain management in children. *Cancer Practice, 2,* 441–445.

The Family Pain Questionnaire (FPQ) is a 16-item ordinal scale that measures the Knowledge and Experience of a family caregiver in managing chronic cancer pain. This tool can be useful in clinical practice as well as for research. This instrument can be administered by mail or in person.

Directions: The caregiver is asked to read each question thoroughly and decide if he/she agrees with the statement or disagrees. The caregiver is then asked to circle a number to indicate the degree to which he/she agrees or disagrees with the statement according to the word anchors on each end of the scale.

The FPQ includes 9 items that measure knowledge about pain and 7 items that measure the caregivers' experience with pain. All of the items have been formatted such that 0 = the most positive outcome and 10 = the most negative outcome. We have found it most helpful to analyze the data by focusing on the subscales as well as the individual items as each item has important implications.

You are welcome to use this instrument in your research/clinical practice to gain information about caregiver knowledge and experience to formulate or evaluate pain management programs. You have permission to duplicate this tool.

This tool is used in conjunction with a version created for use by patients, the Patient Pain Questionnaire (PPQ). The FPQ tool has been tested with established reliability (test retest, internal consistency) and validity (content, construct, concurrent). A series of psychometric analyses were performed on the instrument including content validity (CVI = .90), construct validity (ANOVA, $p. < .05$), concurrent validity ($r = .60, p. < .05$), factor analysis and test–retest reliability ($r = .80$) established with a retest of caregivers ($N = 67$).

FAMILY PAIN QUESTIONNAIRE

Below are a number of statements about cancer pain and pain relief. Please circle a number on the line to indicate your response.

Knowledge

1. Cancer pain can be effectively relieved.

   Agree   0   1   2   3   4   5   6   7   8   9   10   Disagree

2. Pain medicines should be given only when pain is severe.

   Disagree   0   1   2   3   4   5   6   7   8   9   10   Agree

3. Most cancer patients on pain medicines will become addicted to the medicines over time.

   Disagree   0   1   2   3   4   5   6   7   8   9   10   Agree

4. It is important to give the lowest amount of medicine possible to save larger doses for later when the pain is worse.

   Disagree   0   1   2   3   4   5   6   7   8   9   10   Agree

5. It is better to give pain medications around the clock (on a schedule) rather than only when needed.

    Agree   0   1   2   3   4   5   6   7   8   9   10   Disagree

6. Treatments other than medications (such as massage, heat, relaxation) can be effective for relieving pain.

    Agree   0   1   2   3   4   5   6   7   8   9   10   Disagree

7. Pain medicines can be dangerous and can often interfere with breathing.

    Disagree   0   1   2   3   4   5   6   7   8   9   10   Agree

8. Patients are often given too much pain medicine.

    Disagree   0   1   2   3   4   5   6   7   8   9   10   Agree

9. If pain is worse, the cancer must be getting worse.

    Disagree   0   1   2   3   4   5   6   7   8   9   10   Agree

Experience

10. Over the past week, how much pain do you feel your family member has had?

    No Pain   0   1   2   3   4   5   6   7   8   9   10   A Great Deal

11. How much pain is your family member having now?

    No Pain   0   1   2   3   4   5   6   7   8   9   10   A Great Deal

12. How much pain relief is your family member currently receiving?

    A Great Deal   0   1   2   3   4   5   6   7   8   9   10   No Relief

13. How distressing do you think the pain is to your family member?

    Not At All   0   1   2   3   4   5   6   7   8   9   10   A Great Deal

14. How distressing is your family members' pain to you?

    Not At All   0   1   2   3   4   5   6   7   8   9   10   A Great Deal

15. To what extent do you feel you are able to control the patient's pain?

    A Great Deal   0   1   2   3   4   5   6   7   8   9   10   Not At All

16. What do you expect will happen with your family member's pain in the future?

    Will Get Better   0   1   2   3   4   5   6   7   8   9   10   Will Get Worse

---

Used with permission: Betty R. Ferrell, City of Hope National Medical Center, Duarte, California.

The Patient Pain Questionnaire (PPQ) is a sixteen item ordinal scale that measures the Knowledge and Experience of a patient in managing chronic cancer pain. This tool can be useful in clinical practice as well as for research. This instrument can be administered by mail or in person.

Directions: The patient is asked to read each question thoroughly and decide if he/she agrees with the statement or disagrees. The patient is then asked to circle a number to indicate the degree to which he/she agrees or disagrees with the statement according to the word anchors on each end of the scale.

The PPQ includes 9 items that measure knowledge about pain and 7 items that measure the patient's experience with pain. All of the items have been formatted such that 0 = the most positive outcome and 10 = the most negative outcome. We have found it most helpful to analyze the data by focusing on the subscales as well as the individual items as each item has important implications.

You are welcome to use this instrument in your research/clinical practice to gain information about caregiver knowledge and experience to formulate or evaluate pain management programs. You have permission to duplicate this tool.

This tool is used in conjunction with a version created for use by family members, the Family Pain Questionnaire (FPQ). The PPQ tool has been tested with established reliability (test retest, internal consistency) and validity (content, construct, concurrent). A series of psychometric analyses were performed on the PPQ instrument including content validity (CVI = .90), construct validity (ANOVA, $p. < .05$), concurrent validity ($r = .60, p. < .05$), factor analysis and test–retest reliability ($r = .80$) established with a retest of caregivers ($N = 67$). The PPQ was recently revised to the current form and is being used in our current research.

PATIENT PAIN QUESTIONNAIRE

Below are a number of statements about cancer pain and pain relief. Please circle a number on the line to indicate your response.

Knowledge

1. Cancer pain can be effectively relieved.

    Agree   0   1   2   3   4   5   6   7   8   9   10   Disagree

2. Pain medicines should be given only when pain is severe.

    Disagree   0   1   2   3   4   5   6   7   8   9   10   Agree

3. Most cancer patients on pain medicines will become addicted to the medicines over time.

    Disagree   0   1   2   3   4   5   6   7   8   9   10   Agree

4. It is important to give the lowest amount of medicine possible to save larger doses for later when the pain is worse.

    Disagree   0   1   2   3   4   5   6   7   8   9   10   Agree

5. It is better to give pain medications around the clock (on a schedule) rather than only when needed.

   Agree   0   1   2   3   4   5   6   7   8   9   10   Disagree

6. Treatments other than medications (such as massage, heat, relaxation) can be effective for relieving pain.

   Agree   0   1   2   3   4   5   6   7   8   9   10   Disagree

7. Pain medicines can be dangerous and can often interfere with breathing.

   Disagree   0   1   2   3   4   5   6   7   8   9   10   Agree

8. Patients are often given too much pain medicine.

   Disagree   0   1   2   3   4   5   6   7   8   9   10   Agree

9. If pain is worse, the cancer must be getting worse.

   Disagree   0   1   2   3   4   5   6   7   8   9   10   Agree

Experience

10. Over the past week, how much pain have you had?

    No Pain   0   1   2   3   4   5   6   7   8   9   10   A Great Deal

11. How much pain are you having now?

    No Pain   0   1   2   3   4   5   6   7   8   9   10   A Great Deal

12. How much pain relief are you currently receiving?

    A Great Deal   0   1   2   3   4   5   6   7   8   9   10   No Relief

13. How distressing is the pain to you?

    Not At All   0   1   2   3   4   5   6   7   8   9   10   Extremely

14. How distressing is your pain to your family members?

    Not At All   0   1   2   3   4   5   6   7   8   9   10   Extremely

15. To what extent do you feel you are able to control your pain?

    A Great Deal   0   1   2   3   4   5   6   7   8   9   10   Not At All

16. What do you expect will happen with your pain in the future?

    Pain Will Get Better   0   1   2   3   4   5   6   7   8   9   10   Will Get Worse

Used with permission: Betty R. Ferrell, City of Hope National Medical Center, Duarte, California.

63.   Chronic Pain Self-Efficacy Scale

Developed by Karen O. Anderson, Barbara Noel Dowds, Robyn E. Pelletz, W. Thomas Edwards, and Christine Peeters-Asdourian

INSTRUMENT DESCRIPTION, ADMINISTRATION, AND SCORING GUIDELINES

Research to date indicates that SE beliefs are associated with chronic pain patients' level of functioning and response to treatment and therefore are clinically important. The Chronic Pain Self-Efficacy Scale (CPSS) is designed to measure chronic pain patients' perceived SE in coping with the consequences of chronic pain. It is modeled after the Arthritis Self-Efficacy Scale (ASE) with its three subscales related to physical function, controlling other arthritis symptoms, and pain management. Scores for CPSS are derived by summing items (Anderson, Dowds, Pelletz, Edwards, & Peeters-Asdourian, 1995).

PSYCHOMETRIC PROPERTIES

After discussion with patients and pain management specialists, items from the ASE were adapted for use with a chronic pain population, many with low back pain. Factor analysis confirmed three factors: SE for pain management (PSE, alpha = .88), SE for coping with symptoms (CSE, alpha = .90), SE for physical function (FSE, alpha = .87).

Subscale scores were significantly correlated with measures of depression, hopelessness, somatic preoccupation, and adaptation to the chronic pain experience, in the direction predicted by SE theory. Patients with higher CPSS scores reported less severe pain, less interference in their daily lives due to pain, greater perceived life control and less affective distress. Patients with higher levels of functional and coping SE reported higher levels of general activity than did patients with lower FSE and CSE scores. All of these findings support construct validity.

Little evidence about the sensitivity of the CPSS to various interventions is currently available. Social learning theory postulates that successful experiences in pain control, symptom management, and daily function will produce the greatest change in efficacy beliefs. Therefore treatment programs should include coping skills training followed by rehearsal and practice in the patients' daily environments (Anderson, Dowds, Pelletz, Edwards, & Peeters-Asdourian, 1995).

CRITIQUE AND SUMMARY

Only one study developing and using CPSS could be located, and it was carried out at a single institution. Initial study of it shows promise. Future areas of research could include the relationship of efficacy beliefs to the biology of pain, and the role that cognitive factors play in adaptation to chronic pain (Anderson, Dowds, Pelletz, Edwards, & Peeters-Asdourian, 1995).

REFERENCE

Anderson, K. O., Dowds, B. N., Pelletz, R. E., Edwards, W. T., & Peeters-Asdourian, C. (1995). Development and initial validation of a scale to measure self-efficacy beliefs in patients with chronic pain. *Pain, 63,* 77–84.

CHRONIC PAIN SELF-EFFICACY SCALE

10	100
Very Uncertain	Very Certain

Self-efficacy for pain management (PSE)

1. How certain are you that you can decrease your pain quite a bit?
2. How certain are you that your can continue most of your daily activities?
3. How certain are you that you can keep your pain from interfering with your sleep?
4. How certain are you that you can make a small-to-moderate reduction in your pain by using methods other than taking extra medications?
5. How certain are you that you can make a larger reduction in your pain by using methods other than taking extra medications?

Self-efficacy for physical function (FSE)

1. How certain are you that you can walk 1/2 mile on flat ground?
2. How certain are you that you can lift a 10-pound box?
3. How certain are you that you can perform a daily home exercise program?
4. How certain are you that you can perform your household chores?
5. How certain are you that you can shop for groceries or clothes?
6. How certain are you that you can engage in social activities?
7. How certain are you that you can engage in hobbies or recreational activities?
8. How certain are you that you can engage in family activities?
9. How certain are you that you can perform the work duties you had prior to the onset of chronic pain? (For homemakers, please consider your household activities as your work duties.)

Self-efficacy for coping with symptoms (CSE)

1. How certain are you that you can control your fatigue?
2. How certain are you that you can regulate your activity so as to be active without aggravating your physical symptoms (e.g., fatigue, pain)?
3. How certain are you that you can do something to help yourself feel better if you are feeling blue?
4. As compared to other people with chronic medical problems like yours, how certain are you that you can manage your pain during your daily activities?
5. How certain are you that you can manage your physical symptoms so that you can do the things you enjoy doing?
6. How certain are you that you can deal with the frustration of chronic medical problems?
7. How certain are you that you can cope with mild to moderate pain?
8. How certain are you that you can cope with severe pain?

From: Anderson, K. O., Dowds, B. N., Pelletz, R. E., Edwards, W. T., & Peeters-Asdourian, C. (1995). Development and initial validation of a scale to measure self-efficacy beliefs in patients with chronic pain. *Pain, 63,* 77–84. Used with permission.

64. Back Pain Self-Efficacy Scale

Developed by Jennifer B. Levin, Kenneth R. Lofland, Jeffrey E. Cassisi, Amir M. Poreh, and E. Richard Blonsky

INSTRUMENT DESCRIPTION, ADMINISTRATION, AND SCORING GUIDELINES

The Back Pain Self-Efficacy Scale (BPSES) is an adapted version of the Arthritis Self-Efficacy Scale, reviewed elsewhere in this book. Subjects answered each question using a scale ranging from 10 (very uncertain) to 100 (very certain). Scores are summed (Levin, Lofland, Cassisi, Poreh, & Blonsky, 1996).

PSYCHOMETRIC PROPERTIES

Coefficient alpha estimates of internal consistency were .82 for the pain management SE subscale, .91 for the physical function SE subscale, .90 for the controlling other symptoms SE subscale, and .92 for the total BPSES. Test–retest reliability for 16 weeks was .75, .84, .68, and .88.

Patients who reported higher levels on the BPSES also reported higher activity levels, working more hours with lower levels of psychological distress, pain severity, and pain behavior. These findings lend support to BPSES construct validity (Levin, Lofland, Cassisi, Poreh, & Blonsky, 1996).

CRITIQUE AND SUMMARY

Since increasing SE has the potential to decrease medication use and chronic illness behavior, it is important to have instruments that measure its strength.

To form the BPSES the Arthritis SE Scale was altered, substituting the term "back pain" for "arthritis pain." No justification was given as to why this was appropriate, nor were checks on the content validity of the BPSES made. The factor structure was also assumed to be the same. The goal of this approach is to gain some uniformity in the assessment of SE among related populations and the development of norms for different types of chronic pain patients (Levin, Lofland, Cassisi, Poreh, & Blonsky, 1996). Consideration of the tradeoffs between common items and adequate representation of different areas of pain experience should be further explored as well as whether the psychometric properties of the Arthritis SE Scale should be assumed for BPSES.

REFERENCE

Levin, J. B., Lofland, K. R., Cassisi, J. E., Poreh, A. M., & Blonsky, E. R. (1996). The relationship between self efficacy and disability in chronic low back pain patients. *International Journal of Rehabilitation and Health, 2*, 19–28.

BACK-PAIN SELF-EFFICACY SCALE

In the following questions, we'd like to know how your back pain affects you. For each of the following questions, please circle the number which corresponds to your certainty that you can *now* perform the following tasks.

1. How certain are you that you can decrease your pain *quite a bit*?

10	20	30	40	50	60	70	80	90	100
very uncertain				moderately uncertain					very certain

2. How certain are you that you can continue *most* of your daily activities?

10	20	30	40	50	60	70	80	90	100
very uncertain				moderately uncertain					very certain

3. How certain are you that you can keep back pain from interfering with your sleep?

10	20	30	40	50	60	70	80	90	100
very uncertain				moderately uncertain					very certain

4. How certain are you that you can make a *small-to-moderate* reduction in your back pain by using methods other than taking extra medication?

10	20	30	40	50	60	70	80	90	100
very uncertain				moderately uncertain					very certain

5. How certain are you that you can make a *large* reduction in your back pain by using methods other than taking extra medication?

10	20	30	40	50	60	70	80	90	100
very uncertain				moderately uncertain					very certain

We would like to know how confident you are in performing certain daily activities. For each of the following questions, please circle the number which corresponds to your certainty that you can perform the tasks as of *now*, *without* assistive devices or help from another person. Please consider what you *routinely* can do, not what would require a single extraordinary effort.

AS OF NOW, HOW CERTAIN ARE YOU THAT YOU CAN:

1. Walk 100 feet on flat ground in 20 seconds?

10	20	30	40	50	60	70	80	90	100
very uncertain				moderately uncertain					very certain

2. Walk 10 steps downstairs in 7 seconds?

10	20	30	40	50	60	70	80	90	100
very uncertain				moderately uncertain					very certain

3. Get out of an armless chair quickly, without using your hands for support?

10	20	30	40	50	60	70	80	90	100
very uncertain				moderately uncertain					very certain

4. Button and unbutton 3 medium-size buttons in a row in 12 seconds?

10	20	30	40	50	60	70	80	90	100
very uncertain				moderately uncertain					very certain

5. Cut 2 bite-size pieces of meat with a knife and fork in 8 seconds?

10	20	30	40	50	60	70	80	90	100
very uncertain				moderately uncertain					very certain

6. Turn an outdoor faucet all the way on and all the way off?

10	20	30	40	50	60	70	80	90	100
very uncertain				moderately uncertain					very certain

7. Scratch your upper back with both your right and left hands?

10	20	30	40	50	60	70	80	90	100
very uncertain				moderately uncertain					very certain

8. Get in and out of the passenger side of a car without assistance from another person and without physical aids?

10	20	30	40	50	60	70	80	90	100
very uncertain				moderately uncertain					very certain

(continued)

9. Put on a long-sleeve front-opening shirt or blouse (without buttoning) in 8 seconds?

```
10    20    30    40    50    60    70    80    90    100
very                    moderately                   very
uncertain               uncertain                   certain
```

In the following questions, we'd like to know how you feel about your ability to control your back pain. For each of the following questions, please circle the number which corresponds to the certainty that you can *now* perform the following activities or tasks.

1. *How certain* are you that you can control your fatigue?

```
10    20    30    40    50    60    70    80    90    100
very                    moderately                   very
uncertain               uncertain                   certain
```

2. *How certain* are you that you can regulate your activity so as to be active without aggravating your back pain?

```
10    20    30    40    50    60    70    80    90    100
very                    moderately                   very
uncertain               uncertain                   certain
```

3. *How certain* are you that you can do something to help yourself feel better if you are feeling blue?

```
10    20    30    40    50    60    70    80    90    100
very                    moderately                   very
uncertain               uncertain                   certain
```

4. As compared with other people with back pain like yours, *how certain* are you that you can manage back pain during your daily activities?

```
10    20    30    40    50    60    70    80    90    100
very                    moderately                   very
uncertain               uncertain                   certain
```

5. *How certain* are you that you can manage your back symptoms so that you can do the things that you enjoy doing?

```
10    20    30    40    50    60    70    80    90    100
very                    moderately                   very
uncertain               uncertain                   certain
```

6. *How certain* are you that you can deal with the frustration of back pain?

```
10    20    30    40    50    60    70    80    90    100
very                    moderately                   very
uncertain               uncertain                   certain
```

65. Back Beliefs Questionnaire

Developed by T. L. Symonds, A. K. Burton, K. M. Tillotson, and C. J. Main

INSTRUMENT DESCRIPTION, ADMINISTRATION, AND SCORING GUIDELINES

Recent evidence indicates that the influence of psychosocial factors on low-back disability is as great if not greater than ergonomic aspects. The Back Beliefs Questionnaire (BBQ) was developed to identify inappropriate beliefs that foster a reluctance towards early return to activities. Questions focus on various inevitable aspects of low-back trouble (LBT); negative beliefs are represented by low scores (Symonds, Burton, Tillotson, & Main, 1996).

PSYCHOMETRIC PROPERTIES

The instrument was tested with workers in industrial settings. Cronbach's alpha for the entire scale was .84. Factor analysis gave a one-dimensional solution for the inevitability statements with alpha = .7. Workers with LBT and a high rate of absences showed significantly more negative beliefs than did workers with either no LBT, or with LBT but no absences. Workers with current back symptoms showed more negative beliefs on the BBQ compared with those whose symptoms had subsided (Symonds, Burton, Tillotson, & Main, 1996). These findings support validity of the BBQ.

Burton, Waddell, Burtt, and Blair (1996) showed BBQ was sensitive to educational booklets which deviated from traditional biomedical approaches to management of LBT and focused instead on activity and self-coping. Results of a more recent randomized controlled trial (Burton, Waddell, Tillotson, & Summerton, 1999) again showed sensitivity of BBQ to an educational intervention and a reduction in self-reported disability.

CRITIQUE AND SUMMARY

Time to recover from LBT (time off work) is associated with negative beliefs about LBT, and interventions to change those beliefs have been successful (as measured by BBQ) and were associated with less self-reported disability. BBQ is timely because it reflects a distinct change in approach to managing LBT toward continuance of activity and positive coping in order to avoid disability.

REFERENCES

Burton, A. K., Waddell, G., Burtt, R., & Blair, S. (1996). Patient educational material in the management of low back pain in primary care. *Hospital for Joint Diseases Bulletin, 55,* 138–141.

Burton, A. K., Waddell, G., Tillotson, K. M., & Summerton, N. (1999). Information and advice to patients with back pain can have a positive effect. *Spine, 24,* 2484–2491.

Symonds, T. L., Burton, A. K., Tillotson, K. M., & Main, C. J. (1996). Do attitudes and beliefs influence work loss due to low back trouble? *Occupational Medicine, 46,* 25–32.

BACK BELIEFS QUESTIONNAIRE

We are trying to find out what people think about low-back trouble. Please indicate your general views toward back trouble, *even if you have never had any.*

Please answer *ALL* statements and indicate whether you *agree* or *disagree* with each statement by circling the appropriate number on the scale. 1 = COMPLETELY DISAGREE, 5 = COMPLETELY AGREE.

1	2	3	4	5
COMPLETELY DISAGREE				COMPLETELY AGREE

		Disagree				Agree
1	There is no real treatment for back trouble.	1	2	3	4	5
2	Back trouble will eventually stop you from working.	1	2	3	4	5
3	Back trouble means periods of pain for the rest of one's life.	1	2	3	4	5
4	Doctors cannot do anything for back trouble.	1	2	3	4	5
5	A bad back should be exercised.	1	2	3	4	5
6	Back trouble makes everything in life worse.	1	2	3	4	5
7	Surgery is the most effective way to treat back trouble.	1	2	3	4	5
8	Back trouble may mean you end up in a wheelchair.	1	2	3	4	5
9	Alternative treatments are the answer to back trouble.	1	2	3	4	5
10	Back trouble means long periods of time off work.	1	2	3	4	5
11	Medication is the *only* way of relieving back trouble.	1	2	3	4	5
12	Once you have had back trouble there is *always* a weakness.	1	2	3	4	5
13	Back trouble *must* be rested.	1	2	3	4	5
14	Later in life back trouble gets progressively worse.	1	2	3	4	5

The inevitability measure comprises 1 scale using a subset of 9 items.
Items: 1, 2, 3, 6, 8, 10, 12, 13, 14.
The scale is calculated by reversing and summing the 9 scores.
From: Symonds, T. L., Burton, A. K., Tillotson, K. M., & Main, C. J. (1996). Do attitudes and beliefs influence work loss due to low back trouble? *Occupational Medicine, 46,* 25–32. © 1993 University of Huddersfield, UK. Used with permission.

66. Caretaker and Adolescent Confidence in Managing Cystic Fibrosis

Developed by L. Kay Bartholomew, Guy S. Parcel, Paul R. Swank, and Danita I. Czyzewski

INSTRUMENT DESCRIPTION, ADMINISTRATION, AND SCORING GUIDELINES

Self-management refers to the behaviors that patients and family members perform to lessen the impact of a chronic illness. It is different from strict compliance to medical regimens in that it includes the complex cognitive-behavioral skills of self-monitoring, decision making, and communicating about both symptoms and treatment regimens. Behaviors required for cystic fibrosis (CF) self-management are especially complex because the health care of a child with this disease is usually intensive, even when the child is doing well, and includes chest physical therapy and respiratory therapy, diet, and medication. Enhancing self-efficacy (SE) through education may be critical to learning and performing CF home care routines because even good self-management may not be followed by noticeable improvement of physical symptoms or health status, and thus may not be reinforced over long periods (Bartholomew, Parcel, Swank, & Czyzewski, 1993). These instruments test confidence (SE) for adolescents and caretakers in managing cystic fibrosis. The outcome expectation scales measure expectations for positive outcomes as a result of carrying out self-management activities (Bartholomew et al., 1997).

The instrument has a 6th-grade reading level. Scoring is by summing item scores, with the outcomes scores separate (Bartholomew, Parcel, Swank, & Czyzewski, 1993). Scores were not available in published sources.

PSYCHOMETRIC PROPERTIES

Items for the instrument were sampled from 150 self-management performance objectives for CF that represented eight domains of care including aspects of medical care, coping, and communication (Bartholomew, Parcel, Swank, & Czyzewski, 1993). Ratings by a panel of experts and a survey of CF center directors provided evidence for agreement from the practice community that the objectives were important for self-management of CF. This evidence supports content validity.

After pilot work, the instruments were administered to members of 199 families (patients and their primary caretakers) from two CF centers. Twelve of the patients were African-American. Factor analysis yielded solutions reflecting five theorized aspects of self-management for the caretaker instrument: medical judgment and communication, coping, communication, compliance, and acceptance of CF. Cronbach's alphas ranged from .73 to .88. Four factors were found for the adolescent SE instrument: communication with the health care team, acceptance and coping, medical judgment and communication, and medical treatment. Moderate correlations between factors justify their use as subscales representing related yet conceptually consistent domains of SE. Test–retest reliability was not performed because SE is not expected to be a stable trait (Bartholomew, Parcel, Swank, & Czyzewski, 1993).

Both the caretaker version and the adolescent version also include items on outcome expectations that are beliefs about the effect of self-management on the patient's disease process and quality of life. Expectations for positive outcomes from carrying out these activities should also predict self-management behaviors. Results showed that at low levels of outcome expectations, SE was not strongly related to self-management. Cronbach's alpha coefficients of internal consistency for these items was .84 for the caretaker instrument and .75 for the adolescent instrument. Coefficient alphas for the outcome expectation scale were .84 for the caretaker instrument and .88 for the adolescent instrument (Bartholomew et al., 1997).

SE contributed significantly to the prediction of self-management on the part of both caretakers and adolescents with CF, providing evidence of criterion validity (Bartholomew, Parcel, Swank, & Czyzewski, 1993).

These instruments have recently been used to evaluate the efficacy of the Cystic Fibrosis Family Education Program, developed to teach comprehensive self-management skills in CF. This intervention includes skills training practices and success experiences. While outcome expectations were not changed by the intervention, self-efficacy for caregivers with an initial lower level of confidence in their ability to manage CF improved. SE was the most important educational factor predicting self-management behavior (Parcel et al., 1994). This finding also provides some evidence of sensitivity and validity of the Caregiver Confidence instrument.

CRITIQUE AND SUMMARY

Content validity should also be supported by patient experts. In addition, both socioeconomic status and education were high for those in the pilot study. The authors suggest that these instruments can be used to assess educational needs of CF patient caretakers and of the adolescent patients themselves. Interventions can be targeted toward behaviors with the lowest SE scores. The instruments can also be used to monitor over time patients' and caretakers' progress toward becoming confident in their ability and to evaluate the effectiveness of educational interventions designed to increase behavioral capability and SE for CF self-management. Studies documenting the usefulness of these instruments for these purposes should be completed. Evidence that changes in SE can lead to improvements in self-management of CF would be important.

REFERENCES

Bartholomew, L. K., Czyzewski, D. I., Parcel, G. S., Swank, P. R., Sockrider, M. M., Mariotto, M. J., Schidlow, D. V., Fink, R. J., & Seilheimer, D. K. (1997). Self-management of cystic fibrosis: Short-term outcomes of the cystic fibrosis family education program. *Health Education & Behavior, 24,* 652–666.

Bartholomew, L. K., Parcel, G. S., Swank, P. R., & Czyzewski, D. I. (1993). Measuring self-efficacy expectations for the self-management of cystic fibrosis. *Chest, 103,* 1524–1530.

Parcel, G. S., Swank, P. R., Mariotto, M. J., Bartholomew, L. K., Czyzewski, D. E., Sockrider, M. M., & Seilheimer, D. K. (1994). Self-management of cystic fibrosis: A structural model for educational and behavioral variables. *Social Science & Medicine, 38,* 1307–1315.

CARETAKER CONFIDENCE IN MANAGING CYSTIC FIBROSIS SCALE

We are interested in how sure you feel that *you* can do things to manage your child's cystic fibrosis. Please circle the answer that comes closest to describing how sure you feel. Your first reaction to each question should be your answer. Please answer all questions.

In general in your everyday life—How sure are you that *you* can do the following?	Not Sure at All	A Little Sure	Fairly Sure	Mostly Sure	Very Sure
1. Accept that cystic fibrosis may present new problems to your family at any time	1	2	3	4	5
2. Ask other questions when you do not get an answer or do not understand an answer from your child's doctor or nurse	1	2	3	4	5
3. Do chest PT (clapping) the number of times a day that your doctor suggests	1	2	3	4	5
4. Perform breathing treatments (respiratory therapy) as many times a day as your doctor suggests	1	2	3	4	5
5. Accept that cystic fibrosis related problems will demand that you and your family make changes and adjustments	1	2	3	4	5
6. Let your child know that you have understood what he or she has told you	1	2	3	4	5
7. Talk to your child about your feelings	1	2	3	4	5
8. Judge how your child will react when you talk about your feelings	1	2	3	4	5
9. Identify feelings in yourself that you wish to discuss with your child's doctor or nurse	1	2	3	4	5
10. *Figure out* several ways to make yourself feel better when you have a problem or are distressed	1	2	3	4	5
11. Accept cystic fibrosis as your child's diagnosis (acknowledge the effects that cystic fibrosis will have on your child's life)	1	2	3	4	5
12. Decide what you need to talk about with your child's doctor or nurse	1	2	3	4	5
13. Notice changes in cough, sputum, and shortness of breath that might indicate a lower respiratory infection in your child	1	2	3	4	5

(continued)

In general in your everyday life—How sure are you that *you* can do the following?	Not Sure at All	A Little Sure	Fairly Sure	Mostly Sure	Very Sure
14. Use the right words when talking about your child's cystic fibrosis or describing symptoms to your child's doctor or nurse	1	2	3	4	5
15. Judge when a problem has been solved	1	2	3	4	5
16. Correctly perform breathing treatments (for example, measuring and drawing up medication)	1	2	3	4	5
17. Notice whether or not your child's doctor or nurse is understanding what you are saying	1	2	3	4	5
18. *Use* several methods to make yourself feel better when you have a problem or are distressed	1	2	3	4	5
19. Tell when symptoms (for example, coughing, weight loss, and changes in sputum) mean that your child has developed a lower respiratory infection	1	2	3	4	5
20. Perform chest PT (clapping) the way you were shown	1	2	3	4	5
21. Notice signs that you are becoming too stressed or not coping with stress well	1	2	3	4	5

Outcome Expectations

We are interested in how sure you feel that the following things you do to manage your child's cystic fibrosis will be helpful to your child's well-being. Please circle the answer that comes closest to describing how sure you feel that doing these things will delay the progression of cystic fibrosis, will improve how your child feels, or will improve your child's quality of life. Your first reaction to each question should be your answer. Please answer all questions.

Regarding your child's well-being—How sure are you that the following will be helpful?	Not Sure at All	A Little Sure	Fairly Sure	Mostly Sure	Very Sure
22. Making sure that your child's lower respiratory infections are found early and treated	1	2	3	4	5
23. Performing breathing treatments the way your doctor has prescribed	1	2	3	4	5

In general in your everyday life—How sure are you that *you* can do the following?	Not Sure at All	A Little Sure	Fairly Sure	Mostly Sure	Very Sure
24. Performing chest PT (clapping) the way your doctor has prescribed	1	2	3	4	5
25. Making sure that your child eats enough food (gets enough calories)	1	2	3	4	5
26. Making sure that your child takes the right amount of enzymes to control poor digestion	1	2	3	4	5
27. Communicating well with your child's doctor or nurse	1	2	3	4	5
28. Coping well with any problems caused by cystic fibrosis and its management	1	2	3	4	5
29. Making sure your child engages in physical activities several times a week (for example, swimming, running, or bike riding)	1	2	3	4	5

ADOLESCENT CONFIDENCE IN MANAGING CYSTIC FIBROSIS SCALE

We are interested in how sure you feel that you can do things to manage your cystic fibrosis. Please circle the answer that comes closest to describing how sure you feel. Your first reaction to each question should be your answer. Please answer all questions.

In general in your everyday life—How sure are you that you can do the following?	Not Sure at All	A Little Sure	Fairly Sure	Mostly Sure	Very Sure
1. Notice changes in cough, sputum, and shortness of breath that might indicate a lower respiratory infection	1	2	3	4	5
2. Tell when symptoms (for example, coughing, weight loss, and changes in sputum) mean that you have developed a lower respiratory infection	1	2	3	4	5
3. Do chest PT (clapping) the number of times a day that your doctor suggests	1	2	3	4	5
4. Perform breathing treatments (respiratory therapy) as many times a day as your doctor suggests	1	2	3	4	5

(continued)

5.	Watch for signs of changes in your diges-	1	2	3	4	5
	tion (for example, observe stools and ob-					
	serve for bloating)					
6.	Take enzymes when food is eaten	1	2	3	4	5
7.	Notice when you are losing weight	1	2	3	4	5
8.	Notice whether or not you have a good	1	2	3	4	5
	appetite and are eating enough					
9.	Take antibiotics as prescribed	1	2	3	4	5
10.	Perform chest PT (clapping) the way	1	2	3	4	5
	you were shown					
11.	Tell the difference between poor diges-	1	2	3	4	5
	tion due to cystic fibrosis and poor diges-					
	tion due to other stomach problems					
	(such as a "stomach virus" or "flu")					
12.	Eat enough high calorie foods (get	1	2	3	4	5
	enough calories)					
13.	Correctly perform breathing treatments	1	2	3	4	5
	(for example, measuring and drawing up					
	medication)					
14.	Take the right amount of enzymes for	1	2	3	4	5
	the amount and type of food eaten					
15.	Notice changes in your appetite and	1	2	3	4	5
	weight that might indicate a lower respi-					
	ratory infection					
16.	Accept cystic fibrosis as your diagnosis	1	2	3	4	5
	(acknowledge the effects that cystic fibro-					
	sis will have on your life)					
17.	Accept that cystic fibrosis may present	1	2	3	4	5
	new problems to you and your family at					
	any time					
18.	Accept that cystic fibrosis related prob-	1	2	3	4	5
	lems will demand that you and your fam-					
	ily make changes and adjustments					
19.	Identify what problems in your life are	1	2	3	4	5
	causing you to be stressed					
20.	Notice signs that you are becoming too	1	2	3	4	5
	stressed or not coping with stress well					
21.	Recognize when something is going to	1	2	3	4	5
	cause a problem for you or your family					
22.	*Figure out* several ways to solve a	1	2	3	4	5
	problem					
23.	*Figure out* several ways to make your-	1	2	3	4	5
	self feel better when you have a problem					
	or are distressed					
24.	*Try* several ways of solving different	1	2	3	4	5
	problems					
25.	*Use* several methods to make yourself	1	2	3	4	5
	feel better when you have a problem or					
	are distressed					

In general in your everyday life—How sure are you that you can do the following?	Not Sure at All	A Little Sure	Fairly Sure	Mostly Sure	Very Sure
26. Judge when a problem has been solved	1	2	3	4	5
27. Continue to try and solve a problem even after your first try at solving it has been unsuccessful	1	2	3	4	5
28. Decide what you need to talk about with your doctor or nurse	1	2	3	4	5
29. Decide which doctor or nurse to talk with	1	2	3	4	5
30. Ask your doctor or nurse clear questions	1	2	3	4	5
31. Ask other questions when you do not get an answer or do not understand an answer from your doctor or nurse	1	2	3	4	5
32. Use the right words when talking about your cystic fibrosis or describing symptoms to your doctor or nurse	1	2	3	4	5
33. Notice whether or not your doctor or nurse is understanding what you are saying	1	2	3	4	5
34. Identify feelings in yourself that you wish to discuss with your doctor or nurse	1	2	3	4	5
35. Judge how your doctor or nurse will react when you talk about your feelings	1	2	3	4	5
36. Let your doctor or nurse know that you have understood what you have been told	1	2	3	4	5

Outcome Expectations

We are interested in how sure you feel that the following things you do to manage your cystic fibrosis will be helpful to your well-being. Please circle the answer that comes closest to describing how sure you feel that doing these things will delay the progression of cystic fibrosis, will improve how you feel, or will improve your quality of life. Your first reaction to each question should be your answer. Please answer all questions.

Regarding your well-being—How sure are you that the following will be helpful?	Not Sure at All	A Little Sure	Fairly Sure	Mostly Sure	Very Sure
37. Making sure that your lower respiratory infections are found early and treated	1	2	3	4	5
38. Performing breathing treatments the way your doctor has prescribed	1	2	3	4	5
39. Performing chest PT (clapping) the way your doctor has prescribed	1	2	3	4	5
40. Making sure that you eat enough food (get enough calories)	1	2	3	4	5
41. Making sure that you take the right amount of enzymes to control poor digestion	1	2	3	4	5
42. Communicating well with your doctor or nurse	1	2	3	4	5
43. Coping well with any problems caused by cystic fibrosis and its management	1	2	3	4	5
44. Making sure you engage in physical activities several times a week (for example, swimming, running, or bike riding)	1	2	3	4	5

67. Endoscopy Confidence Questionnaire

Developed by Suzanne M. Gattuso, Mark D. Litt,
and Terence E. Fitzgerald

INSTRUMENT DESCRIPTION, ADMINISTRATION, AND SCORING GUIDELINES

High levels of anxiety related to invasive medical and dental procedures have been associated with a variety of adverse effects including negative affective responses, prolonged and more difficult recoveries, and increased need for pain medication. These findings have prompted the development of numerous preparatory interventions designed to help patients cope with invasive and stressful procedures. It has been suggested that successful coping after preparatory interventions results from changes in certain cognitive mechanisms such as perceived self-efficacy. Self-efficacy (one's confidence in the ability to behave in a particular way) is situation specific and thus likely to be a good predictor of behavior. Self-efficacy also appears to be manipulable and applicable to clinical intervention (Gattuso, Litt, & Fitzgerald, 1992).

The Endoscopy Confidence Questionnaire (ECQ) is a nine-item scale to assess patients' estimates of confidence in their ability to engage in six specific behaviors that contribute to successful coping with endoscopy. Scale score is an average of the ratings for the items; mean scores ranged from 3.8 to 4.8 preintervention, and 4.5 to 4.9 postintervention (Gattuso, Litt, & Fitzgerald, 1992).

PSYCHOMETRIC PROPERTIES

The ECQ was used in an intervention study with 48 male patients in a Veterans Administration Hospital. Internal reliability alphas for the ECQ preintervention and postintervention were .90 and .92, respectively. Changes in self-efficacy judgments predicted changes in affective distress over the same period, and this effect was most pronounced after an intervention intended to raise self-efficacy. The ECQ was sensitive to this intervention (Gattuso, Litt, & Fitzgerald, 1992). A subsequent randomized controlled trial by different authors using a modified ECQ showed that teaching patients cognitive exercises including visualization was associated with improved scores while providing information about the procedure alone did not improve self-confidence. While this study produced no new psychometric information about ECQ, scores are provided with additional information about the kind of intervention to which the ECQ is sensitive (Hackett, Lane, & McCarthy, 1998).

SUMMARY AND CRITIQUE

Self-confidence has been found to influence a patient's tolerance of an endoscopic procedure and can be influenced by instruction. The ECQ offers an opportunity to assess self confidence. There is little discussion of content validity for ECQ, although some evidence of construct validity and adequate reliability. Additional testing of the ECQ with a broader population will be necessary.

REFERENCES

Gattuso, S. M., Litt, M. D., & Fitzgerald, T. E. (1992). Coping with gastrointestinal endoscopy: Self-efficacy enhancement and coping style. *Journal of Consulting and Clinical Psychology, 60,* 133–139.

Hackett, M. L., Lane, M. R., & McCarthy, D. C. (1998). Upper gastrointestinal endoscopy: Are preparatory interventions effective? *Gastrointestinal Endoscopy, 48,* 341–347.

ENDOSCOPY CONFIDENCE QUESTIONNAIRE (ECQ)

For each of the questions below, please *circle the number* which represents the best description of your feelings *right now:*

1. How confident are you that you can swallow the tube without difficulty during the upcoming examination?

1	2	3	4	5	6	7
Not at All Confident			Somewhat Confident			Very Confident

2. How confident are you that you can keep your body still during the examination?

1	2	3	4	5	6	7
Not at All Confident			Somewhat confident			Very Confident

3. How well do you think you can relax your body during the examination?

1	2	3	4	5	6	7
Not at All			Somewhat			Completely

4. How comfortable do you think you will be during the examination?

1	2	3	4	5	6	7
Not at All Comfortable			Somewhat Comfortable			Extremely Comfortable

5. How easily do you think you will swallow the tube during the examination?

1	2	3	4	5	6	7
Not at All Easy			Somewhat Easy			Extremely Easy

6. How much medication (sedative) do you think you will need to relax during the examination?

1	2	3	4	5	6	7
A Great Deal of Medication			Some Medication			No Medication

(continued)

7. How confident are you that you can complete this examination without any medication to help you relax?

1	2	3	4	5	6	7
Not at All Confident			Somewhat Confident			Extremely Confident

8. How much time do you think the examination will take?

1	2	3	4	5	6	7
More Time than Usual			About the same Time as Usual			Less Time than Usual

9. Overall, how confident are you that you will get through the examination without any difficulty?

1	2	3	4	5	6	7
Not at All Confident			Somewhat Confident			Extremely Confident

68.   Crohn's and Colitis Knowledge Score

Developed by Jayne A. Eaden, Keith Abrams, and John F. Mayberry

INSTRUMENT DESCRIPTION, ADMINISTRATION, AND SCORING GUIDELINES

The Crohn's and Colitis Knowledge Score (CCKnowScore) contains eight questions related to general irritable bowel disease (IBD) knowledge, five related to medication, four to anatomy, five to disease complications, and two related to diet. One point is scored for each correct answer. Readability was grade 4.4 (Eaden, Abrams, & Mayberry, 1999).

PSYCHOMETRIC PROPERTIES

Areas to be covered by CCKnowScore were key elements in the educational booklets used in the authors' clinics and reviewed by experts (content validity). Junior doctors had higher scores than did staff nurses, who in turn did better than did ward clerks (known groups). Cronbach's alpha was .95 (Eaden, Abrams, & Mayberry, 1999).

CRITIQUE AND SUMMARY

This is one of few published measurement instruments for persons with inflammatory bowel disease and their families. Psychometric properties so far studied do not establish links with significant disease outcomes.

REFERENCE

Eaden, J. A., Abrams, K., & Mayberry, J. F. (1999). The Crohn's and Colitis Knowledge Score: A test for measuring patient knowledge in inflammatory bowel disease. *American Journal of Gastroenterology, 94,* 3560–3566.

THE CCKNOW SCORE

Testing Your Knowledge of Crohn's and Colitis

This questionnaire will help your doctors and nurses know on which topics you may need more information. This will help make your treatment more effective. Please tick only one answer for each question. Thank you.

1. The intestines play an important role in the body but they only work during meal times:
   a) True
   b) False
   c) Don't know

2. People with inflammatory bowel disease are never allowed to eat dairy products:
   a) True
   b) False
   c) Don't know

3. Elemental feeds are sometimes used to treat Crohn's disease and ulcerative colitis. They:
   a) Always contain a lot of fibre
   b) Are very easy to digest
   c) Come in the form of tablets
   d) Don't know

4. Proctitis:
   a) Is a form of colitis that affects the rectum or back passage only
   b) Is a form of colitis that affects the whole of the large bowel
   c) Don't know

5. When a patient with inflammatory bowel disease passes blood in their stool it means:
   a) They definitely have bowel cancer
   b) They are having a flare-up of their disease
   c) Don't know

6. Patients with inflammatory bowel disease are probably cured if they have been symptom-free for 3 years:
   a) True
   b) False
   c) Don't know

7. Inflammatory bowel disease runs in families:
   a) True
   b) False
   c) Don't know

8. If patients with inflammatory bowel disease are not careful with their personal hygiene they can pass on their disease to friends and members of the family:
   a) True
   b) False
   c) Don't know

9. Patients with inflammatory bowel disease can get inflammation in other parts of the body as well as the bowel:
   a) True
   b) False
   c) Don't know

10. A fistula:
    a) Is an abnormal track between 2 pieces of bowel or between the bowel and skin
    b) Is a narrowing of the bowel which may obstruct the passage of the contents
    c) Don't know

11. The terminal ileum:
    a) Is a section of the bowel just before the anus
    b) Is a section of the bowel just before the large intestine
    c) Don't know

12. During a flare-up of inflammatory bowel disease:
    a) The platelet count in the blood rises
    b) The albumin level in the blood rises
    c) The white cell count in the blood falls
    d) Don't know

13. Steroids (such as prednisolone/prednisone/budesonide/hydrocortisone):
    a) Can only be taken by mouth
    b) Can be given in the form of an enema into the back passage
    c) Cannot be given directly into the vein
    d) Don't know

14. Steroids usually cause side effects:
    a) only after they have been taken for a long time and in high doses
    b) Immediately and even after small doses
    c) Which are not permanent and all disappear after treatment is stopped
    d) Don't know

15. Immunosuppressive drugs are given to inflammatory bowel disease patients to:
    a) Prevent infection in the bowel by bacteria
    b) Reduce inflammation in the bowel
    c) Don't know

16. Sulphasalazine:
    a) Controls the level of sulphur in the bloodstream
    b) Can be used to reduce the frequency of flare ups
    c) Cannot be used to prevent flare ups
    d) Don't know

17. An example of an immunosuppressive drug used in inflammatory bowel disease is:
    a) Sulphasalazine
    b) Mesalazine
    c) Azathioprine
    d) Don't know

18. If a woman has Crohn's disease:
    a) She may find it more difficult to become pregnant

(continued)

    b)   She should not have children
    c)   Her pregnancy will always have complications
    d)   She should stop all medication during her pregnancy
    e)   Don't know

19. Patients who smoke are more likely to have:
    a)   Ulcerative colitis
    b)   Crohn's disease
    c)   Don't know

20. Which one of the following statements is false?
    a)   Ulcerative colitis can occur at any age
    b)   Stress and emotional events are linked with the onset of ulcerative colitis
    c)   Ulcerative colitis is least common in Europeans and North Americans
    d)   Patients with ulcerative colitis have an increased risk of developing bowel cancer
    e)   Don't know

21. The examination of the large bowel with a flexible camera is called a:
    a)   Barium enema
    b)   Biopsy
    c)   Colonoscopy
    d)   Don't know

22. Male patients who take sulphasalazine:
    a)   Have reduced fertility levels that are reversible
    b)   Have reduced fertility levels that are not reversible
    c)   The drug does not have any effect on male fertility
    d)   Don't know

23. The length of the small bowel is approximately:
    a)   2 feet
    b)   12 feet
    c)   20 feet
    d)   Don't know

24. The function of the large bowel is to absorb:
    a)   Vitamins
    b)   Minerals
    c)   Water
    d)   Don't know

25. Another name for an ileorectal anastomosis operation with formation of a reservoir is:
    a)   Purse
    b)   Pouch
    c)   Stoma
    d)   Don't know

26. If a part of the bowel called the terminal ileum is removed during surgery the patient will have impaired absorption of:
    a)   Vitamin C
    b)   Vitamin A
    c)   Vitamin B12
    d)   Don't know

27. Patients with IBD need to be screened for cancer of the colon. Which one of the following statements about screening is false?
Screening should be offered to all patients with ulcerative colitis:
   a) Which affects only the rectum
   b) Which has lasted for 8–10 years
   c) Which started before the age of 50
   d) Don't know

28. There are millions of tiny "hairs" in the small bowel to increase the absorptive surface. They are called:
   a) Villi
   b) Enzymes
   c) Bile salts
   d) Crypts
   e) Don't know

29. Which one of the following is not a common symptom of inflammatory bowel disease?
   a) Abdominal pain
   b) Change in bowel habit
   c) Headache
   d) Fever
   e) Don't know

30. If a child has inflammatory bowel disease, he/she probably will not:
   a) live beyond the age of 45
   b) be as tall as his or her friends
   c) be as intelligent as his or her friends
   d) Don't know

From: Eaden, J. A., Abrams, K., & Mayberry, J. F. (1999). The Crohn's Colitis Knowledge Score: A test for measuring patient knowledge in inflammatory bowel disease. *American Journal of Gastroenterology, 94,*3560–3566. Used with permission.

69. Irritable Bowel Syndrome Misconceptions Scale

Developed by Christine P. Dancey, Rachel Fox, and Gerald M. Devins

INSTRUMENT DESCRIPTION, ADMINISTRATION, AND SCORING GUIDELINES

Irritable bowel syndrome (IBS) is a common chronic disorder that individuals must learn to manage. Medical understanding of the triggers, causes, and successful treatment is less certain than for other chronic conditions, and the nature, severity, and frequency of symptoms varies considerably. Therefore, particular care must be taken to assure that there is agreement on what is a misconception.

Each item of the Irritable Bowel Syndrome Misconceptions Scale (IBS-MS) has a 7-point scale from strongly disagree (scored 7) to strongly agree with items reverse scored. A higher score indicates more misconceptions (Dancey, Fox, & Devins, 1999).

PSYCHOMETRIC PROPERTIES

Items were judged by researchers, gastroenterologists, nurses, and workers in the IBS Network, in an effort to assure content validity. Validity was also supported by the fact that gastroenterologists scored the lowest (fewest misconceptions), students scored the highest (most misconceptions), and people with IBS scored in between. Internal consistency reliability (Cronbach's alpha) was .84. Test–retest reliability after 3 months was .73. Item discrimination was judged by the authors to be satisfactory (Dancey, Fox, & Devins, 1999).

CRITIQUE AND SUMMARY

It would have been helpful for IBS-MS items to be chosen based on some sense of what is important to persons with the syndrome. Much more work needs to be done to further establish reliability, validity and sensitivity to instruction of this instrument. No other instruments addressing this common problem were found despite a reasonable expectation that education could be helpful to these individuals.

REFERENCE

Dancey, C. P., Fox, R., & Devins, G. M. (1999). The measurement of irritable bowel syndrome (IBS)-related misconceptions in people with IBS. *Journal of Psychosomatic Research, 47,* 269–276.

IRRITABLE BOWEL SYNDROME MISCONCEPTION SCALE

Item number	Item
1	The bowel is described in terms of the small and large bowel (c)
2	A feeling of incomplete evacuation after a bowel movement is a common symptom of IBS (c)
3[a]	Children and teenagers do not suffer from IBS (i)
4	A core symptom of IBS is bloating (c)
5	Antidepressants may be prescribed for IBS (c)
6[a]	It is not unusual for IBS sufferers to have blood in their stool (i)
7	In America and the UK women are twice as likely to receive a diagnosis of IBS (c)
8[a]	IBS is known to lead to other diseases such as Crohn's disease, colitis, and bowel cancer (i)
9[a]	Rapid weight loss is recognized as one of the core symptoms of IBS (i)
10	Antidepressants can have side effects that may include blurred vision, skin irritations, fatigue, insomnia, and gastric irritations (c)
11	Abdominal distension is another name for a bloated belly (c)
12	Bulking agents are designed to soften the stool making it easier to pass (c)
13	The colon is part of the large bowel (c)
14	Gas-producing vegetables such as beans and broccoli can make IBS symptoms worse (c)
15[a]	Inflammatory bowel disease is another name for irritable bowel syndrome (i)
16[a]	IBS is a diagnosis given to adults only (i)
17	A bout of gastroenteritis is a possible trigger of IBS symptoms (c)

[a]Items reverse scored.
c, "correct" response; i, "incorrect" response.
From Dancey, C. P., Fox, R., & Devins, G. M. (1999). The measurement of irritable bowel syndrome (IBS)-related misconceptions in people with IBS. *Journal of Psychosomatic Research, 47,* 269–276. Reprinted with permission from Elsevier Science.

70. Osteoporosis Health Belief, Self-Efficacy, and Knowledge Tests

Developed by Katherine K. Kim, Mary Horan, Phyllis Gendler, and Minu Patel

INSTRUMENT DESCRIPTION, ADMINISTRATION, AND SCORING GUIDELINES

This set of three instruments developed to measure important aspects of osteoporosis self-care is in the early stages of development.

The Osteoporosis Health Belief Scale (OHBS) is based on the health belief model (HBM) and is especially designed to assess beliefs related to exercise and calcium intake in the elderly. Questions have a readability level of 5th grade. The revised OHBS included here is scored by awarding 1 for "strongly disagree" to 5 for "strongly agree." Because there are six items in each subscale, the possible score for each ranges from 6 to 30. The instrument can be administered in 20 minutes (Kim, Horan, Gendler, & Patel, 1991).

HBM elements include susceptibility (perceived risk of developing osteoporosis); seriousness (perception of threat from having osteoporosis including to physical health, role and social status, and ability to complete desired tasks); benefits (belief in the effectiveness of specific behaviors to prevent the occurrence of the disease); barriers (beliefs about the negative components of the behaviors that would be undertaken to prevent the disease); and health motivation (general tendency for an individual to engage in health behaviors). Self-efficacy (SE) is now also part of the model, which predicts that health behaviors are more likely to occur if an individual believes in personal susceptibility to the condition, believes that having the condition would have serious consequences, recognizes the impact of health motivation, perceived barriers, and benefits, and feels self-confident (SE) in taking the specific health actions necessary to prevent osteoporosis (Kim, Horan, Gendler, & Patel, 1991).

Osteoporosis Self-Efficacy Scale (OSES) items represent the three theoretical dimensions of efficacy expectation: initiation, maintenance, and persistence in performing the activity (Horan, Kim, Gendler, Froman, & Patel, 1998). The scale is scored by measuring distance of the patient's mark from the left anchor in millimeters; thus, the range is 0 to 100. There are two subscales. OSES Exercise includes items 1 to 10 and OSES Calcium includes items 11 to 21. The score for each subscale is obtained by totaling item scores and calculating a mean. The questions were worded at a sixth-grade readability level as determined by the Flesch formula (Horan, Kim, Gendler, Froman, & Patel, 1998).

Osteoporosis Knowledge Test (OKT) also has two subscales: OKT Exercise (items 1 to 16) and OKT Calcium (items 1 to 9 and 17 to 24). Correct answers are summed (Kim, K., personal communication, March 1996).

PSYCHOMETRIC PROPERTIES

OHBS was revised based on a pilot study of 16 elderly individuals. The tools were then administered to 150 individuals recruited from senior citizen centers (80% female). This group had a mean age of 74 years and were neither cognitively impaired, nor reported that they had osteoporosis. A review of the literature and input from nurses around elements of the HBM were used to generate items (Kim, Horan, Gendler, & Patel, 1991).

OHBS items form six subscales supported by factor analysis: susceptibility (items 1 to 6, alpha = .82, test–retest .84); seriousness (items 7 to 12, alpha = .71, test–retest .79); benefits from exercise (items 13 to 18, alpha = .81, test–retest .63); benefits from calcium intake (items 19 to 24, alpha = .80, test–retest .52); barriers exercise (items 25 to 30, alpha = .82, test–retest .80); barriers calcium intake (items 31 to 36, alpha = .74, test–retest .68); and health motivation (items 37 to 42, alpha = .73, test–retest .67). Discriminant classification of the OHBS exercise scores correctly classified 66% of cases of self-reported low and high levels of exercise, and 69% of those with self-reported low and high calcium intake, in evaluation of concurrent validity (Kim, personal communication, March 1996).

Horan and colleagues (1998) evaluated a revised OSES and found two factors (OSE-Exercise and OSE-Calcium) with internal consistency estimates of .94 and .93. Convergent and discriminant validity analysis as well as hierarchical regression analysis to explain self reports of physical activity and calcium intake were supportive. Details may be found in Horan, Kim, Gendler, Froman, and Patel (1998).

OKT Exercise subscale internal consistency reliability coefficient was .69; OKT Calcium subscale internal consistency reliability coefficient was .72. Validity of the OKT was evaluated by factor analysis and discriminant function analysis (Kim, personal communication, March 1996). Details in published form could not be located.

Both the OHBS and the OSES were used in a study of stages of readiness for osteoporosis prevention in 452 women ages 35 to 45. Osteoporosis-specific beliefs showed little relationship to women's decisions to exercise. Compared with those who were not engaged in adopting exercise precautions, those who were so engaged had higher OSES scores (Blalock et al., 1996). Such a finding is consistent with self-efficacy theory and, therefore, supportive of validity. Blalock and colleagues (1996) also found that for both calcium and exercise as measured by the OHBS, perceived benefits were higher among currently engaged women compared with never-engaged women but with no differences between these groups on perceived barriers.

CRITIQUE AND SUMMARY

The focus of these instruments is preventive behavior on the part of elderly subjects within the context of the HBM. The process for establishing content was not described in detail. Self-report measures for exercise and calcium intake may themselves suffer from limitations of reliability and validity, and may not constitute strong measures of concurrent validity for the OHBS. Ability of the HBM to predict health actions has been widely studied and is variable. Therefore, early findings that the OHBS was marginally related to decision to take the preventive actions may reflect limitations of the model. Nursing interventions related to osteoporosis prevention have consisted primarily of educational programs aimed at changing dietary and exercise habits, and at removing perceived barriers to these actions

(Kim, Horan, Gendler, & Patel, 1991). It is therefore important to have evidence of these scales' sensitivity to instruction.

REFERENCES

Blalock, S. J., DeVellis, R. F., Giorgino, B., DeVellis, B. M., Gold, D. T., Dooley, M. A., Anderson, J. J. B., & Smith, S. L. (1996). Osteoporosis prevention in premenopausal women: Using a stage model approach to examine the predictors of behavior. *Health Psychology, 15,* 84–93.

Horan, M. L., Kim, K. K., Gendler, P., Froman, R. D., & Patel, M. D. (1998). Development and evaluation of the Osteoporosis Self-Efficacy Scale. *Research in Nursing and Health, 21,* 395–403.

Kim, K. K., Horan, M. L., Gendler, P., & Patel, M. K. (1991). Development and evaluation of the Osteoporosis Health Belief Scale. *Research in Nursing and Health, 14,* 115–163.

OSTEOPOROSIS HEALTH BELIEF SCALE

(Interviewer: Read the following instruction *slowly*)

Osteoporosis (os-teo-po-ro-sis) is a condition in which the bones become excessively thin (porous) and weak so that they are fracture prone (they break easily).

I am going to ask you some questions about your beliefs about osteoporosis. There are no right or wrong answers. Everyone has different experiences that will influence how they feel. After I read each statement, tell me if you STRONGLY DISAGREE, DISAGREE, are NEUTRAL, AGREE, or STRONGLY AGREE with the statement. I am going to show you a card with these five choices. When I read each statement, tell me which one of the five is your choice.

It is important that you answer according to your actual beliefs and not according to how you feel you should believe or how you think we want you to believe. We need the answers that best explain how *you* feel.

(Interviewer: Before administration of the scale, check whether the participant can read the five choices on the card. If the person is unable to read them, you need to read the five choices after each statement.)

Strongly Disagree 1	Disagree 2	Neutral 3	Agree 4	Strongly Agree 5		
SD	D	N	A	SA	1.	Your chances of getting osteoporosis are high.
SD	D	N	A	SA	2.	Because of your body build, you are more likely to develop osteoporosis.
SD	D	N	A	SA	3.	It is extremely likely that you will get osteoporosis.
SD	D	N	A	SA	4.	There is a good chance that you will get osteoporosis.
SD	D	N	A	SA	5.	You are more likely than the average person to get osteoporosis.
SD	D	N	A	SA	6.	Your family history makes it more likely that you get osteoporosis.
SD	D	N	A	SA	7.	The thought of having osteoporosis scares you.
SD	D	N	A	SA	8.	If you had osteoporosis you would be crippled.

(continued)

_____

Scoring Instructions. The Osteoporosis Health Belief Scale (OHBS) is scored by awarding 5 for responses of "strongly agree" to 1 for "strongly disagree" for each item. The OHBS has 7 subscores. Because there are 6 items in each subscale, the possible score for each ranges from 6 to 30.

Susceptibility	OHB01-OHB06	Barriers Exercise	OHB25-OHB30
Seriousness	OHB07-OHB12	Barriers Calcium Intake	OHB31-OHB36
Benefits Exercise	OHB13-OHB18	Health Motivation	OHB37-OHB42
Benefits Calcium Intake	OHB19-OHB24		

Strongly Disagree 1	Disagree 2	Neutral 3	Agree 4	Strongly Agree 5	
SD	D	N	A	SA	9. Your feelings about yourself would change if you got osteoporosis.
SD	D	N	A	SA	10. It would be very costly if you got osteoporosis.
SD	D	N	A	SA	11. When you think about osteoporosis you get depressed.
SD	D	N	A	SA	12. It would be very serious if you got osteoporosis.
SD	D	N	A	SA	13. Regular exercise prevents problems that would happen from osteoporosis.
SD	D	N	A	SA	14. You feel better when you exercise to prevent osteoporosis.
SD	D	N	A	SA	15. Regular exercise helps to build strong bones.
SD	D	N	A	SA	16. Exercising to prevent osteoporosis also improves the way your body looks.
SD	D	N	A	SA	17. Regular exercise cuts down the chances of broken bones.
SD	D	N	A	SA	18. You feel good about yourself when you exercise to prevent osteoporosis.

(Interviewer: Read the following instruction *slowly*)

For the following 6 questions, when I say "taking in enough calcium" it means taking enough calcium by eating calcium-rich foods and/or taking calcium supplements.

SD	D	N	A	SA	19. Taking in *enough calcium* prevents problems from osteoporosis.
SD	D	N	A	SA	20. You have lots to gain from taking in *enough calcium* to prevent osteoporosis.
SD	D	N	A	SA	21. Taking in *enough calcium* prevents painful osteoporosis.
SD	D	N	A	SA	22. You would not worry as much about osteoporosis if you took in *enough calcium*.
SD	D	N	A	SA	23. Taking in *enough calcium* cuts down on your chances of broken bones.
SD	D	N	A	SA	24. You feel good enough about yourself when you take in *enough calcium* to prevent osteoporosis.
SD	D	N	A	SA	25. You feel like you are not strong enough to exercise regularly.
SD	D	N	A	SA	26. You have no place where you can exercise.

Strongly Disagree 1	Disagree 2	Neutral 3	Agree 4	Strongly Agree 5	
SD	D	N	A	SA	27. Your spouse or family discourages you from exercising.
SD	D	N	A	SA	28. Exercising regularly would mean starting a new habit which is hard for you to do.
SD	D	N	A	SA	29. Exercising regularly makes you uncomfortable.
SD	D	N	A	SA	30. Exercising regularly upsets your every day routine.
SD	D	N	A	SA	31. Calcium-rich foods cost too much.
SD	D	N	A	SA	32. Calcium-rich foods do not agree with you.
SD	D	N	A	SA	33. You do not like calcium-rich foods.
SD	D	N	A	SA	34. Eating calcium-rich foods means changing your diet which is hard to do.
SD	D	N	A	SA	35. In order to eat more calcium-rich foods you have to give up other foods that you like.
SD	D	N	A	SA	36. Calcium-rich foods have too much cholesterol.
SD	D	N	A	SA	37. You eat a well-balanced diet.
SD	D	N	A	SA	38. You look for new information related to health.
SD	D	N	A	SA	39. Keeping healthy is very important for you.
SD	D	N	A	SA	40. You try to discover health problems early.
SD	D	N	A	SA	41. You have a regular health check-up even when you are not sick.
SD	D	N	A	SA	42. You follow recommendations to keep you healthy.

OSTEOPOROSIS SELF-EFFICACY SCALE

We are interested in learning how confident you feel about doing the following activities. We all have different experiences, which will make us more or less confident in doing the following things. Thus, there are no right or wrong answers to this questionnaire. It is your opinion that is important. In this questionnaire, EXERCISE means activities such as walking, swimming, golfing, biking, aerobic dancing.

Place your "X" anywhere on the answer line that you feel best describes your confidence level.

If it were recommended that you do any of the following THIS WEEK, how confident or certain would you be that you could:

1. begin a new or different exercise program

   Not at All ———————————————————————————————— Very
   Confident   Confident

2. change your exercise habits

   Not at All ———————————————————————————————— Very
   Confident   Confident

3. put forth the effort required to exercise

   Not at All ———————————————————————————————— Very
   Confident   Confident

4. do exercises even if they are difficult

   Not at All ———————————————————————————————— Very
   Confident   Confident

5. maintain a regular exercise program

   Not at All ———————————————————————————————— Very
   Confident   Confident

6. exercise for the appropriate length of time

   Not at All ———————————————————————————————— Very
   Confident   Confident

Scoring instructions. When scoring the OSES, first with a ruler, measure from the left anchor on the visual analogue in millimeters to the line where the subject has marked, on each item. The line from "Not at All Confident" to "Very Confident" should measure exactly 10 cm (100 mm). The subject's score on each item should be measured to the nearest millimeter. Thus the range for each item is 0–100. The OSES has two subscales. Exercise includes OSE01-OSE06 for the 12 item OSES, and OSE01-OSE10 for the 21 item OSES. Calcium includes OSE07-OSE12 for the 12 item OSES and OSE11-OSE21 for the 21 item OSES. In order to calculate the scores for each subscale (calcium and exercise), first add the scores for each item within the respective subscale, then divide the total score for each subscale (calcium and exercise) by the number of items in the respective scale to obtain the individual subscale score. The total possible for each subscale ranges from 0 to 100.

7. do exercises even if they are tiring

Not at All ————————————————————————————————— Very
Confident   Confident

8. stick to your exercise program

Not at All ————————————————————————————————— Very
Confident   Confident

9. exercise at least three times a week

Not at All ————————————————————————————————— Very
Confident   Confident

10. do the type of exercise that you are supposed to do

Not at All ————————————————————————————————— Very
Confident   Confident

11. begin to eat more calcium rich foods

Not at All ————————————————————————————————— Very
Confident   Confident

12. increase your calcium intake

Not at All ————————————————————————————————— Very
Confident   Confident

13. consume adequate amounts of calcium rich foods

Not at All ————————————————————————————————— Very
Confident   Confident

14. eat calcium rich foods on a regular basis

Not at All ————————————————————————————————— Very
Confident   Confident

15. change your diet to include more calcium rich foods

Not at All ————————————————————————————————— Very
Confident   Confident

16. eat calcium rich foods as often as you are supposed to do

Not at All ————————————————————————————————— Very
Confident   Confident

(continued)

17. select appropriate foods to increase your calcium intake

Not at All ——————————————————————————————— Very
Confident   Confident

18. stick to a diet which gives an adequate amount of calcium

Not at All ——————————————————————————————— Very
Confident   Confident

19. obtain foods that give an adequate amount of calcium

Not at All ——————————————————————————————— Very
Confident   Confident

20. remember to eat calcium rich foods

Not at All ——————————————————————————————— Very
Confident   Confident

21. take calcium supplements if you don't get enough calcium from your diet

Not at All ——————————————————————————————— Very
Confident   Confident

OSTEOPOROSIS KNOWLEDGE TEST

(Interviewer: Read the following instruction *slowly*.)

Osteoporosis (os-teo-po-ro-sis) is a condition in which the bones become very brittle and weak so that they break easily.
I am going to read a list of things which may or may not affect a person's chance of getting osteoporosis. After I read each one, tell me if you think the person is:

    MORE LIKELY TO GET OSTEOPOROSIS, or
    LESS LIKELY TO GET OSTEOPOROSIS, or
    IT HAS NOTHING TO DO WITH GETTING OSTEOPOROSIS.

I am going to show you a card with these 3 choices. When I read each statement, tell me which one of the 3 will be your best answer. (Test administrator. *Do not read ''don't know'' choice*. If the participants say ''don't know,'' circle this option.)

	More Likely	Less Likely	Neutral	Don't Know
1. Eating a diet *low* in milk products	(ML)	LL	NT	DK
2. Being menopausal; ''change of life''	(ML)	LL	NT	DK
3. Having big bones	ML	(LL)	NT	DK
4. Eating a diet high in dark green leafy vegetables	ML	(LL)	NT	DK
5. Having a mother or grandmother who has osteoporosis	(ML)	LL	NT	DK
6. Being a white woman with fair skin	(ML)	LL	NT	DK
7. Having ovaries surgically removed	(ML)	LL	NT	DK
8. Taking cortisone (steroids, e.g., Prednisone) for long time	(ML)	LL	NT	DK
9. Exercising on a regular basis	ML	(LL)	NT	DK

(continued)

(Interviewer: Read the following instruction *slowly*)

For the next group of questions, you will be asked to choose one answer from several choices. Be sure to choose only one answer. If you think there is more than one answer, choose the best answer. If you are not sure, just say "I don't know."

10.   Which of the following exercises is the *best way* to reduce a person's chance of getting osteoporosis?
    A.   Swimming.
    Ⓑ.   Walking briskly.
    C.   Doing kitchen chores, such as washing dishes or cooking.
    D.   Don't know

11.   Which of the following exercises is the *best way* to reduce a person's chance of getting osteoporosis?
    Ⓐ.   Bicycling.
    B.   Yoga.
    C.   Housecleaning.
    D.   Don't know

12.   *How many days a week* do you think a person should exercise to strengthen the bones?
    A.   1 day a week.
    B.   2 days a week.
    Ⓒ.   3 or more days a week.
    D.   Don't know

13.   What is the *least amount of time* a person should exercise on each occasion to strengthen the bones?
    A.   Less than 15 minutes.
    Ⓑ.   20 to 30 minutes.
    C.   More than 45 minutes.
    D.   Don't know

14.   Exercise makes bones strong, but it must be *hard enough to make breathing*:
    A.   Just a little faster.
    B.   So fast that talking is not possible.
    Ⓒ.   *Much faster*, but talking is possible.
    D.   Don't know

15.   Which of the following exercises is the *best way* to reduce a person's chance of getting osteoporosis?
    Ⓐ.   Jogging or running for exercise.
    B.   Golfing using golf cart.
    C.   Gardening.
    D.   Don't know

16.   Which of the following exercises is the *best way* to reduce a person's chance of getting osteoporosis?
    A.   Bowling.
    B.   Doing laundry.
    Ⓒ.   Aerobic dancing.
    D.   Don't know

(Interviewer: Read the following statement *slowly*)

Calcium is one of the nutrients our body needs to keep bones strong.

17. Which of these is a good source of calcium?
   A. Apple.
   Ⓑ. Cheese.
   C. Cucumber.
   D. Don't know

18. Which of these is a good source of calcium?
   A. Watermelon.
   B. Corn.
   Ⓒ. Canned sardines.
   D. Don't know

19. Which of these is a good source of calcium?
   A. Chicken.
   Ⓑ. Broccoli.
   C. Grapes.
   D. Don't know

20. Which of these is a good source of calcium?
   Ⓐ. Yogurt.
   B. Strawberries.
   C. Cabbage.
   D. Don't know

21. Which of these is a good source of calcium?
   Ⓐ. Ice cream.
   B. Grapefruit.
   C. Radishes.
   D. Don't know

22. Which of the following is the recommended amount of calcium intake for an adult?
   A. 100 mg–300 mg daily.
   B. 400 mg–600 mg daily.
   Ⓒ. 800 mg or more daily.
   D. Don't know

23. How much milk must an adult drink to meet the recommended amount of calcium?
   A. 1/2 glass daily.
   B. 1 glass daily.
   Ⓒ. 2 or more glasses daily.
   D. Don't know

24. Which of the following is the *best reason* for taking a calcium supplement?
   A. If a person skips breakfast.
   Ⓑ. If a person does not get enough calcium from diet.
   C. If a person is over 45 years old.
   D. Don't know

Kim, K., Horan, M., & Gendler, P. (1991). Reproduction without authors' express written consent is not permitted. Permission to use this test may be obtained from one of the authors at Grand Valley State University, Allendale, MI 49401.

71. Osteoporosis Questionnaire

Developed by Ketan C. Pande, Dominic de Takats, John A. Kanis, Veronica Edwards, Pauline Slade, and Eugene V. McCloskey

INSTRUMENT DESCRIPTION, ADMINISTRATION, AND SCORING GUIDELINES

The Osteoporosis Questionnaire (OPQ) assesses patient knowledge in areas of general information, risk factors, consequences and treatment. Readability analysis found OPQ was easier than standard writing. Score is the sum of correct answers (Pande et al., 2000).

PSYCHOMETRIC PROPERTIES

Clinicians managing patients with osteoporosis identified facts they would hope their patients would know, and information pamphlets were analyzed in support of content validity. Criterion validity was supported in the finding that members of the osteoporosis awareness charity scored higher than first time attendees (contrasted groups). Internal consistency was .84 (Pande et al., 2000).

CRITIQUE AND SUMMARY

OPQ is expected to be useful in assessment of individuals and in evaluation of patient education programs on the subject. Although there is no gold standard for appropriate patient knowledge in osteoporosis, further work on relating knowledge level to clinically relevant outcomes would be useful.

REFERENCE

Pande, K. C., deTakats, D., Kanis, J. A., Edwards, V., Slade, P., & McCloskey, E. V. (2000). Development of a questionnaire (OPQ) to assess patients' knowledge about osteoporosis. *Maturitas, 237,* 75–81.

This questionnaire has been designed to assess the amount of knowledge you have about osteoporosis. You are not expected to know the answers to all the questions. If you do not know the answer or are unsure about it, please mark "Do not know." You do not need to write your name. The information obtained will be treated in the strictest confidence and used only for research. Please put a tick (/) in the box against the one answer you think is the most correct. THERE IS ONLY ONE CORRECT ANSWER.

Number of patients (%) providing a correct response is given next to each item.

1. A woman cannot take hormone replacement therapy (HRT) if she: (68)
   - ☐ Is above 60 years of age
   - ☒ Has breast cancer
   - ☐ Has hot flashes
   - ☐ Don't know

2. Early menopause is a risk factor for osteoporosis because of: (72)
   - ☐ Psychological distress
   - ☒ Lack of sex hormones
   - ☐ Neither of the above
   - ☐ Don't know

3. An excessive intake of which of the following is most likely to cause osteoporosis: (70)
   - ☐ Leafy green vegetables
   - ☐ Multivitamins
   - ☒ Alcohol
   - ☐ Does not know

4. Excessive dieting: (70)
   - ☒ Can cause osteoporosis
   - ☐ Is good for your bones
   - ☐ Has no effect on bones
   - ☐ Don't know

5. Side effects of HRT include: (24)
   - ☒ Clots in the leg veins
   - ☐ Low back pain
   - ☐ Vaginal dryness
   - ☐ Don't know

6. More women than men are reported to have osteoporosis because: (72)
   - ☒ They actually do get osteoporosis more than men do
   - ☐ Men are not aware of it
   - ☐ Women are more concerned about their health problems than men
   - ☐ Don't know

7. Osteoporosis is more likely to develop in people who: (72)
   - ☒ Exercise regularly
   - ☐ Exercise occasionally
   - ☐ Do not exercise at all
   - ☐ Don't know

8. Which of the following types of exercise will NOT strengthen bones much in osteoporosis: (38)
   - ☒ Swimming
   - ☐ Running
   - ☐ Walking
   - ☐ Do not know

9. What is the LEAST likely cause of osteoporosis: (54)
   - ☒ Weather changes
   - ☐ Genetic factors
   - ☐ Lack of exercise
   - ☐ Do not know

10. Osteoporosis and osteoarthritis are: (72)
    - ☐ Different names for the same disease
    - ☐ Differ only in the parts of the body that are affected
    - ☒ Are different conditions with few similarities
    - ☐ Do not know

11. The condition characterized by fragile brittle bones is commonly known as: (76)
    - ☐ Arthritis
    - ☒ Osteoporosis
    - ☐ Spondylitis
    - ☐ Do not know

12. The following is NOT a common complaint in patients with osteoporosis: (76)
    - ☐ Low back pain
    - ☐ Loss of height
    - ☒ Swelling of the feet
    - ☐ Don't know

13. A woman over 60 years is LEAST likely to develop: (24)
    - ☐ Osteoporosis
    - ☐ Arthritis
    - ☒ Bone cancer
    - ☐ Don't know

(continued)

14. All types of hormone replacement therapy (HRT): (72)
    - ☒ Help prevent progress of osteoporosis
    - ❑ Cause regular menstrual bleeding
    - ❑ Have no effect on bones
    - ❑ Don't know

15. Our bones are strongest at the following age: (38)
    - ❑ Below 20 years
    - ☒ Between 20 and 50 years
    - ❑ Over 50 years
    - ❑ Don't know

16. Having broken your wrist: (38)
    - ❑ Your chance of breaking the other wrist is lower
    - ☒ You are more likely to break the other wrist
    - ❑ The chances of further fractures remains unchanged
    - ❑ Don't know

17. If your mother or father have had osteoporosis: (68)
    - ☒ You are more likely to suffer from it
    - ❑ It does not affect your chance of suffering from it
    - ❑ You are less likely to suffer from it
    - ❑ Don't know

18. If you have an overactive thyroid: (20)
    - ❑ It does not affect the bones
    - ☒ You are more likely to suffer from osteoporosis
    - ❑ You are less likely to suffer from osteoporosis
    - ❑ Don't know

19. Muscle weakness: (56)
    - ❑ Does not affect your chance of breaking bones
    - ❑ Has no effect on the chance of falling over
    - ☒ Makes you more likely to break bones
    - ❑ Don't know

20. You are more likely to fall over if you take: (42)
    - ☒ Sleeping tablets, e.g., Diazepam
    - ❑ Hormone replacement therapy
    - ❑ Aspirin
    - ❑ Don't know

From: Pande, K. C., deTakats, D., Kanis, J. A., Edwards, V., Slade, P., & McCloskey, E. V. (2000). Development of a questionnaire (OPQ) to assess patients' knowledge about osteoporosis. *Maturitas, 237,* 75–81. Used with permission from Elsevier Science.

72.   Facts on Osteoporosis Quiz

Developed by Rita L. Ailinger, Doreen C. Harper, and Howard A. LaSus

INSTRUMENT DESCRIPTION, ADMINISTRATION, AND SCORING GUIDELINES

Orem's self-care theory provides the framework for this instrument. Three objectives guided item development: indicating known facts about osteoporosis, recognizing preventive health behaviors for osteoporosis, and identifying major risk factors associated with osteoporosis (Ailinger & Emerson, 1998).

Correct items are given a score of 1 and those answered incorrectly or with "don't know" are given a score of 0, and a percentage score calculated. Items 2, 4, 6–11, 15 and 16 are true. Total possible score is 20 with higher scores indicating more knowledge of osteoporosis. FOOQ has a sixth grade readability level and takes 5 minutes to complete (Ailinger, Harper, & Lasus, 1998).

PSYCHOMETRIC PROPERTIES

Two nurse investigators funded by the National Institutes of Health for clinical trials on osteoporosis considered the items. A content validity index of .92 was obtained, items were culled, and those remaining were tested with a convenience sample of nursing and nonnursing students and a community group. Respondents exposed to another person with osteoporosis had higher levels of knowledge (known groups). Internal consistency was .83 in the student and community group and .84 in an ethnically diverse community group.

CRITIQUE AND SUMMARY

FOOQ can be used as a screening tool in osteoporosis health promotion/disease prevention programs and by laywomen as a self-care knowledge quiz (Ailinger, Harper, & Lasus, 1998). Initial work on validity and reliability has been completed although evidence of sensitivity to educational interventions has yet to be established.

REFERENCES

Ailinger, R. L., & Emerson, J. (1998). Women's knowledge of osteoporosis. *Applied Nursing Research, 11,* 111–114.

Ailinger, R. L., Harper, D. C., & Lasus, H. A. (1998). Bone up on osteoporosis. *Orthopaedic Nursing, 7*(5), 66–73.

FACTS ON OSTEOPOROSIS QUIZ

Osteoporosis refers to weakened bone strength. It is commonly called "brittle bones" because this disease increases the risk of bone fractures. Completely fill in the circle of the appropriate answer.

		True	False	Don't Know
1	Physical activity increases the risk of osteoporosis.	Ⓣ	Ⓕ	Ⓓ
2	High impact exercise (weight training) improves bone health.	Ⓣ	Ⓕ	Ⓓ
3	Most people gain bone mass after 30 years of age.	Ⓣ	Ⓕ	Ⓓ
4	Low-weight women have osteoporosis more than heavy women.	Ⓣ	Ⓕ	Ⓓ
5	Alcoholism is not linked to the occurrence of osteoporosis.	Ⓣ	Ⓕ	Ⓓ
6	The most important time to build bone strength is between 9 and 17 years of age.	Ⓣ	Ⓕ	Ⓓ
7	Normally, bone loss speeds up after menopause.	Ⓣ	Ⓕ	Ⓓ
8	High caffeine combined with low calcium intake increases the risk of osteoporosis.	Ⓣ	Ⓕ	Ⓓ
9	There are many ways to prevent osteoporosis.	Ⓣ	Ⓕ	Ⓓ
10	Without preventive measures 20% of women older than 50 years will have a fracture due to osteoporosis in their lifetime.	Ⓣ	Ⓕ	Ⓓ
11	There are treatments for osteoporosis after it develops.	Ⓣ	Ⓕ	Ⓓ
12	A lifetime of low intake of calcium and vitamin D does not increase the risk of osteoporosis.	Ⓣ	Ⓕ	Ⓓ
13	Smoking does not increase the risk of osteoporosis.	Ⓣ	Ⓕ	Ⓓ
14	Walking has a great effect on bone health.	Ⓣ	Ⓕ	Ⓓ
15	After menopause, women not on estrogen need about 1500 mg of calcium (for example, 5 glasses of milk) daily.	Ⓣ	Ⓕ	Ⓓ
16	Osteoporosis affects men and women.	Ⓣ	Ⓕ	Ⓓ
17	Early menopause is not a risk factor for osteoporosis.	Ⓣ	Ⓕ	Ⓓ
18	Replacing hormones after menopause cannot slow down bone loss.	Ⓣ	Ⓕ	Ⓓ
19	Children 9 to 17 years of age get enough calcium from one glass of milk each day to prevent osteoporosis.	Ⓣ	Ⓕ	Ⓓ
20	Family history of osteoporosis is not a risk factor for osteoporosis.	Ⓣ	Ⓕ	Ⓓ

73. Hormone Replacement Therapy Self-Efficacy Scale

Developed by Nagia Ali

INSTRUMENT DESCRIPTION, ADMINISTRATION, AND SCORING GUIDELINES

Women frequently discontinue hormone replacement therapy (HRT) because of fear of cancer. Taking or discontinuing HRT might be expected to be related to self-efficacy (SE) beliefs and outcome expectations. Items were developed from SE theory, literature review, and focus groups with past and current users of the therapy. Scores are summed with a possible range for efficacy beliefs of 8–40 and for outcome beliefs of 6–30 (Ali, 1998).

PSYCHOMETRIC PROPERTIES

Content validity was judged by experts in SE and HRT. Study of psychometric characteristics was based on a convenience sample of past or current users of HRT. The item pool contained two factors: factor 1 efficacy beliefs (items 1–8, alpha = .86), efficacy beliefs and factor 2 outcome beliefs (items 9–14, alpha = .78). This finding is congruent with self-efficacy theory, providing support for construct validity. Cronbach's alpha for the whole scale was .87 (Ali, 1998).

CRITIQUE AND SUMMARY

This instrument is in the early stages of development. Basic psychometric properties were studied in an all-Caucasian, highly educated convenience sample of 116 women. Study in other populations is important. Test–retest reliability has not yet been studied, and studies of the instrument's predictive validity would seem to be especially important. SE beliefs and outcome expectations can be influenced by intervention targeted at each women's pattern. Women who are candidates for benefiting from the long-term effects of the therapy and who agree to take it might be the focus of such an intervention (Ali, 1998).

REFERENCE

Ali, N. S. (1998). The Hormone Replacement Therapy Self-Efficacy Scale. *Journal of Advanced Nursing, 28,* 1115–1119.

HORMONE REPLACEMENT THERAPY SELF-EFFICACY SCALE

Directions: For each of the following statements, please circle the one that best describes your feelings about hormone replacement therapy (**HRT**).

	Strongly Agree (SA)	Agree (A)	Undecided (U)	Disagree (D)	Strongly Disagree (SD)
1. I believe that **HRT** reduces hot flashes.	SA	A	U	D	SD
2. I am unsure of the safety of **HRT**.	SA	A	U	D	SD
3. I will retry to take **HRT** if I missed.	SA	A	U	D	SD
4. I can't complete the whole course of **HRT**.	SA	A	U	D	SD
5. I am motivated to take **HRT**.	SA	A	U	D	SD
6. I am unsure that **HRT** prevents heart disease.	SA	A	U	D	SD
7. I believe that **HRT** prevents further bone loss.	SA	A	U	D	SD
8. Even if I try hard, I will not be able to continue using **HRT**.	SA	A	U	D	SD
9. I am able to deal with side-effects of **HRT**.	SA	A	U	D	SD
10. I believe **HRT** maintains my feelings of well-being.	SA	A	U	D	SD
11. I believe that **HRT** helps improve my intimate relations with my significant other.	SA	A	U	D	SD
12. I believe that **HRT** promotes my quality of life.	SA	A	U	D	SD
13. I am persistent in using **HRT**.	SA	A	U	D	SD
14. I can succeed in continued use of **HRT**.	SA	A	U	D	SD

Hormone Replacement Therapy Self-Efficacy Scale

Scoring Instructions:

Items are scored as

> Strongly agree (SA) = 5
> Agree (A) = 4
> Undecided (U) = 3
> Disagree (DA) = 2
> Strongly Disagree (SD) = 1

The two subscale subscores are obtained by calculating the means to each subscale item. The items included on each scale are as follows:

Efficacy Beliefs in Hormone Replacement Therapy   2, 3, 4, 5, 8, 9, 13, 14

Items that should be reversed in scoring are 2, 4, 8

The higher the score, the greater the tendency to be self-efficacious in continued use of HRT

Outcome Expectations in Hormone Replacement Therapy   1, 6, 7, 10, 11, 12

Only one item should be reversed in scoring, 6

The higher the score, the greater the tendency to perceive greater positive outcomes to using HRT.

74. Preoperative Self-Efficacy Scale

Developed by Sharon Oetker-Black

INSTRUMENT DESCRIPTION, ADMINISTRATION, AND SCORING GUIDELINES

Preoperative instruction about deep breathing and coughing, leg exercises/position change, ambulation, hydration, pain management, and knowledge about the procedures and processes related to surgery have been found to decrease postoperative complications and the length of hospitalization. Self-efficacy is hypothesized to be one of the mechanisms by which this effect is created.

The Preoperative Self-Efficacy Scale (PSES) measures behaviors important to postoperative self-care in four subscales established through factor analysis: deep breathing (items 1 to 3), turning (items 4 to 6), mobility (items 7 to 12), and pain relaxation (items 13 to 15) (Oetker-Black, 1996). Each subscale is summated and behaviorally specific. Increased self-efficacy is linked to an increased likelihood that patients will enact behaviors. Therefore, patients with low self-efficacy may need additional patient teaching to increase their confidence in their ability to perform behaviors postoperatively. Patients took 10 to 15 minutes to complete the questionnaire (Oetker-Black, Hart, Hoffman, & Geary, 1992).

PSYCHOMETRIC PROPERTIES

The PSES was first tested with 68 patients undergoing cholecystectomy. Content validity was supported by professional experts' judgments about how each item fit the conceptual definitions of efficacy expectations and postoperative behaviors. Cronbach's alpha was .78. Scores were related significantly to deep breathing, ambulation, and recollection of preoperative events, which are postoperative behaviors designed to minimize complications and facilitate recovery, providing support for validity (Oetker-Black, Hart, Hoffman, & Geary, 1992).

A second study (Oetker-Black & Taunton, 1994) involved 200 adult surgical patients excluding those undergoing open-heart and orthopedic procedures because of the potential limitations of their postoperative activities. The best items were retained based on item means, standard deviations, ranges, item subscale score correlations, alpha if deleted, and factor loadings, with 16 items remaining. Cronbach's alpha was .74. Face validity was assessed with patients who found the scale clear and readable, content validity by experts in self-efficacy and nursing, and construct validity was assessed by testing the hypothesis that those patients who already had received preoperative instruction would score higher than those who had not. This hypothesis was not supported, perhaps in part because it was difficult to control for previous surgical experience.

A third study was carried out with 85 adult patients scheduled for unilateral knee replacements under general anesthesia. Means after completion of the hospital's routine preoperative teaching, ranged from 5.8 for turning self in bed every hour to 8.5 for remembering one third of preoperative activities. Most items had an optimal range of 10. These means indicate that patients were moderately confident (0 = no confidence, 10 = total confidence) about their ability to perform the postoperative behaviors listed on the questionnaire. Cronbach's alphas for the four subscales were recalling activities self-efficacy (SE), .90; breathing deeply SE, .84; turning SE, .97; and mobility SE, .98 (Oetker-Black & Kauth, 1995).

A fourth study tested PSES with 75 women having total abdominal hysterectomies (Oetker-Black, 1996). Scores on the PSES after completion of routine preoperative instruction ranged from 4.9 for turning self every hour to 8.6 for ambulating 10 feet. Factor analysis showed the same factors as described previously, with Cronbach's alphas of .94 for mobility, .97 for turning, .96 for relaxation techniques, and .95 for breathing.

A fifth study has now tested PSES with 60 patients undergoing laparoscopic cholecystectomy (Oetker-Black, Teeters, Curr, & Rininger, 1997). Through factor analysis four factors were identified: mobility (alpha = .96), turning (alpha = .94), relaxation techniques (alpha = .98), and breathing (alpha = .93). These are consistent with previous findings. In the study one group was given usual care preoperative instruction while the other received this treatment supplemented with an efficacy-enhancing teaching protocol incorporating the concepts of performance accomplishments, vicarious learning, and verbal persuasion to individually prepare patients for their impending surgeries. No significant differences between the groups were found on any of the subscales. These findings may be due to lack of consistency or strength of the intervention (Oetker-Black, Teeters, Curr, & Rininger, 1997) or to lack of sensitivity of the PSES.

CRITIQUE AND SUMMARY

Development of the PSES should enable nurses to more effectively assess patients' levels of need for preoperative teaching and to more systematically evaluate the effectiveness of preoperative teaching in preparing patients for the surgical experience (Oetker-Black & Taunton, 1994). Instructional techniques can be tailored to improving SE (use of mastery and vicarious experiences, modeling of desired behaviors, and persuasion) in the areas where a particular patient shows low SE.

Although norms have not been established, scores on items in the present version of the PSES were reported in study 3 summarized earlier. Studies using PSES have been carried out only on adults; socioeconomic or minority status were not reported, although mean educational level was 12 to 13.5 years. Further studies need to control for both the experience of past surgeries and determine whether the PSES is sensitive to the effects of instruction. In addition, more research is needed to determine what types of preoperative instruction will motivate postoperative patients to perform behaviors, especially those that cause pain. The authors also believe that new items that deal with relaxation techniques need to be written and tested. Although there is a core of behaviors that are common across surgeries (Oetker-Black & Kauth, 1995), it will be important to note whether the specific scale items match with those required of your patient. Sensitivity of PSES to intervention must be established. Finally, future studies need to evaluate the relationship between preoperative PSES scores and actual postoperative behavior in mobility, turning, relaxation, and breathing (Oetker-Black, Teeters, Curr, & Rininger, 1997).

REFERENCES

Oetker-Black, S. L. (1996). Generalizability of the Preoperative Self-Efficacy Scale. *Applied Nursing Research, 9,* 40–44.

Oetker-Black, S. L., Hart, F., Hoffman, J., & Geary, S. (1992). Preoperative self-efficacy and postoperative behaviors. *Applied Nursing Research, 5,* 134–139.

Oetker-Black, S. L., & Kauth, C. (1995). Evaluating a revised self-efficacy scale for preoperative patients. *Association of Operating Room Nurses Journal, 62,* 244–250.

Oetker-Black, S. L., & Taunton, R. L. (1994). Evaluation of a self-efficacy scale for preoperative patients. *Association of Operating Room Nurses Journal, 60,* 43–50.

Oetker-Black, S., Teeters, D., Curr, P., & Rininger, S. (1997). Self-efficacy enhanced preoperative instruction. *Association of Operating Room Nurses Journal, 66,* 854–864.

PREOPERATIVE SELF-EFFICACY SCALE

DIRECTIONS: This questionnaire should take no more than 10–15 minutes to complete.

Each of the statements below is written so patients can describe their perceptions of their confidence in performing certain behaviors that they are commonly expected to do after surgery.

Please *circle the number* that identifies how confident you are *right now* of your ability to perform each of the behaviors. Remember there are no right or wrong answers but it is very important that you answer the questions honestly.

Example: How confident are you right now that you will be able to exercise your leg once every hour in bed the day of surgery?

   0   1   2   3   4   5   6   7   8   9   10

No Confidence   Total Confidence

---

1.   How confident are you right now that you will be able to do deep breathing exercises three times an hour after surgery?

   0   1   2   3   4   5   6   7   8   9   10

No Confidence   Total Confidence

2.   How confident are you right now that you will be able to do deep breathing exercises six times an hour after surgery?

   0   1   2   3   4   5   6   7   8   9   10

No Confidence   Total Confidence

3.   How confident are you right now that you will be able to do deep breathing exercises ten times an hour after surgery?

   0   1   2   3   4   5   6   7   8   9   10

No Confidence   Total Confidence

4.   How confident are you right now that you will be able to turn yourself from side to side in bed every three hours the day of surgery?

   0   1   2   3   4   5   6   7   8   9   10

No Confidence   Total Confidence

5.   How confident are you right now that you will be able to turn yourself from side to side in bed every two hours the day of surgery?

   0   1   2   3   4   5   6   7   8   9   10

No Confidence   Total Confidence

(continued)

6. How confident are you right now that you will be able to turn yourself from side to side in bed every hour the day of surgery?

   0   1   2   3   4   5   6   7   8   9   10

No Confidence   Total Confidence

7. How confident are you right now that you will be able to get into a chair with assistance one time the day of surgery?

   0   1   2   3   4   5   6   7   8   9   10

No Confidence   Total Confidence

8. How confident are you right now that you will be able to get into a chair with assistance two times the day of surgery?

   0   1   2   3   4   5   6   7   8   9   10

No Confidence   Total Confidence

9. How confident are you right now that you will be able to get into a chair with assistance three times the day of surgery?

   0   1   2   3   4   5   6   7   8   9   10

No Confidence   Total Confidence

10. How confident are you right now that you will be able to walk 5 minutes with assistance the first day after surgery?

   0   1   2   3   4   5   6   7   8   9   10

No Confidence   Total confidence

11. How confident are you right now that you will be able to walk 10 minutes with assistance the first day after surgery?

   0   1   2   3   4   5   6   7   8   9   10

No Confidence   Total Confidence

12. How confident are you right now that you will be able to walk 15 minutes with assistance the first day after surgery?

   0   1   2   3   4   5   6   7   8   9   10

No Confidence   Total Confidence

13. How confident are you right now that you will be able to do relaxation exercises one time when you experience pain?

   0   1   2   3   4   5   6   7   8   9   10

No Confidence   Total Confidence

14. How confident are you right now that you will be able to do relaxation exercises often when you experience pain?

    0 1 2 3 4 5 6 7 8 9 10

    No Confidence   Total Confidence

15. How confident are you right now that you will be able to do relaxation exercises every time you experience pain?

    0 1 2 3 4 5 6 7 8 9 10

    No Confidence   Total Confidence

Before finishing this questionnaire, please fill in all of the blank spaces in this section.

1. What is your age? _____

2. How many years of education have you completed? _____

3. What is your approximate annual family income before taxes? _____

4. Have you ever had surgery before? Yes ____ No ____

▼ *If yes, what type of surgery?* _____

▼ *If yes, did you receive information on how to care for yourself after surgery? (check one)*

 Yes ____ No ____

5. Have you received any information on how to care for yourself after surgery during this hospital visit?

 Yes ____ No ____

Thank you for completing this questionnaire.

Today's Date _____

Date of Scheduled Surgery _____

Home Address _____

_____

_____

_____

Home Phone Number _____

Work Phone Number _____

75.   The Amsterdam Preoperative Anxiety and Information Scale

Developed by Nelly Moerman, Frits S. A. M. vanDam, Martin J. Muller, and Hans Oosting

INSTRUMENT DESCRIPTION, ADMINISTRATION, AND SCORING GUIDELINES

Providers of anesthesia care face several challenges in preoperative psychological preparation. First, because it is known that anxious patients respond differently to anesthesia than do nonanxious patients, it is useful to identify anxious individuals. Second, patients cope with a threatening situation differently—some (monitors) want to know as much as possible and search for information, whereas others (blunters) have no need for information and try to avoid it. Parental anxiety is directly correlated with children's preoperative anxiety and also may limit the informed-consent process (Miller, Wysocki, Cassady, Cancel, & Izenberg, 1999). The Amsterdam Preoperative Anxiety and Information Scale (APAIS) was developed to assess these needs.

The anxiety scale (items 1, 2, 4, 5) yields a score ranging from 4 (not anxious) to 20 (highly anxious). The Need for Information scale (items 3 and 6) had a scoring range from 2 to 10. Patients with a score of 2–4 on this scale can be considered "blunters" and those with a score of 8–10 can be considered "monitors." APAIS can be completed in about 2 minutes (Moerman, van Dam, Muller, & Oosting, 1996).

PSYCHOMETRIC PROPERTIES

Factor analysis showed that the four items representing fear of anesthesia and of the surgery formed one factor (anxiety) with an internal consistency reliability of .86, and the two items representing the need for information had a reliability of .72. Results of the factor analysis were replicated by Miller and colleagues (1999), with alphas of .82, .75, and .87 for the total scale. Test–retest reliability was .92 for the total scale, .91 for the anxiety factor, and .62 for the information items.

Correlation of the Spielberger State-Trait Anxiety Inventory (STAI)—long considered the gold standard—and the anxiety subscale of APAIS was .74 and the need for information subscale .16. Patients with previous operative experience had a lower score on the information scale than did those who had not been operated on before. These relationships are as would be expected. In the parental study cited below, APAIS items were much more closely correlated with STAI than were information items, supporting concurrent validity (Moermann, vanDam, Muller, & Oosting, 1996).

One study has reviewed the usefulness of APAIS in clinical practice. Parents of children scheduled to undergo ambulatory surgical procedures under general anesthesia being shown a videotape about pediatric anesthesia had lower APAIS scores than did parents shown a videotape with no medical content (Cassady, Wysocki, Muller, Cancel, & Izenberg, 1999). This shows APAIS is sensitive to intervention.

CRITIQUE AND SUMMARY

The purpose of the APAIS is to screen preoperatively for anxiety and information requirements in order to identify those in need of extra support. Patients with high information requirements turned out to be the ones who were most anxious. The authors recommend that patients with a score of 11–13 on the anxiety scale be considered anxiety cases, and that patients with an information score of 5 or higher should be given information on the topics on which they wish to be informed. A score below 5 should be a signal to provide no more information than is legally required (Moermann, van Dam, Muller, & Oosting, 1996).

Parental anxiety has been identified as a risk factor for preoperative anxiety and postoperative maladaptive behavior in children. The study by Cassady and others (1999) extends information about APAIS beyond the adult surgical patients on which it was developed. Studies are now needed to examine the effects of such preparation on the day of surgery. In addition, low reliabilities on the information subscale need to be addressed.

REFERENCES

Cassady, J. F., Jr., Wysocki, T. T., Miller, K. M., Cancel, D. D., & Izenberg, N. (1999). Use of a preanesthetic video for facilitation of parental education and anxiolysis before pediatric ambulatory surgery. *Anesthesia & Analgesia, 88,* 246–250.

Miller, K. M., Wysocki, T., Cassady, J. F., Cancel, O., & Izenberg, N. (1999). Validation of measures of parents' preoperative anxiety and anesthesia knowledge. *Anesthesia Analgesia, 88,* 251–257.

Moerman, N., vanDam, F. S. A. M., Muller, M. J., & Oosting, H. (1996). The Amsterdam Preoperative Anxiety and Information Scale (APAIS). *Anesthesia & Analgesia, 82,* 445–451.

THE AMSTERDAM PREOPERATIVE ANXIETY
AND INFORMATION SCALE (APAIS)

1.   I am worried about the anesthetic.

2.   The anesthetic is on my mind continually.

3.   I would like to know as much as possible about the anesthetic.

4.   I am worried about the procedure.

5.   The procedure is on my mind continually.

6.   I would like to know as much as possible about the procedure.

The measure of agreement with these statements should be graded on a 5-point Likert scale from 1 = not at all to 5 = extremely.

From: Moermann, Nelly van Dam, Frits S. A. M., Muller, Martin J., & Oosting, Hans. (1996). The Amsterdam Preoperative Anxiety and Information Scale (APAIS). *Anesthesia Analgesia, 82,* 445–451. Lippincott, Williams, & Wilkins ©. Used with permission.

76. Perceived Personal Control Questionnaire

Developed by Michal Berkenstadt, Shoshana Shiloh, Gad Barkai, Mariassa Bat-Miriam Katznelson, and Bolesslav Goldman

INSTRUMENT DESCRIPTION, ADMINISTRATION, AND SCORING GUIDELINES

Perceived personal control is thought to be an important outcome of genetic counseling because it has been found to be central to coping with health threats and to adapting to a broad spectrum of health problems. A definition of personal control is the belief that one has at one's disposal a response that can influence the aversiveness of an event. Genetic counseling can be regarded as a control-enhancing intervention (Shiloh, Berkenstadt, Miran, Katznelson, & Goldman, 1997).

The Perceived Personal Control questionnaire (PPC) asks counselees their perception of how much control they believe they have about their genetic problem. The scale is made up of nine items representing three dimensions of control: cognitive, behavioral, and decisional. A total score and three subscales ranging from 0–2 represent the sum of raw scores divided by the number of questions (Berkenstadt, Shiloh, Barkai, Katznelson, & Goldman, 1997).

PSYCHOMETRIC PROPERTIES

The reliability (Cronbach's alpha) of the total PPC was .86. Factor analysis yielded the three predetermined scales (cognitive, behavioral, and decisional), thus validating the structure of the PPC concept.

Although no control group was involved, comparisons of mean PPC scores before and after counseling showed significant increase on all subscales and on total score, supporting its sensitivity to intervention. Study of interventions designed to increase perceptions of control would further clarify the relationship. Higher postcounseling PPC was found among counselees who had been given a definite diagnosis and a specific recurrence risk, and had been offered prenatal diagnosis. Postcounseling PPC also correlated with knowledge, satisfaction, counseling evaluations, and expectation fulfillment. The most significant predictor of PPC was the possibility to determine a recurrence risk of the problem in future pregnancies. All of these findings are in the expected direction (Berkenstadt, Shiloh, Barkai, Katznelson, & Goldman, 1999).

CRITIQUE AND SUMMARY

Most empirical studies of the outcomes of genetic counseling focus on measures of learning such as recall of diagnosis and recurrence risk presented in counseling and to decisions reached after counseling. The authors correctly assert that these outcomes only partially cover the goals and impacts of genetic counseling on counselees' adjustments to their genetic problems. Additional studies are needed to validate the scale's clinical power and to reveal more factors that influence the degree of PPC gained in counseling. The authors' goal is to develop PPC to become a standard tool for enabling comparisons of counseling methods and populations (Berkenstadt, Shiloh, Barkai, Katznelson, & Goldman, 1999).

REFERENCES

Berkenstadt, M., Shiloh, S., Barkai, G., Katznelson, M., & Goldman, B. (1999). Perceived personal control (PPC): A new concept in measuring outcome of genetic counseling. *American Journal of Medical Genetics, 82,* 53–59.

Shiloh, S., Berkenstadt, M., Miran, N., Katznelson, M. B., & Goldman, B. (1997). Mediating effects of perceived control in coping with a health threat: The case of genetic counseling. *Journal of Applied Social Psychology, 27,* 1146–1173.

PERCEIVED PERSONAL CONTROL QUESTIONNAIRE

To what extent do you agree with the following statements?

$$0 \;=\; \text{DO NOT AGREE}$$
$$1 \;=\; \text{SOMEWHAT AGREE}$$
$$2 \;=\; \text{COMPLETELY AGREE}$$

_____ I think I understand what problem brought me to genetic counseling.

_____ I feel I know the meaning of the problem for my and my family's future.

_____ I think I know what caused the problem.

_____ I feel I have the tools to make decisions that will influence my future.

_____ I feel I can make a logical evaluation of the various options available to me in order to choose one of them.

_____ I feel I can make decisions that will change my family's future.

_____ I feel there are certain things I can do to prevent the problem from recurring.

_____ I feel I know what to do to ease the situation.

_____ I think I know what should be my next steps.

From Berkenstadt, M., Shiloh, S., Barkai, G., Katznelson, M., & Goldman, B. (1999). Perceived personal control (PPC): A new concept in measuring outcome of genetic counseling. *American Journal of Medical Genetics, 82,* 53–59. Reprinted by permission of Wiley-Liss, Inc., a subsidiary of John Wiley & Sons, Inc.

77. Macular Degeneration Self-Efficacy Scale

Developed by Barbara L. Brody, Rebecca A. Williams, Ronald B. Thomas, Robert M. Kaplan, Ray M. Chu, and Stuart I. Brown

INSTRUMENT DESCRIPTION, ADMINISTRATION, AND SCORING GUIDELINES

One out of five persons age 65 or older can expect to have some vision loss as a result of age-related macular degeneration, making it the leading cause of incurable blindness and low vision in older adults. Because the negative impact of the disease occurs in patients who still retain functional vision, a self-management program focused on increased self-efficacy (SE) could be expected to be effective.

The 14 items on the Macular Degeneration Self-Efficacy Scale (MDSES) are rated on a scale from 1 to 100 with high scores indicating confidence in accomplishing the task related to vision loss (Brody et al., 1999).

PSYCHOMETRIC PROPERTIES

Previous research has revealed that people with low vision may be isolated and experience decreased activity. The current study involved elderly persons with age-related macular degeneration (AMD). Factor analysis identified three subscales: knowledge SE, activity SE, and communication SE. Alphas for the total and subscales ranged from .60–.74, test–retest reliability for the total score over 2 days = .84, and over 6 weeks = .89. Test–retest reliability for the subscales ranged from .79–.88 over 2 days and .59 for the activity SE subscale to .83 for the knowledge SE subscale over 6 weeks (Brody et al., 1999).

Validity of the MDSES was supported by significant improvement in mood, increase in number of vision aids used, and increase in some activities among those receiving the intervention; this would be expected by SE theory. MDSES was sensitive to an intervention designed specifically to build SE in comparison with waitlisted controls randomly assigned. This intervention included cognitive elements, behavioral skills training, and modeling of adaptive behaviors (Brody et al., 1999).

CRITIQUE AND SUMMARY

The progressive deterioration of vision caused by macular degeneration causes great distress, and since medical treatments to slow this disease are limited, training to optimize function and quality of life are important. SE theory-based interventions would be expected to be helpful. MDSES performance to date should be tested with larger and diverse samples (Brody et al., 1999).

REFERENCE

Brody, B. L., Williams, R. A., Thomas, R. G., Kaplan, R. M., Chu, R. M., & Brown, S. I. (1999). Age-related macular degeneration: A randomized clinical trial of a self-management intervention. *Annals of Behavioral Medicine, 21,* 322–329.

MACULAR DEGENERATION (AMD) SELF-EFFICACY QUESTIONNAIRE

Subject # _____   Interviewer _____   Interview Date _____

I will read to you a series of questions which will ask how certain you are under different circumstances. The answers you may select range from 1 to 100 with 1 being very uncertain and 100 being very certain.

Q1. How certain are you that you know what macular degeneration is?

1	10	20	30	40	50	60	70	80	90	100

Very Uncertain   Moderately Uncertain   Very Certain

Q2. How certain are you that you can explain what is known about macular degeneration to a relative or friend so they can better understand your condition?

1	10	20	30	40	50	60	70	80	90	100

Very Uncertain   Moderately Uncertain   Very Certain

Q3. If you cannot see the face of a friend clearly, how certain are you that you can comfortably ask for the friend's name?

1	10	20	30	40	50	60	70	80	90	100

Very Uncertain   Moderately Uncertain   Very Certain

Q4. How certain are you that you can maintain a simple exercise program which is tailored to your needs?

1	10	20	30	40	50	60	70	80	90	100

Very Uncertain   Moderately Uncertain   Very Certain

Q5. How certain are you that you can comfortably communicate questions or concerns about your macular degeneration to your doctor?

1	10	20	30	40	50	60	70	80	90	100

Very Uncertain   Moderately Uncertain   Very Certain

Q6. How certain are you that you can find out where to get more information about services for people with low vision?

1	10	20	30	40	50	60	70	80	90	100

Very Uncertain   Moderately Uncertain   Very Certain

Q7. How certain are you that you can find transportation to an appointment or event whenever you need to?

1	10	20	30	40	50	60	70	80	90	100

Very Uncertain   Moderately Uncertain   Very Certain

Q8. How certain do you feel that you can call someone on the phone for any reason? (or can you use the telephone?)

1	10	20	30	40	50	60	70	80	90	100

Very Uncertain   Moderately Uncertain   Very Certain

Q9. How certain are you that you know about most of the different types of low-vision aids that are available?

1	10	20	30	40	50	60	70	80	90	100

Very Uncertain   Moderately Uncertain   Very Certain

Q10. How certain are you that you can comfortably leave your house on your own?

1	10	20	30	40	50	60	70	80	90	100

Very Uncertain   Moderately Uncertain   Very Certain

Q11. How certain are you that you can get involved in some new activities such as cultural events or recreation, for example?

1	10	20	30	40	50	60	70	80	90	100

Very Uncertain   Moderately Uncertain   Very Certain

Q12. How certain are you that you can maintain contact with persons with macular degeneration who share similar interests as yourself?

1	10	20	30	40	50	60	70	80	90	100

Very Uncertain   Moderately Uncertain   Very Certain

Q13. How certain are you that you can feel comfortable participating in a social gathering with a few friends? (How many people?)

1	10	20	30	40	50	60	70	80	90	100

Very Uncertain   Moderately Uncertain   Very Certain

Q14. How certain are you that you can participate in some of the same hobbies and activities you enjoyed before you developed macular degeneration?

1	10	20	30	40	50	60	70	80	90	100

Very Uncertain   Moderately Uncertain   Very Certain

Macular Degeneration (AMD) Self-Efficacy Questionnaire Scoring

There are three subscales:

$$\text{Knowledge} = \frac{q1 + q2 + q6 + q9 + q12}{5}$$

$$\text{Communication} = \frac{q5 + q7 + q10 + q11 + q14}{5}$$

$$\text{Activities} = \frac{q3 + q4 + q8 + q13}{4}$$

$$\text{TOTAL SCORE} = \frac{q1 \text{ through } q14}{14}$$

78.   COPD Self-Efficacy Scale

Developed by Joan K. Wigal, Thomas L. Creer, and Harry Kotses

INSTRUMENT DESCRIPTION, ADMINISTRATION, AND SCORING GUIDELINES

The episodic bouts of severe shortness of breath that many patients with chronic obstructive pulmonary disease (COPD) have frequently lead them to lose confidence in their ability to undertake certain activities without experiencing dyspnea, even though they may be physically able to do so. This avoidance hinders their ability to successfully manage activities of daily living as well as leisure time physical activities.

The COPD Self-Efficacy Scale (CSES) provides a list of activities the person with COPD rates according to the level of confidence that she can manage without breathing difficulty. Its purpose is to identify areas of poor SE and to assess changes in SE during activities of daily living (Zimmerman, Brown, & Bowman, 1996).

Scores are obtained by adding item responses for each subscale to obtain a total score and dividing by the number of items to obtain a mean score. Higher scores mean more confidence in ability to manage or avoid breathing difficulties in the situations presented.

PSYCHOMOTOR PROPERTIES

Internal consistency reliability was .95, and for the five subscales identified through factor analysis: negative affect = .95, intense emotional arousal = .90, physical exertion = .89, weather or environment = .87, and behavioral risk factors = .74. Test–retest reliability was = .77 (Wigal, Creer, & Kotses, 1991). CSES has been shown to be sensitive to participation in a group self-management program (Zimmerman, Brown, & Bowman, 1996) and an outpatient rehabilitation program which included education and exercise training in methods known to increase SE. Neither of these studies included a control group. In the latter, higher CSES scores were positively correlated with lowered perceptions of dyspnea and greater distances walked in twelve minutes (Scherer & Schmeider, 1997). Tu and colleagues (1997) found a strong correlation between CSES and a measure of mastery of COPD.

CRITIQUE AND SUMMARY

Participation in self-management programs that increase areas of low SE identified by CSES may help patients sustain functional levels (Zimmerman, Brown, & Bowman, 1996). Subsequent users depended on initial psychometric work; it should be studied on other diverse populations.

REFERENCES

Scherer, Y. K., & Schmider, L. E. (1997). The effect of a pulmonary rehabilitation program on self-efficacy perception of dyspnea and physical endurance. *Heart & Lung, 26,* 15–22.

Tu, S., McDonell, M. B., Spertus, J. A., Steel, B. G., & Fihn, S. D. (1997). A new self-administered questionnaire to monitor health-related quality of life in patients with COPD. *Chest, 112,* 614–622.

Wigal, J. K., Creer, T. L., & Kotses, H. (1991). The COPD Self-Efficacy Scale. *Chest, 99,* 1193–1196.

Zimmerman, B. W., Brown, S. T., & Bowman, J. M. (1996). A self-management program for chronic obstructive pulmonary disease: Relationship to dyspnea and self-efficacy. *Rehabilitation Nursing, 21,* 253–257.

THE COPD SELF-EFFICACY SCALE

Read each numbered item below, and determine how confident you are that you could manage breathing difficulty or avoid breathing difficulty in that situation. Use the following scale as a basis for your answers:

(a) = Very confident
(b) = Pretty confident
(c) = Somewhat confident
(d) = Not very confident
(e) = Not at all confident

(I)   1. When I become too tired.

(W)   2. When there is humidity in the air.

(W)   3. When I go into cold weather from a warm place.

(I)   4. When I experience emotional stress or become upset.

(P)   5. When I go up stairs too fast.

(N)   6. When I try to deny that I have respiratory difficulties.

(W)   7. When I am around cigarette smoke.

(I)   8. When I become angry.

(P)   9. When I exercise or physically exert myself.

(I)   10. When I feel distressed about my life.

(N) 11. When I feel sexually inadequate or important.

(N) 12. When I am frustrated.

(P) 13. When I lift heavy objects.

(I)   14. When I begin to feel that someone is out to get me.

(I)   15. When I yell or scream.

(N) 16. When I am lying in bed.

(W) 17. During very hot or very cold weather.

(I)   18. When I laugh a lot.

(B) 19. When I do not follow a proper diet.

(N) 20. When I feel helpless.

(N) 21. When I drink alcoholic beverages.

(W) 22. When I get an infection (throat, sinus, colds, the flu, etc.).

(N) 23. When I feel detached from everyone and everything.

(N) 24. When I experience anxiety.

(W) 25. When I am around pollution.

(B) 26. When I overeat.

(N) 27. When I feel down or depressed.

(B)   28. When I breathe improperly.

(P)   29. When I exercise in a room that is poorly ventilated.

(I)   30. When I am afraid.

(N)   31. When I experience the loss of a valued object or a loved one.

(N)   32. When there are problems in the home.

(N)   33. When I feel incompetent.

(P)   34. When I hurry or rush around.

Subscales:

N = Negative affect
I = Intense emotional arousal
P = Physical exertion
W = Weather/environment
B = Behavioral risk factors

From: Wigal, J. K., Creer, T. L., & Kotses, H. (1991). The COPD Self-Efficacy Scale. *Chest, 99,* 1193–1196. Used with permission.

79. Assessment of Information Provided

Developed by Jacqueline J. Medland and
Carol Estwing Ferrans

INSTRUMENT DESCRIPTION, ADMINISTRATION, AND SCORING GUIDELINES

It is well recognized that family members of intensive care unit (ICU) patients need information, and that it is essential to their satisfaction with care. Assessment of Information Provided (AIP) was developed to measure family members' perceptions of the information provided by nursing staff. Responses are summed with the lowest possible score being 29 and the highest, 174, the latter indicating respondents' information needs were well met (Medland & Ferrans, 1998).

PSYCHOMETRIC PROPERTIES

Authors indicate that items were based on an extensive literature review of the information needs of family members of ICU patients, supporting content validity. Internal consistency reliability was .94–.96. The instrument was sensitive to a structured communication intervention in which the nurse had a discussion with a family 24 hours postadmission, providing a pamphlet and daily phone notification regarding the patient's condition. Change in the control group's scores (occasionally given a less comprehensive ICU information pamphlet, report from ward clerk for telephone inquiries as fair, serious, or critical sometimes augmented by discussion with nurse) were not statistically significant. In addition, the number of calls received from control group family members was significantly greater than those received from family members in the experimental group, and their satisfaction was lower, supporting validity of AIP (Medland & Ferrans, 1998).

CRITIQUE AND SUMMARY

More structured description of content validity would be helpful as would other evidence of validity. In addition, AIP has been developed and used in only one medical ICU (Medland & Ferrans, 1998).

REFERENCE

Medland, J. J., & Ferrans, C. E. (1998). Effectiveness of a structured communication program for family members of patients in an ICU. *American Journal of Critical Care, 7*, 24–29.

ASSESSMENT OF INFORMATION PROVIDED (AIP)

Each of the following statements are regarding information given to you by the nurses about your relative in the Intensive Care Unit. Choose the answer that best describes how you feel about the statement. PLEASE ANSWER ALL OF THE QUESTIONS. If none of the answers fit exactly, pick the answer that comes closest to how you feel. If the question asks about something that was not done, should it have been done?

Mark your answer by circling the number that corresponds to the column heading. *For example:* The waiting room had comfortable chairs. If you strongly disagree, circle number 1. If you moderately disagree, circle number 2.

The doctors, nurses, and staff in your unit will never see your answers or know what you've said. PLEASE GIVE YOUR HONEST ANSWERS. There are no right or wrong answers. BOTH POSITIVE AND NEGATIVE ANSWERS ARE HELPFUL TO US.

	Strongly Disagree	Moderately Disagree	Slightly Disagree	Slightly Agree	Moderately Agree	Strongly Agree
1. The nurse seemed knowledgeable.	1	2	3	4	5	6
2. The nurse found someone to answer my questions when she was unable to.	1	2	3	4	5	6
3. The nurse assured me that I would be notified of any changes in my relative's condition.	1	2	3	4	5	6
4. The nurse gave us suggestions on what to do at my relative's bedside. (For example, you may hold his/her hand.)	1	2	3	4	5	6
5. The nurse gave me specific facts about my relative's progress.	1	2	3	4	5	6
6. The nurse assured me that the best possible care was being given to my relative.	1	2	3	4	5	6

(continued)

405

	Strongly Disagree	Moderately Disagree	Slightly Disagree	Slightly Agree	Moderately Agree	Strongly Agree
7. The nurse told me exactly what was being done for my relative.	1	2	3	4	5	6
8. The nurse informed me daily of my relative's condition.	1	2	3	4	5	6
9. The nurse answered my questions.	1	2	3	4	5	6
10. The nurse seemed to answer my questions honestly.	1	2	3	4	5	6
11. The nurse explained medical terms in a way I could understand.	1	2	3	4	5	6
12. The nurse talked *with* me, not *at* me.	1	2	3	4	5	6
13. The nurse told me why things were being done for my relative.	1	2	3	4	5	6
14. The nurse explained the equipment being used for my relative.	1	2	3	4	5	6
15. The nurse provided me with the Intensive Care Unit's phone number.	1	2	3	4	5	6
16. The nurse informed me of other support service available in the hospital (e.g., chaplain).	1	2	3	4	5	6
17. The nurse and the doctor gave me similar information regarding my relative.	1	2	3	4	5	6
18. The nurse arranged for the physician to speak to me.	1	2	3	4	5	6
19. If I was not allowed to visit during the posted visiting hours, the nurse explained why not.	1	2	3	4	5	6
20. The nurse explained the reason for limited visiting hours.	1	2	3	4	5	6

	Strongly Disagree	Moderately Disagree	Slightly Disagree	Slightly Agree	Moderately Agree	Strongly Agree
21. The nurse provided me with an information booklet about the unit.	1	2	3	4	5	6
22. The nurse encouraged questions from me.	1	2	3	4	5	6
23. The nurse explained information given to me by the doctor.	1	2	3	4	5	6
24. The nurse tried to find out what I knew about my relative's condition before she explained new information to me.	1	2	3	4	5	6
25. The nurse caring for my relative introduced herself to me.	1	2	3	4	5	6
26. The nurse made herself available to answer questions.	1	2	3	4	5	6
27. The nurse allowed an adequate amount of time to speak with me regarding my relative.	1	2	3	4	5	6
28. I felt comfortable talking with the nurse.	1	2	3	4	5	6
29. The nurse never made me seem like a burden when I phoned or asked questions.	1	2	3	4	5	6

80. Benign Prostatic Hyperplasia Knowledge Questionnaire

Developed by Michael J. Barry, Daniel Cherkin, Yu Chiao Chang, Floyd J. Fowler, Jr., and Steven Skates

INSTRUMENT DESCRIPTION, ADMINISTRATION, AND SCORING GUIDELINES

Men with benign prostatic hyperplasia (BPH) face a choice of "watchful waiting" or active medical or surgical treatment. The BPH Knowledge Questionnaire (BPH Knowledge) was developed as one outcome measure of a prospective randomized trial of a shared decision-making program. Correct responses are scored +1, incorrect −1, and "not sure" 0. Total score range is −20 to +20 (Barry, Cherkin, Chang, Fowler, & Skates, 1997).

PSYCHOMETRIC PROPERTIES

BPH Knowledge was developed by a professional expert panel. Cronbach's alpha was .68. Criterion validity was supported by the fact that nurses had a significantly higher mean score than did patients. Sensitivity of the instrument is supported by the fact that the experimental group receiving a computer and interactive video shared decision making program had a significantly higher knowledge score than did control patients who received a brochure (Barry, Cherkin, Chang, Fowler, & Skates, 1997), supporting sensitivity of the instrument.

CRITIQUE AND SUMMARY

Subjects in this single study at one institution were predominantly Caucasian and well educated; BPH Knowledge should be tested in other groups. While only preliminary information on psychometric properties is available, the potential impact of a correct knowledge base from which to approach shared decision making should be clinically relevant and justifies further testing of the instrument.

REFERENCE

Barry, M. J., Cherkin, D., Chang, Y. C., Fowler, F. J., & Skates, S. (1997). A randomized trial of a multimedia shared decision making program for men facing a treatment decision for benign prostatic hypertrophy. *Disease Management & Clinical Outcomes, 1,* 5–14.

BPH KNOWLEDGE QUESTIONNAIRE

(F) 1. The prostate is a small gland that helps purify the urine.

(T) 2. Symptoms of benign prostatic hyperplasia (BPH) can become less bothersome over time without treatment.

(T) 3. An enlarged prostate gland can cause a change in urination, such as a weak urine stream.

(F) 4. Men bothered by uncomplicated BPH generally have a choice between prostate surgery and simply following their condition with their doctor ("watchful waiting").

(F) 5. Most men with benign prostatic hyperplasia (BPH) who decide against surgery are treated with drugs.

(T) 6. When a man cannot urinate at all due to a large prostate, a tube must be passed through the penis into the bladder to drain the urine.

(F) 7. The standard prostate operation for BPH lowers your future risk of prostate cancer.

(T) 8. Men with BPH who choose not to have prostate surgery should see their doctors once a year or so to check on the condition of their prostate.

(F) 9. Most men have persistent trouble with dripping urine or wet pants after prostate surgery.

(T) 10. Some men who have prostate surgery for BPH eventually need another operation because the prostate tissue grows back over time.

(F) 11. Most sexually active men have difficulty getting sexual erections after surgery for benign prostatic hyperplasia (BPH).

(T) 12. Retrograde ejaculation means the semen goes into the bladder during a sexual climax.

(F) 13. Only a few men who have prostate surgery have retrograde ejaculation after the operation.

Response frame for questions 1–13:
1 True   2 False   3 Not sure

14. When your doctor checks the prostate gland with a gloved finger, he or she can:
    ① Feel some prostate cancers
    2 Check the kidneys
    3 Both of the above
    4 Not sure

15. Benign prostatic hyperplasia (BPH) occasionally causes:
    1 Damage to the kidneys
    2 Damage to the bladder
    ③ Both of the above
    4 Not sure

16. Men who have benign prostatic hyperplasia (BPH) have a higher risk of which of the following conditions:
    1 Prostate cancer
    ② Urinary tract infections
    3 Both of the above
    4 Not sure

17. The main purpose of surgery for benign prostatic hyperplasia (BPH) is:
    ① To reduce bothersome urinary symptoms
    2 To reduce the risk of death from BPH
    3 To find small prostate cancers
    4 Not sure

(continued)

18. Men who have small prostate cancers found when an operation is done for BPH:
    1 Almost always need to be treated
    ② Usually do *not* die from prostate cancer
    3 Both of the above
    4 Not sure

19. Some men who follow "watchful waiting" for their prostate condition:
    1 Will eventually need an operation because they can't urinate at all
    2 Will eventually need an operation because their symptoms get worse
    ③ Both of the above
    4 Not sure

20. The most common kind of prostate surgery requires:
    1 An incision (a cut) made in the abdomen (belly)
    ② A lighted scope passed through the penis
    3 Both of the above
    4 Not sure

From: Barry, M. J., Cherkin, D., Chang, Y. C., Fowler, F. J., & Skates, S. (1997). A randomized trial of a multimedia shared decision making program for men facing a treatment decision for benign prostatic hyperplasia. *Disease Management & Clinical Outcomes, 1,* 5–14. Used with permission.

Correct answers are indicated.

81. Knowledge About Schizophrenia Questionnaire

Developed by Haya Ascher-Svanum

INSTRUMENT DESCRIPTION, ADMINISTRATION, AND SCORING GUIDELINES

The Knowledge About Schizophrenia Questionnaire (KASQ) was developed to assess patients' knowledge about their illness and its management. Patient education focusing on these issues is becoming more prevalent due to growing emphasis on psychosocial rehabilitation and the standards mandated by the Joint Commission on Accreditation of Healthcare Organizations (JCAHO) (Ascher-Svanum, 1999).

Correct answers are summed, with a total possible score of 25. A study of patients in didactic and decision forms of patient education found mean scores pre- and post-intervention between 13 and 19 (Ascher-Svanum & Whitesel, 1999).

PSYCHOMETRIC PROPERTIES

Items were developed to reflect content areas covered in a psychoeducation program for patients diagnosed as having schizophrenia and judged by four educators as having done so. Content focuses on diagnosis and medical management of schizophrenia, including its prevalence, etiology, course, prognosis, nondrug treatment, stress factors, and legal issues.

KASQ was tested with 136 adult inpatients with a diagnosis of schizophrenia or schizoaffective disorder and who were prescribed antipsychotic medications. Studies with subgroups found coefficient alpha of .89 and .85 and test–retest reliability coefficient over three weeks of .83. In two small studies KASQ was found to be sensitive to instruction while the control group's mean scores did not change significantly (Ascher-Svanum, 1999). A significant association has been found between educational level and gaining at least twenty percent on the KASQ score, which indicates some support for validity (Ascher-Svanum & Whitesel, 1999).

CRITIQUE AND SUMMARY

Because KASQ was initially constructed to evaluate a particular educational program, investigation of its content validity and thus its wider usability remains to be completed. Description of outcome behaviors desired and obtained in the educational program were not detailed in the published sources describing development and use of KASQ.

REFERENCES

Ascher-Svanum, H. (1999). Development and validation of a measure of patients' knowledge about schizophrenia. *Psychiatric Services, 50,* 561–563.

Ascher-Svanum, H., & Whitesel, J. (1999). A randomized controlled study of two styles of group patient education about schizophrenia. *Psychiatric Services, 50,* 926–930.

THE KNOWLEDGE ABOUT SCHIZOPHRENIA QUESTIONNAIRE (KASQ)

1. How many people have schizophrenia?
   a. One person in every 1,000.
   b. One person in every 100.
   c. Two persons in every 10.
   d. Twenty persons in every 100.

2. How do we know if someone has schizophrenia?
   a. By asking the person about unusual thoughts, delusions, hallucinations, or if he/she feels like things are no longer real.
   b. By taking X-rays of the head (like CT scan).
   c. By determining whether the person is working or not.
   d. By using special blood tests.
   e. All of the above.

3. Which areas of a patient's life does schizophrenia affect?
   a. Thinking.
   b. Feeling.
   c. Behaving.
   d. None of the above.
   e. All of the above.

4. A delusion is:
   a. Seeing things that are not really there.
   b. Not a symptom of schizophrenia.
   c. A feeling of sadness.
   d. A belief that seems very real even though it is totally false and not shared by other people.

5. A visual hallucination is:
   a. Not a symptom of schizophrenia.
   b. Seeing things that are not really there.
   c. A type of delusion.
   d. A symptom that psychiatry cannot treat.

6. Which of the following is a possible cause of schizophrenia?
   a. Being mistreated by a parent in childhood.
   b. Receiving poor education.
   c. A disorder of brain chemistry combined with life stressors.
   d. None of the above.

7. A person with schizophrenia:
   a. Can be rapidly cured by hypnosis.
   b. Will always experience a worsening of the illness over a lifetime.
   c. Is very likely to be helped by the right medicines.
   d. Will get better eventually without help.

8. Schizophrenia is:
   a. Like having multiple personalities.

(continued)

    b.   A mental illness that causes people to become confused and have difficulty deciding what is real.
    c.   Likely to be caused by using LSD or marijuana.
    d.   A contagious disease.
    e.   All of the above.

  9. Which of the following makes schizophrenia worse?
    a.   Stress with family members.
    b.   Having nothing to do with one's free time.
    c.   Taking street drugs.
    d.   Drinking alcohol.
    e.   All of the above.

10. Common side effects of antipsychotic drugs are:
    a.   Drowsiness.
    b.   Sensitivity to sunburn.
    c.   Restless legs or shakiness.
    d.   All of the above.
    e.   None of the above.

11. Ways of coping with and reducing side effects include:
    a.   Waiting awhile.
    b.   Reducing the dosage on doctor's advice.
    c.   Changing to a medication without the annoying side effects on the doctor's advice.
    d.   All of the above.
    e.   None of the above.

12. A person suffering from schizophrenia nearly always has:
    a.   Difficulty deciding what is real and what is not real.
    b.   An abnormal heart beat.
    c.   A fear of heights.
    d.   A tendency to behave violently.
    e.   Two or more personalities.

13. A person suffering from schizophrenia:
    a.   Sees things that others do not see.
    b.   Hears voices when there is nobody around.
    c.   Believes that thoughts are being put into his/her mind by other people.
    d.   Believes that he/she is someone very important (like Jesus, Virgin Mary).
    e.   All of the above.

14. A person with schizophrenia who is under pressure should:
    a.   Take an extra dose of medication (without consulting the doctor).
    b.   Spend several days in bed and rest.
    c.   Discuss his/her difficulties with a doctor or therapist.
    d.   Ignore it because time will heal all problems.

15. Which is the most important treatment of schizophrenia?
    a.   Electro-shock treatment (ECT).
    b.   Medication.
    c.   Occupational therapy.
    d.   Recreational therapy.

16. Antipsychotic medications do not cure schizophrenia, but they do:
    a.   Damage the brain.

    b. Result in addiction to the drug.

    c. Take all your problems away.

    d. Help control the symptom of the illness.

17. What are the chances of complete recovery from schizophrenia?

    a. 100 percent.

    b. 0 percent.

    c. 33 percent.

    d. 50 percent.

18. Which symptoms of schizophrenia tend not to be improved by antipsychotics?

    a. Feeling bored.

    b. Hallucinations.

    c. Delusions.

    d. Problems in thinking.

19. Antipsychotics are known to be:

    a. Easy to overdose on, possibly resulting in death.

    b. Addictive over time.

    c. Unsafe medications.

    d. Effective in controlling symptoms of schizophrenia.

20. If an adult psychiatric patient is committed by court (temporary or regular commitment), he or she:

    a. Can give a 24-hour notice and then leave the hospital.

    b. Cannot refuse psychiatric treatment.

    c. Can refuse treatment but first needs to petition the court about it.

    d. Is more likely to receive electro-shock treatment (ECT).

21. An adult who is admitted voluntarily to the psychiatric hospital:

    a. Has very few legal rights.

    b. Has no right to refuse psychiatric treatment.

    c. Cannot be placed in seclusion or restraint.

    d. Can leave the hospital 24 hours after his/her request reaches the hospital's superintendent.

22. Electro-shock therapy (ECT) is rarely used in the treatment of schizophrenia, but when it is used, it is:

    a. Very painful.

    b. Painless and safe.

    c. Very time-consuming and much slower to help than medicines.

    d. Quite unsafe.

23. Tardive Dyskinesia is:

    a. A type of skin problem.

    b. A type of medicine for schizophrenia.

    c. A very rare but serious side effect of antipsychotic medicines.

    d. A problem of all people with schizophrenia.

24. If a person who has been diagnosed with schizophrenia continues to take medicines as prescribed by the doctor, he or she:

    a. Is likely to have more severe symptoms during a relapse (recurrence of the illness).

    b. Does not change at all the chances of being rehospitalized for schizophrenia.

(continued)

    c.   Is more likely to be rehospitalized because of medicine's side effects.

    d.   Double the chances of staying out of the hospital (of not having a relapse).

25. Persons with schizophrenia are more likely to have:
    a.   A close relative with schizophrenia.
    b.   A punitive and domineering mother.
    c.   Allergic reactions to starches and sweets.
    d.   Fear of heights.

Answers: 1B; 2A; 3E; 4D; 5B; 6C; 7C; 8B; 9E; 10D; 11D; 12A; 13E; 14C; 15B; 16D; 17C; 18A; 19D; 20C; 21D; 22B; 23C; 24D; 25A.

82. Eating Styles Questionnaire

Developed by Margaret K. Hargreaves, David G. Schlundt, Maciej S. Buchowski, Robert E. Hardy, Susan R. Rossi, and Joseph S. Rossi

INSTRUMENT DEVELOPMENT, ADMINISTRATION, AND SCORING GUIDELINES

The purpose of the Eating Styles Questionnaire (ESQ) is to represent behaviors associated with reduced fat dietary intake. This issue is of particular concern with African-American populations, who have been found to preferentially select high-fat, low-fiber diets. Changing these diets may decrease this population's risk for diabetes, hypertension, and some cancers. The authors believe ESQ is culturally sensitive. Its format also allows people to see the changes they have already made and those necessary to further lower fat intake.

ESQ is scored by summing the ratings across the 16 items; scores can range from 16 to 80 (Hargreaves et al., 1999).

PSYCHOMETRIC PROPERTIES

ESQ items were based on behaviors that best discriminated between groups far along in changing their eating behaviors and those who were not contemplating change. The instrument was tested on a well-educated, middle-aged, middle-income population of African-American women. Mean ESQ score for this population was 47 + or minus 12.6. Coefficient alpha for the total score was .90. The correlation between ESQ total score and percentage of energy from fat was −.65 and with fiber intake −.40, representing good validity for prediction of dietary fat and moderate validity for dietary fiber (Hargreaves et al., 1999).

Also supportive of validity is the fact that groups at various stages of change according to the transtheoretical model (TTM) differed significantly on total ESQ score and on 14 of the 16 items. TTM posits that individuals pass through five stages of change in adopting healthful behaviors: precontemplation (no intention to change), contemplation (seriously considering change), preparation (taking steps to change), action (actively involved in meaningful change), and maintenance (maintaining meaningful change). Assigning individuals correctly to stage of change is important because each stage requires different interventions to move the individual to the next stage. An ESQ cutoff score of 50 was used to assign the participant to the preparation stage and a score of 57 to the action stage (Hargreaves et al., 1999).

CRITIQUE AND SUMMARY

Apparently testing of the sensitivity of ESQ and its tie to TTM with varying interventions is not yet available. Within this model ESQ is particularly important because it provides a more objective way to describe actual behavior than does asking individuals to indicate their stage of change regarding dietary fat and fiber. Whether the ESQ will prove a useful tool in applying TTM to other population groups in different geographic regions is not known, and cutoff scores would also need to be studied in these populations.

Studies of the usefulness of ESQ with other theoretical models of behavior change could not be located.

REFERENCE

Hargreaves, M. K., Schlundt, D. G., Buchowski, M. S., Hardy, R. E., Rossi, S. R., & Rossi, J. S. (1999). Stages of change and the intake of dietary fat in African-American women: Improving stage assessment using the Eating Styles Questionnaire. *Journal of the American Dietetic Association, 99,* 1392–1399.

EATING STYLES QUESTIONNAIRE

How often does each statement describe your behavior?

	Never (1)	Rarely (2)	Sometimes (3)	Usually (4)	Always (5)
1. I avoid eating hamburgers, fried chicken, french fries, and other high-fat foods at fast-food restaurants.					
2. When I eat at a restaurant, I look for low-fat foods to order.					
3. I choose snack foods that are low in fat or fat free.					
4. When I want to eat meat, I choose baked, broiled, or boiled chicken without skin instead of red meat.					
5. I avoid eating red meat (beef, ham, liver, or pork).					
6. When I eat red meat (beef, hamburgers, ham, hot dogs, or pork), I choose lean cuts or trim off the fat (answer always if you never eat red meat).					
7. When I eat lunch meats (bologna, sliced ham, sliced turkey, salami), I often choose cuts that are low in fat or fat free (answer always if you never eat lunch meats).					
8. I avoid using butter, margarine, gravy, regular mayonnaise, and salad dressings made with oil.					
9. I eat 5 or more servings of fruits and vegetables every day.					
10. When I have a choice between a regular product and one that is low in fat or fat free, I choose the low-fat or fat free product.					
11. When I buy dairy products (milk, yogurt, cheese, ice cream), I buy items that are low in fat or fat free.					
12. I eat a serving of bread, rolls, bagels, rice, pasta, grits, oatmeal, or cereal at every meal.					

(continued)

	Never (1)	Rarely (2)	Sometimes (3)	Usually (4)	Always (5)
13. I eat a green salad every day.					
14. When I eat greens and other vegetables, I never use fatback, butter, or other fats for seasoning.					
15. When I eat grits, I avoid adding butter or margarine.					
16. I avoid eating nut breads, biscuits, or croissants and choose breads that are low in fat or fat free instead.					

From: Hargreaves, M. K., Schlundt, D. G., Buchowski, M. S., Hardy, R. E., Rossi, S. R., & Rossi, J. S. (1999). Stages of change and the intake of dietary fat in African-American women: Improving stage assignment using the Eating Styles Questionnaire. Reprinted by permission from *Journal of the American Dietetic Association, 99,* 1392–1399.

83.   Brief Medication Questionnaire

Developed by Bonnie L. Svarstad, Betty A. Chewning, Betsy L. Sleath, and Cecelia Claesson

INSTRUMENT DESCRIPTION, ADMINISTRATION, AND SCORING GUIDELINES

Patient lack of adherence to drug regimens is a widespread problem that is costly both economically and in terms of health outcomes. Because patients are reluctant to admit nonadherence unless clinicians make specific efforts to monitor it on a regular basis, screening tools are important. Accurate information about adherence is also important in targeting interventions, interpreting drug effects, and measuring the outcomes of patient education and disease management programs.

The Brief Medication Questionnaire (BMQ) is a self-report tool for screening adherence and barriers to adherence. It includes a 5-item Regimen Screen that asks patients how they took each medication in the past week scored 0 if the report indicates no nonadherence and 1 if it does. A 2-item Belief Screen asks about drug effects and bothersome features, both of which have been linked in past studies to nonadherence. Patients receive a score of 1 if they respond "not well" or "don't know" when asked how the medication works for them and if the medication is identified as bothersome. Item scores are summed with positive scores indicating one or more belief barriers (range 0–2).

A 2-item Recall Screen measures potential difficulties remembering all doses. Patients receive a score of 0 if they have a single dose regimen and report that it's not hard to remember all pills, 1 if they have a multiple dose regimen or report it is hard to remember all the pills, and 2 if both indicators are present. BMQ is designed to avoid known reporting errors.

PSYCHOMETRIC PROPERTIES

BMQ was studied with patients using catopril and enalapril. The Medication Event Monitoring System (MEMS) with a microprocessor in the bottle cap to record time and date of bottle opening was used as the "gold standard" of adherence measurement. A positive BMQ screen indicated the patient reported some nonadherence or barrier to adherence. A positive Regimen Screen had very good sensitivity and positive predictive value for repeat nonadherence but not for sporadic nonadherence. Similar findings were obtained for the Belief Screen. The Recall Screen had poor sensitivity for repeat nonadherence and good sensitivity with sporadic nonadherence. The reported rate of dose omission using the Regimen Screen was highly correlated with the MEMS recorded rate. These findings support validity of BMQ (Svarstad, Chewning, Sleath, & Claesson, 1999).

CRITIQUE AND SUMMARY

Initial work on BMQ validity is encouraging. Its approach demonstrates that sensitivity levels vary by type of nonadherence and type of screening tool. Sporadic nonadherence is usually unintended and infrequent, whereas repeat nonadherence probably reflects deliberate changes in the regimen made by patients who have unresolved concerns or doubts about the drug and how it is affecting them.

Larger studies in other settings are needed as is research to assess BMQ's ability to predict future behavior and to assess issues of interviewer reliability (Svarstad, Chewning, Sleath, & Claesson, 1999) and sensitivity to particular kinds of instructional/counseling interventions.

REFERENCE

Svarstad, B. L., Chewning, B. A., Sleath, B. L., & Claesson, C. (1999). The brief medication questionnaire: A tool for screening patient adherence and barriers to adherence. *Patient Education & Counseling, 37,* 113–124.

BRIEF MEDICATION QUESTIONNAIRE (PART A)

1. Please list below all of the medications you took in the PAST WEEK. For each medication you list, please answer each of the questions in the box below.

IN THE PAST WEEK:						
a. Medication name and strength	b. How many days did you take it?	c. How many times per day did you take it?	d. How many pills did you take each time?	e. How many times did you miss taking a pill?	f. For what reason were you taking it?	g. How well does the medicine work for you? 1 = well 2 = okay 3 = not well

_____ _____ _____ _____ _____ _____
_____ _____ _____ _____ _____ _____
_____ _____ _____ _____ _____ _____
_____ _____ _____ _____ _____ _____

2. Do any of your medications bother you in any way? YES _____ NO _____

   a. IF YES, please name the medication and check below how much it bothers you.

   How much did it bother you?

Medication name	A lot	Some	A little	Never	In what way did it bother you?
_____	____	____	____	____	_____
_____	____	____	____	____	_____
_____	____	____	____	____	_____

3. Below is a list of problems that people sometimes have with their medicines. Please check how hard it is for you to do each of the following:

	Very hard	Somewhat hard	Not hard at all	COMMENT (Which medicine)
a. *Open or close* the medication bottle	____	____	____	_____
b. *Read the print* on the bottle	____	____	____	_____
c. *Remember* to take all the pills	____	____	____	_____
d. *Get* your refills in time	____	____	____	_____
e. *Take so many pills* at the same time	____	____	____	_____

Scoring Procedures for BMQ Part A

Screen	Scoring

Regimen Screen (Questions 1a–1e)

Did R fail to list the prescribed drug in the initial (spontaneous) report?	1 = yes 0 = no
Did R stop or interrupt therapy due to a late refill or other reason?	1 = yes 0 = no
Did R report any missed days or doses?	1 = yes 0 = no
Did R reduce or cut down the prescribed amount per dose?	1 = yes 0 = no
Did R take any extra doses or more medication than prescribed?	1 = yes 0 = no
Did R report "don't know" in response to any questions?	1 = yes 0 = no
Did R refuse to answer any questions?	1 = yes 0 = no

NOTE: Score of ≥1 indicates positive screen for potential nonadherence.

Belief Screen (Questions 1g and 2–2a)

Did R report "not well" or "don't know" in response to Q 1g?	1 = yes 0 = no
Did R name the prescribed drug as a drug that bothers him/her?	1 = yes 0 = no

NOTE: Score of ≥1 indicates positive screen for belief barriers

Recall Screen (Questions 1c and 3c)

Did R receive a multiple dose regimen (2 or more times/day)?	1 = yes 0 = no
Did R report "very hard" or "somewhat hard" in response to Q 3c?	1 = yes 0 = no

NOTE: Score of ≥1 indicates positive screen for recall barriers

R= respondent.

Section I

Health Promotion, Disease Prevention, and Increasing Quality of Life

A small cluster of instruments can perhaps best be considered related to health promotion, disease prevention, and quality of life. Several instruments related to HIV are included in this section.

---

84.   Falls Efficacy Scale

Developed by Mary E. Tinetti, Donna Richman, and Lynda Powell

INSTRUMENT DEVELOPMENT, ADMINISTRATION, AND SCORING GUIDELINES

Falls Efficacy Scale (FES) was developed to measure fear of falling defined as "low perceived self-efficacy at avoiding falls during ten essential, nonhazardous activities of daily living." Fear of falling may result in a self-imposed decline in activity and function not necessitated by physical disability or injury. It occurs in 50% to 60% of elderly who have fallen as well as in those who have not, and deterioration in the physical ability to balance may result from activity restriction mediated through fear of falling (Powell & Myers, 1995). It is hoped that the scale may identify elderly persons likely to become dependent on family, friends, or agencies. Falls are the most prevalent form of injury among old people; 30% of community elderly persons fall each year. Falls and their sequelae represent one group of potentially modifiable factors contributing to functional decline (Tinetti, Mendes de Leon, Doucette, & Baker, 1994), and fear of falling or low confidence may represent a remediable independent contributor to functional decline (Tinetti & Powell, 1993).

The FES score is the sum of item scores (range from 0 to 100), with a lower score reflecting lower efficacy (Tinetti, Richman, & Powell, 1990).

PSYCHOMETRIC PROPERTIES

Items were generated by asking physical therapists, occupational therapists, rehabilitation nurses, and physicians to name the most important activities essential to independent living that would be safe and nonhazardous to most elderly persons. The consensus established in identifying these activities supported the validity of the items. In two pretests, the FES was administered to a total of 74 persons, with an average age of 79 years. Test–retest reliability was .71, and Cronbach's alpha .91. There was sufficient variability to suggest that the instrument may measure the continuum of self-imposed activity restriction among elderly fallers (Tinetti, Richman, & Powell, 1990).

The FES score was associated with a measure of relevant skills, such as gait, and with past experience, such as difficulty in getting up after a fall, both of which would be predicted by theory. Convergent validity of the instrument was suggested by the finding that total score increased progressively among respondents who denied fear of falling, those who acknowledged fear but denied avoiding activities, and those who reported avoiding activities. The same trend of increase in efficacy score was found among individual activities as well (Tinetti & Powell, 1993). In a second study of community-dwelling elderly, fall-related efficacy was a potent independent correlate of activities of daily living and physical functioning. This suggests that clinical programs should attempt simultaneously to improve physical skills and confidence (Tinetti et al., 1995).

Powell and Myers (1995) describe the development of the Activities-Specific Balance Confidence Scale, a more situation-specific measure of balance confidence than the FES, and which includes a wider continuum of activity difficulty and more detailed activity descriptors. Items include "reach at eye level" and "escalator not holding rail." These authors found a Cronbach's alpha of .90 for the FES administered to an independent sample of community-living seniors. Scores on the FES in this sample were more variable than in the study by Tinetti, Richman, and Powell (1990), where the range was restricted. Utility of the FES as a discriminative index was also supported based on significantly different scores in the expected direction, for high- and low-mobility groups. Mean score on the FES was 26.9 (*SD* 18.6), similar to a previously found mean score of 25.11 (*SD* 12.26). Taking a bath or shower was the item associated with the lowest self-efficacy. Scalability analysis supported the hierarchical nature of the FES (Tinetti, Richman, & Powell, 1990).

The FES has also been used in other studies including the multicenter trial Frailty and Injuries: Cooperative Studies of Intervention Techniques (FICSIT), modified to use a four-category scoring system because respondents had difficulty with the 10 levels of response categories (Buchner et al., 1993). FICSIT is a series of clinical trials of biomedical, behavioral, and environmental interventions to reduce the risks of frailty and fall-related injury among the elderly.

A study that is part of the FICSIT delivered a multifactorial intervention to reduce the risk of falling among elderly people living in the community. Because the risk of falling increased with the number of risk factors present, such a multifactorial strategy of risk abatement may decrease the risk of falling. After assessment of the risk factors, interventions including education about use of sedative-hypnotic agents, gait training, and training in transfer skills were given. The intervention group had significantly fewer falls with a longer time until the first fall than did the control group. The mean change in the scores on the FES differed significantly in favor of the intervention group. At reassessment 4 months later, a significantly smaller percentage of the intervention group than of the control group continued to use at least four prescription medications, to transfer unsafely to bathtub or toilet, or to have impairment in balance or gait, all being risk factors for falling. Thus, the FES was sensitive to an education program (Tinetti et al., 1995).

Several additions to FES and results of its use in interventions have been published in the past few years. Since FES incorporates only indoor activities, Hill and others (1996) added four outdoor activities as a subscale: using public transport, crossing roads, light gardening or hanging out the washing, and using front or rear steps at home. These activities are commonly reported by fallers as inducing greater fear of falling. The addition of these items from the Modified Falls Efficacy Scale (MFES) is expected to be helpful in identifying fear of falling in active community-dwelling older people. MFES demonstrated a Cronbach's alpha of .95 with the two subscales (indoor and outdoor activity) verified by factor analysis. Validity was also supported by significant differences in the expected direction on MFES by individuals referred to a falls and balance clinic and a healthy older group.

In an investigation of women (who are at greater risk of injury due to falls and are overrepresented in the senior population, Gill, Williams, Williams, and Hale (1998) added to the FES two items on stair climbing and descent and four items on getting back up and avoiding injury after a fall going up or down stairs. These additional items were called stair fall efficacy and had a Cronbach's alpha of .86. This expanded scale was one of several variables that distinguished fallers from nonfallers.

A randomized single-blind controlled trial testing the efficacy of a community-based group intervention showed reduction of fear of falling (and showed sensitivity of FES) and associated restrictions in activity levels among older adults in public housing. The intervention targeted fear of falling and included: restructuring misconceptions to promote a view of falls risk and fear of falls as controllable, setting realistic goals for increasing activity, changing the environment to decrease falls risk, and promoting physical exercise to increase strength and balance. Videotapes, lecture, group discussion, mutual problem solving, role playing, exercise training, assertiveness training, home assignments, and behavioral contracting were used—a potent instructional program although elements aimed at increased self-efficacy were not well identified. FES was modified to use a 1 (not at all sure) to 4 (very sure) scoring procedure and showed Cronbach alphas of .90–.93. The intervention was not associated with increased falls even though activity levels increased (Tennstedt et al., 1998).

Petrella, Payne, Myers, Overend, and Chesworth (2000) found the FES to be more sensitive to change than was the activities-specific Balance Confidence Scale in a prospective cohort study of a hip fracture rehabilitation program. And two prospective studies (Cumming, Salkeld, Thomas, & Szonyi, 2000; Mendes de Leon, Seeman, Baker, Richardson, & Tinetti, 1996) found that those with low FES had an increased risk of falling compared with those with high FES scores, and greater declines in ability to perform ADLs. Among nonfallers, being afraid of falling was predictive of admission to an aged care institution. All of these relationships are in the expected direction and support validity of FES.

CRITIQUE AND SUMMARY

An accurate measure of self-efficacy to avoid falls, with good predictive validity, used as one element of an assessment and intervention program, could have enormous impact, simply because falls in the elderly are so common and costly. FES may identify persons likely to become dependent on family, friends, or agencies. Preliminary findings suggest that the FES can be used to measure the impact of fear of falling on behavior and function, and in monitoring response to therapy. A program of intervention would, no doubt, assure adequate transfer and gait skills, decrease fall risks, and increase fall self-efficacy. Neither falling nor fear of falling should be considered inevitable accompaniments of aging. The FES can also be useful in research to show whether depression, anxiety trait, physical ability, and fear of falling exert an independent effect on functional decline (Tinetti & Powell, 1993; Tinetti, Richman, & Powell, 1990).

Powell and Myers (1995) found problems with a ceiling effect, particularly for higher mobility participants, perhaps because FES items are limited to relatively nonhazardous activities. Further evidence of both concurrent and predictive validity would be helpful.

REFERENCES

Buchner, D. M., Hornbrook, M. C., Kutner, N. G., Tinetti, M. E., Ory, M. G., Mulrow, C. D., Schechtman, K. B., Gerety, M. B., Fiatarone, M. A., Wolf, S. L., Rossiter, J., Artken, C., Kanten, K., Lipsitz, L. A., Sattin, R. W., DeNino, L. A., & the FICSIT Group. (1993). Development of the common data base for the FICSIT trials. *Journal of the American Geriatrics Society, 41,* 297–308.

Cumming, R. G., Salkeld, G., Thomas, M., & Szonyi, G. (2000). Prospective study of the impact of fear of falling on activities of daily living: SF-36 scores and nursing home admission. *Journals of Gerontology, 55a,* M299–M305.

Gill, D. L., Williams, K., Williams, L., & Hale, W. A. (1998). Multidimensional correlates of falls in older women. *International Journal of Aging & Human Development, 47,* 35–51.

Mendes de Leon, C. F., Seeman, T. E., Baker, D. I., Richardson, E. D., & Tinetti, M. E. (1996). Self efficacy, physical decline and change in functioning in community-living elders: A prospective study. *Journal of Gerontological Science, 51,* S183–S190.

Petrella, R. J., Payne, M., Myers, A., Overend, T., & Chesworth, B. (2000). Physical function and fear of falling after hip fracture rehabilitation in the elderly. *American Journal of Physical Medicine & Rehabilitation, 79,* 154–160.

Powell, L. E., & Myers, A. M. (1995). The Activities-Specific Balance Confidence Scale. *Journals of Gerontology: Medical Sciences, 50A,* M28–M34.

Tennstedt, S., Howland, J., Lachman, M., Peterson, E., Kasten, L., & Jetta, A. (1998). A randomized, controlled trial of a group intervention to restrict fear of falling and associated activity restriction in older adults. *Journals of Gerontology, 53B,* P384–P392.

Tinetti, M. E., Mendes de Leon, C. F., Doucette, J. T., & Baker, D. I. (1994). Fear of falling and fall-related efficacy in relationship to functioning among community-living elders. *Journals of Gerontology: Medical Sciences, 49,* M140–M147.

Tinetti, M. E., & Powell, L. (1993). Fear of falling and low self-efficacy: A cause of dependence on elderly persons [Special issue]. *Journals of Gerontology, 48,* 35–38.

Tinetti, M. E., Richman, D., & Powell, L. (1990). Falls efficacy as a measure of fear of falling. *Journals of Gerontology: Psychological Sciences, 45,* P239–P243.

Tinetti, M. E., Baker, D. I., McAvay, G., Claus, E. B., Garrett, P., Gottschalk, M., Koch, M. L., Trainor, K., & Horwitz, R. I. (1995). A multifactorial intervention to reduce the risk of falling among elderly people living in the community. *New England Journal of Medicine, 331,* 821–827.

FALLS EFFICACY (FE)

On a scale from 0 to 10 with zero meaning not confident/sure at all, 5 being fairly confident/sure, and 10 being completely confident/sure, how confident/sure are you that you can do each of the following without falling:

IF "R" PHYSICALLY UNABLE TO DO ACTIVITY CONTINUE TO PROBE FOR A RESPONSE AND ASK IF THEY WERE ABLE.

(REPEAT FOR EACH ACTIVITY) How confident/sure are you that you can (ASK ACTIVITY BELOW) without falling?

		Not confident/ sure at all				Fairly confident/sure				Completely confident/sure		REF	DK	
+	1.	Clean house (e.g., sweep or dust)	00	01	02	03	04	05	06	07	08	09	10	97	98	(8)
+	2.	Get dressed and undressed	00	01	02	03	04	05	06	07	08	09	10	97	98	(10)
+	3.	Prepare simple meals (not involving carrying hot or heavy objects)	00	01	02	03	04	05	06	07	08	09	10	97	98	(12)
+	4.	Take a bath or shower	00	01	02	03	04	05	06	07	08	09	10	97	98	(14)
+	5.	Simple shopping	00	01	02	03	04	05	06	07	08	09	10	97	98	(16)
+	6.	Get in and out of a chair	00	01	02	03	04	05	06	07	08	09	10	97	98	(18)
+	7.	Go up and down stairs	00	01	02	03	04	05	06	07	08	09	10	97	98	(20)
+	8.	Walk around the neighborhood	00	01	02	03	04	05	06	07	08	09	10	97	98	(22)
+	9.	Reach into cabinets or closets	00	01	02	03	04	05	06	07	08	09	10	97	98	(24)
+	10.	Hurry to answer the telephone	00	01	02	03	04	05	06	07	08	09	10	97	98	(26)

+Do not ask proxy and/or nursing home respondent.

Tinetti, M. E., Richman, D., & Powell, L. (1990). Falls efficacy as a measure of fear of falling. *Journals of Gerontology: Psychological Sciences, 45,* 239–243. Copyright, The Gerontological Society of America.

85. HIV Prevention Attitude Scale

**Developed by Mohammad R. Torabi
and William L. Yarber**

INSTRUMENT DESCRIPTION, ADMINISTRATION, AND SCORING GUIDELINES

For the human immunodeficiency virus (HIV) infection and the acquired immunodeficiency syndrome, prevention education is a major control measure. Needs assessments and evaluation of educational programs require appropriate instruments, both for populations and individuals. Adolescents are believed to be particularly at risk because they underestimate their risk, miscalculate their vulnerability, or feel impervious to negative outcomes. Little research is available to guide program developers regarding the content, timing, or format for risk reduction interventions targeting teenagers (St. Lawrence, Jefferson, Alleyne, & Brasfield, 1995).

The HIV Prevention Attitude Scale (HIVPAS) is based on a multidimensional concept of attitude including cognitive (belief), affective (feeling), and conative (intention to act). Beliefs express one's perceptions of concepts toward an attitudinal object; feelings are described as an expression of liking or disliking relative to an attitudinal object; and intention to act is an expression of what the individual says he or she would do in a given situation. Average time to respond to the questions is 12 minutes. Scoring guidelines may be seen at the end of each form. Minimum and maximum possible points for each form are 15 to 75, with higher scores indicating more positive attitudes toward HIV and HIV prevention (Torabi & Yarber, 1992).

PSYCHOMETRIC PROPERTIES

Items were generated from a two-way table of specifications with the three components of attitude (belief, feeling, and intention to act) as the horizontal dimension, and nature of HIV and HIV transmission and prevention as the vertical dimension. This structure and items were developed from a review of the literature. Items were reviewed by a jury of health educators, students, measurement specialists, and federal government HIV officials, for clarity and content validity, and refined. The 50-item scale was administered to a representative sample of 210 students in intact classes in a midwestern high school. The group was 18% minority. From the first administration, 30 maximally discriminating items with the highest internal consistency and that fulfilled the table of specifications were selected for alternative forms.

The revised alternative forms of 15 comparable items each were then administered to a sample of 600 students from midwestern high schools, with 95% being White. Item correlation with total scale scores ranged from .39 to .63. Alternative parallel forms are shown subsequently. The percentage distributions of the responses by alternatives for both forms were described as reasonably spread and comparable, with means and standard deviations for total and subscale scores practically the same. Average scores with this administration were about 59 points. Reliability coefficients using Cronbach's alpha and split-half methods were .78 and .76 for Form A, and .77 and .69 for Form B. Test–retest reliability for the alternative forms with a 1-week interval was .60. Factor analyses of both forms identified reasonably comparable factor structures of myths about transmission, myths about infected people, communication for prevention, and methods of prevention, supporting content validity and comparability. For Form A, mean total scores were 59 ($SD = 7.7$), and for Form B, the mean was 59.4 ($SD = 7.7$). The authors indicate that it is premature to use the factors as subscales (Torabi & Yarber, 1992).

St. Lawrence and colleagues (1994) administered the HIV Prevention Attitude Scale before and after a five-session HIV risk reduction intervention to substance dependent adolescents ($N = 19$) court referred into a residential drug treatment facility. The intervention was similar to that reported in St. Lawrence, Jefferson, Alleyne, and Brasfield (1995). No control group was available, and statistical analysis was not done. The scale showed a Cronbach's alpha of .82 for this sample, with score means and standard deviations of 55.4 and 8.6 preintervention, and 60.3 and 11.5 postintervention. Following intervention, the participants reporting sexual activity in high-risk contexts decreased as did records of sexually transmitted disease treatment. The durability of the changes is not known.

A subsequent study with 34 similarly situated adolescents (16% African-American) found behavioral skills training superior to standard education presented didactically and through interactive game formats. The behavioral skills training included skill rehearsal in correct condom use, interpersonal communication skills, problem solving, and self-management strategies. [Group leaders modeled the specific skills and their use in situations that might arise following behavior skills training (pretraining mean 55.4, posttraining mean 63.0, statistically significant change).] Cronbach's alpha was .82 for this sample (St. Lawrence et al., 1995).

More recent studies have tested HIVPAS with a broader range of populations. St. Lawrence and colleagues (1997) found the instrument sensitive to interventions based on social cognitive theory and on the theory of gender and power and sustained through six months for women in correctional institutions. Social cognitive theory interventions provided specific skills training regarding social and technical competency, and problem-solving and self-management strategies for risk reduction, using instruction, modeling, and skill rehearsal. The Cronbach's alpha for Form A of HIVPAS was .82. In a subsequent study with African American women, HIVPAS was adapted to a fourth grade reading level and had a Cronbach's alpha of .73 (St. Lawrence et al., 1998).

Peer-led education among tenth grade students showed a modest increase in HIVPAS scores in comparison with a control group (Smith, Dane, Archer, Devereaux, & Katner, 2000). Other studies focused specifically on nonhealth outcomes are not included in this review.

CRITIQUE AND SUMMARY

This scale is focused on HIV prevention attitudes among adolescents and is intended as an evaluation tool for educational approaches to HIV control. The availability of alternative forms is especially useful for pretest-posttest evaluation models. Evidence of content validity came from a jury of experts, table of specifications, and factor analysis procedures. There is also evidence of form comparability and reliability (Torabi & Yarber, 1992).

The original evidence of validity and reliability was obtained from samples of predominantly white in-school students. The two studies of substance-dependent adolescents in a residential drug treatment facility provide information about the scale's performance with a different population, although with small sample sizes. Scores for all groups were generally in the same range. No data relating scale scores to behavior or practices are available (criterion-related validity). Data regarding concurrent validity were available. No predictive validity data could be located. There is consistent evidence of the scale's sensitivity to intervention with a larger response to behavioral skills training, theoretically consistent with the kind of intervention that should create attitude change. New information about the use of this scale with minority and incarcerated populations is appropriate as these groups are disproportionately affected by AIDS and HIV infection.

REFERENCES

St. Lawrence, J. S., Eldridge, G. D., Reitman, D., Little, C. E., Shelby, M. C., & Brasfield, T. L. (1998). Factors influencing condom use among African American women: Implications for risk reduction interventions. *American Journal of Community Psychology, 26,* 7–27.

St. Lawrence, J. S., Eldridge, G. D., Shelby, M. C., Little, C. E., Brasfield, T. L., & O'Bannon, R. E. III (1997). HIV risk reduction for incarcerated women: A comparison of brief interventions based on two theoretical models. *Journal of Consulting & Clinical Psychology, 65,* 504–509.

St. Lawrence, J. S., Jefferson, K. W., Alleyne, E., & Brasfield, T. L. (1995). Comparison of education versus behavioral skills training interventions in lowering sexual HIV-risk behavior of substance-dependent adolescents. *Journal of Consulting and Clinical Psychology, 63,* 154–157.

St. Lawrence, J. S., Jefferson, K. W., Banks, P. G., Cline, T. R., Alleyne, E., & Brasfield, T. L. (1994). Cognitive-behavioral group intervention to assist substance-dependent adolescents in lowering HIV infection risk. *AIDS Education and Prevention, 6,* 425–435.

Smith, M. U., Dane, F. C., Archer, M. E., Devereaux, R. S., & Katner, H. P. (2000). Students together against negative decisions (STAND): Evaluation of a school-based sexual risk reduction intervention in the rural South. *AIDS Education and Prevention, 12,* 49–70.

Torabi, M. R., & Yarber, W. (1992). Alternate forms of HIV Prevention Attitude Scales for teenagers. *AIDS Education and Prevention, 4,* 172–182.

ALTERNATE FORMS OF HIV PREVENTION ATTITUDE SCALE

Form A

DIRECTIONS: Please read each statement carefully. *Record your immediate reaction to the statement by blackening the proper oval on the answer sheet.* There is no right or wrong answer for each statement, so mark your own response. Use the below key:

KEY:

A = strongly agree
B = agree
C = undecided
D = disagree
E = strongly disagree

Example: Doing something to prevent getting HIV is the responsibility of each person.

A   B   C   D   E

RECORD ANSWER ON COMPUTER ANSWER SHEET

1. I would feel very uncomfortable being around someone with HIV.

2. I feel that HIV is a punishment for immoral behavior.

3. If I were having sex, it would be insulting if my partner insisted we use a condom.

4. I dislike the idea of limiting sex to just one partner to avoid HIV infection.

5. I would dislike asking a possible sex partner to get the HIV antibody test.

6. It would be dangerous to permit a student with HIV to attend school.

7. It is easy to use the prevention methods that reduce one's chance of getting HIV.

8. It is important to talk to a sex partner about HIV prevention before having sex.

9. I believe that sharing IV drug needles has nothing to do with HIV.

10. HIV education in schools is a waste of time.

11. I would be supportive of persons with HIV.

12. Even if a sex partner insisted, I would not use a condom.

13. I intend to talk about HIV prevention with a partner if we were to have sex.

14. I intend not to use drugs so I can avoid HIV.

15. I will use condoms when having sex if I'm not sure if my partner has HIV.

Scoring instructions: Calculate the total points for each form using the following point values:
Form A, for items number 7, 8, 11, 13, 14, 15, strongly agree = 5 points, agree = 4, undecided = 3, disagree = 2, strongly disagree = 1, for the remaining items of Form A use strongly agree = 1, agree = 2, undecided = 3, disagree = 4, strongly disagree = 5.

From Torabi, M. R., & Yarber, W. (1992). Alternate Forms of HIV Prevention Attitude Scales for Teenagers. *AIDS Education and Prevention, 4*, 172–182. Reprinted App. A—Alternate Forms of HIV Prevention Attitude Scale Form A with permission.

ALTERNATE FORMS OF HIV PREVENTION ATTITUDE SCALE

Form B

DIRECTIONS: Please read each statement carefully. *Record your immediate reaction to the statement by blackening the proper oval on the answer sheet.* There is no right or wrong answer for each statement, so mark your own response. Use the below key:

KEY:

A = strongly agree
B = agree
C = undecided
D = disagree
E = strongly disagree

Example: Doing something to prevent getting HIV is the responsibility of each person.

A   B   C   D   E

RECORD ANSWER ON COMPUTER ANSWER SHEET

1. I am certain that I could be supportive of a friend with HIV.

2. I feel that people with HIV got what they deserve.

3. I am comfortable with the idea of using condoms for sex.

4. I would dislike the idea of limiting sex to just one partner to avoid HIV infection.

5. It would be embarrassing to get the HIV antibody test.

6. It is meant for some people to get HIV.

7. Using condoms to avoid HIV is too much trouble.

8. I believe that AIDS is a preventable disease.

9. The chance of getting HIV makes using IV drugs stupid.

10. People can influence their friends to practice safe behavior.

11. I would shake hands with a person having HIV.

12. I will avoid sex if there is a slight chance that the partner might have HIV.

13. If I were to have sex I would insist that a condom be used.

14. If I used IV drugs, I would not share the needles.

15. I intend to share HIV facts with my friends.

Scoring instructions: Calculate the total points for each form using the following point values:
For items number 1, 3, 8, 9, 10, 11, 12, 13, 14, 15, strongly agree = 5, agree = 4, undecided = 3, disagree = 2, strongly disagree = 1, for the remaining items of Form B use strongly agree = 1, agree = 2, undecided = 3, disagree = 4, strongly disagree = 5.

From Torabi, M. R., & Yarber, W. (1992). Alternate Forms of HIV Prevention Attitude Scales for Teenagers. *AIDS Education and Prevention, 4*, 172–182. Reprinted App. B—Alternate Forms of HIV Prevention Attitude Scale Form B with permission.

86. HIV Knowledge Questionnaire

Developed by Michael P. Carey, Dianne Morrison-Beedy, and Blair T. Johnson

INSTRUMENT DESCRIPTION, ADMINISTRATION, AND SCORING GUIDELINES

The HIV Knowledge Questionnaire (HIV-KQ) taps knowledge of transmission, risk reduction, prevention methods, and consequences of infection. The score is the number of correct answers. The instrument requires a sixth grade education and seven minutes to complete (Carey, Morrison-Beedy, & Johnson, 1997).

PSYCHOMETRIC PROPERTIES

Definition of the domain to be tested and content validity was derived from existing measures, experts, and focus groups of low-income women (Carey, Gordon, Morrison-Beedy, & McLean, 1997). Alpha was .91 and test–retest reliability at 1 week .83, 7 weeks .91, and 12 weeks .90. Factor analysis showed a single factor labeled "HIV Knowledge." Additional evidence of validity was found with known groups—HIV experts, well-educated college students, and community samples differed on HIV-KQ scores in the expected directions. The instrument showed sensitivity to a psychoeducational intervention in comparison with a control (Carey et al., 2000). Discriminant evidence of validity was obtained through nonsignificant relationships between HIV-KQ and unrelated measures, and convergent evidence with other measures of HIV knowledge and educational attainment (Carey, Morrison-Beedy, & Johnson, 1997).

CRITIQUE AND SUMMARY

HIV-KQ is well done psychometrically.

REFERENCES

Carey, M. P., Braaten, L. S., Maisto, S. A., Gleason, J. R., Forsyth, A. D., Durant, L. E., & Jaworski, B. C. (2000). Using information, motivational enhancement, and skills training to reduce the risk of HIV infection for low-income urban women: A second randomized clinical trial. *Health Psychology, 19,* 3–11.

Carey, M. P., Gordon, C. M., Morrison-Beedy, D., & McLean, D. A. (1997). Low-income women and HIV risk reduction: Elaborations from qualitative research. *AIDS & Behavior, 1,* 163–168.

Carey, M. P., Morrison-Beedy, D., & Johnson, B. T. (1997). The HIV-Knowledge Questionnaire: Development and evaluation of a reliable, valid and practical self-administered questionnaire. *AIDS and Behavior, 1,* 61–74.

HIV KNOWLEDGE QUESTIONNAIRE (HIV-K-Q)*

For each statement, please circle True (T), False (F), or I Don't Know (DK). If you do not know, please do not guess; instead, please circle "DK."

	True	False	Don't Know
1. HIV and AIDS are the same thing.	T	Ⓕ	DK
2. There is a cure for AIDS.	T	Ⓕ	DK
3. A person can get HIV from a toilet seat.	T	Ⓕ	DK
4. Coughing and sneezing DO NOT spread HIV.	Ⓣ	F	DK
5. HIV can be spread by mosquitoes.	T	Ⓕ	DK
6. AIDS is the cause of HIV.	T	Ⓕ	DK
7. A person can get HIV by sharing a glass of water with someone who has HIV.	T	Ⓕ	DK
8. HIV is killed by bleach.	Ⓣ	F	DK
9. It is possible to get HIV when a person gets a tattoo.	Ⓣ	F	DK
10. A pregnant woman with HIV can give the virus to her unborn baby.	Ⓣ	F	DK
11. Pulling out the penis before a man climaxes/cums keeps a woman from getting HIV during sex.	T	Ⓕ	DK
12. A woman can get HIV if she has anal sex with a man.	Ⓣ	F	DK
13. Showering, or washing one's genitals/private parts, after sex keeps a person from getting HIV.	T	Ⓕ	DK
14. Eating healthy foods can keep a person from getting HIV.	T	Ⓕ	DK
15. All pregnant women infected with HIV will have babies born with AIDS.	T	Ⓕ	DK
16. Using a latex condom or rubber can lower a person's chance of getting HIV.	Ⓣ	F	DK
17. A person with HIV can look and feel healthy.	Ⓣ	F	DK
18. People who have been infected with HIV quickly show serious signs of being infected.	T	Ⓕ	DK
19. A person can be infected with HIV for 5 years or more without getting AIDS.	Ⓣ	F	DK
20. There is a vaccine that can stop adults from getting HIV.	T	Ⓕ	DK

(continued)

	True	False	Don't Know
21. Some drugs have been made for the treatment of AIDS.	(T)	F	DK
22. Women are always tested for HIV during their pap smears.	T	(F)	DK
23. A person *cannot* get HIV by having oral sex, mouth-to-penis, with a man who has HIV.	T	(F)	DK
24. A person can get HIV even if she or he has sex with another person only one time.	(T)	F	DK
25. Using a lambskin condom or rubber is the best protection against HIV.	T	(F)	DK
26. People are likely to get HIV by deep kissing, putting their tongue in their partner's mouth, if their partner has HIV.	T	(F)	DK
27. A person can get HIV by giving blood.	T	(F)	DK
28. A woman cannot get HIV if she has sex during her period.	T	(F)	DK
29. You can usually tell if someone has HIV by looking at them.	T	(F)	DK
30. There is a female condom that can help decrease a woman's chance of getting HIV.	(T)	F	DK
31. A natural skin condom works better against HIV than does a latex condom.	T	(F)	DK
32. A person will NOT get HIV if she or he is taking antibiotics.	T	(F)	DK
33. Having sex with more than one partner can increase a person's chance of being infected with HIV.	(T)	F	DK
34. Taking a test for HIV one week after having sex will tell a person if she or he has HIV.	T	(F)	DK
35. A person can get HIV by sitting in a hot tub or a swimming pool with a person who has HIV.	T	(F)	DK
36. A person can get HIV through contact with saliva, tears, sweat, or urine.	T	(F)	DK
37. A person can get HIV from a woman's vaginal secretions/wetness from her vagina.	(T)	F	DK
38. A person can get HIV if having oral sex, mouth on vagina, with a woman.	(T)	F	DK
39. If a person tests positive for HIV, then the test site will have to tell all of his or her partners.	T	(F)	DK
40. Using Vaseline or baby oil with condoms lowers the chance of getting HIV.	T	(F)	DK

	True	False	Don't Know
41. Washing drug use equipment/"works" with cold water kills HIV.	T	(F)	DK
42. A woman can get HIV if she has vaginal sex with a man who has HIV.	(T)	F	DK
43. Athletes who share needles when using steroids can get HIV from the needles.	(T)	F	DK
44. Douching after sex will keep a woman from getting HIV.	T	(F)	DK
45. Taking vitamins keeps a person from getting HIV.	T	(F)	DK

*Keyed with answers.
Revised 5/1/96.

From: Carey, M. P., Morrison-Beedy, D., & Johnson, B. T. (1997). The HIV-Knowledge Questionnaire: Development and evaluation of a reliable, valid, and practical self-administered questionnaire. *AIDS and Behavior, 1,* 61–74. Used with permission from Plenum Publishers.

87. AIDS Knowledge Questionnaire

Developed by the Centers for Disease Control and Prevention

INSTRUMENT DESCRIPTION, ADMINISTRATION, AND SCORING GUIDELINES

Measures of AIDS-related knowledge that have good psychometric properties are needed to evaluate the impact of educational interventions, particularly among impoverished populations. Being informed about AIDS is a necessary if not sufficient precursor of risk reduction or avoidance (Leake, Nyamanthi, & Gelberg, 1997). The psychometric properties of a subset of 21 AIDS knowledge items from the questionnaire developed by the Centers for Disease Control & Prevention (CDC) National Health Interview supplement survey form the core of this instrument.

An overall knowledge score of 0–21 is formed by summing the number of correct responses to all items and for subscales 0–9. Higher scores indicate greater knowledge. The instruments are available in Spanish.

PSYCHOMETRIC PROPERTIES

Leake, Nyamanthi, and Gelberg (1997) studied women and their friends ($N = 486$) in homeless shelters and residential drug recovery programs in the skid row area of Los Angeles. They believe the scale has face validity for this population. Content validity was supported by an expert panel (Nyamanthi, Keenan, & Bayley, 1998).

Factor analysis offered good support for the construction of an overall scale composed of all items. A two-factor solution of cognitive knowledge (alpha = .80) and concern about AIDS transmission (alpha = .92) allows use of subscales to measure these separate dimensions. Internal consistency for the total scale was .89. The overall scale and two subscales had positive although low correlations with educational level, offering some support for convergent validity; variation in educational level was limited in this sample.

Scores improved markedly in the subsample reinterviewed six months after receiving AIDS education known to be effective with these populations. Although this study lacked a control group (Leake, Nyamanthi, & Gelberg, 1997), a later study of two forms of educational intervention also showed dramatic improvement in AIDS knowledge (Nyamanthi, Flaskerud, Keenan, & Leake, 1998). In a related study, Nyamanthi, Keenan, and Bailey (1998) found significantly greater AIDS knowledge among former alcohol or drug users than among current or never-user groups, supporting validity of the scale. It is likely that many of these women participated in recovery programs that incorporated AIDS prevention classes.

CRITIQUE AND SUMMARY

Study of this instrument in its revised form has largely taken place among homeless and drug abusing women, a population with tremendous needs for AIDS knowledge and other skills to decrease their vulnerability to this disease. Psychometric properties of this scale have been well studied although largely in one geographic area (Los Angeles).

An immediate retest to establish stability of the scale should be accomplished. Those studying this scale recommend that the subscales be used with poorly acculturated populations. These groups are known to exaggerate HIV transmissibility and this belief may predispose them to refrain from protective behaviors. It would be useful to assess the effects of educational interventions aimed at correcting these misbeliefs (Leake, Nyamanthi, & Gelberg, 1997).

REFERENCES

Leake, B., Nyamanthi, A., & Gelberg, L. (1997). Reliability, validity and composition of a subset of the Centers for Disease Control and Prevention acquired immunodeficiency syndrome knowledge questionnaire in a sample of homeless and impoverished adults. *Medical Care, 35,* 747–755.

Nyamanthi, A., Flaskerud, J., Keenan, C., & Leake, B. (1998). Effectiveness of a specialized versus traditional AIDS education program attended by homeless and drug-addicted women alone or with supportive persons. *AIDS Education and Prevention, 10,* 433–446.

Nyamanthi, A., Keenan, C., & Bayley, L. (1998). Differences in personal, cognitive, psychological, and social factors associated with drug and alcohol use and nonuse by homeless women. *Research in Nursing and Health, 21,* 525–532.

AIDS KNOWLEDGE QUESTIONNAIRE

Items	Definitely True	Probably True	Probably False	Definitely False	Don't Know
1. AIDS can reduce the body's natural protection against disease. (K)					
2. AIDS can damage the brain. (K)					
3. AIDS is caused by an infectious virus. (K)					
4. Teenagers cannot get AIDS.					
5. A person can be infected with the AIDS virus and not have the disease AIDS. (K)					
6. Looking at a person is enough to tell if he or she has AIDS.					
7. A person who has the AIDS virus can look and feel well. (K)					
8. A pregnant woman who has the AIDS virus can give the virus to her baby. (K)					
9. There is a vaccine available to the public that protects a person from getting the AIDS virus.					
10. There is no cure for AIDS at present. (K)					

A person can get AIDS or the AIDS virus infection from:

11. Living near a home or hospital for AIDS patients. (T)					
12. Working near someone with the AIDS virus. (T)					

Items	Definitely True	Probably True	Probably False	Definitely False	Don't Know
13. Eating in a restaurant where the cook has the AIDS virus. (T)					
14. Shaking hands, touching, or kissing on the cheek someone who has the AIDS virus. (T)					
15. Sharing plates, forks, or glasses with someone who has the AIDS virus. (T)					
16. Using public toilets. (T)					
17. Sharing needles for drug use with someone who has the AIDS virus. (K)					
18. Being near someone who coughs or sneezes and has the AIDS virus. (T)					
19. Attending school with a child who has the AIDS virus. (T)					
20. From mosquitos or other insects. (T)					
21. Having sex with a person who has the AIDS virus. (K)					

K = Knowledge subscale; T = Transmission subscale.

From Leake, B., Nyamanthi, A., & Gelberg, L. (1997). Reliability, validity, and composition of a subset of the Centers for Disease Control and Prevention Acquired Immunodeficiency Syndrome Knowledge Questionnaire in a sample of homeless and impoverished adults. *Medical Care, 35,* 747–755. Used with permission.

88. Levels of Institutionalization Scales for Health Promotion Programs: A Measure of How Well-Established a Health Promotion Program Is in an Institution

Developed by Robert M. Goodman, Kenneth R. McLeroy, Allan B. Steckler, and Rick H. Hoyle

INSTRUMENT DESCRIPTION, ADMINISTRATION, AND SCORING GUIDELINES

In optimum circumstances, innovations such as health promotion programs are conceived, born, and nurtured within host organizations, then mature, produce desired outcomes, and live for a long and productive period. They settle into their host organizations through mutual adaptation. An innovation need not be novel but merely new to the innovating organization.

Adoption and implementation of innovative programs have been much better studied than has institutionalization (the attainment of longevity); therefore, we are left without guidelines for positioning meritorious programs for survival so that their benefits will be available to clients. Different tasks distinguish these phases. Implementation focuses on immediate programmatic needs such as client recruitment; institutionalization is more politically oriented, such as seeking permanent funding (Goodman & Steckler, 1989). Patient education programs are examples of innovations that must progress through institutionalization. The reasons that some of them fail to thrive have been neither well documented nor understood (Goodman & Steckler, 1989).

A model for the institutionalization of health promotion programs was developed from theory and a study of multiple programs in schools in Virginia. Institutionalization involves passages in procedure or structure, such as transition from outside to local funding, standardization of program job descriptions, and the number of budget cycles survived. A program achieving four or fewer passages and cycles was rated as low for institutionalization, 5 to 8 as low to moderate, 9 to 12 as moderate to high, and more than 12 as a highly institutionalized program (Goodman & Steckler, 1989).

Passages and cycles occurred within the context of six factors associated with program institutionalization: (a) standard operating routines, such as regular reports to supervisors about the program that provided them with enough information to assess the program's costs and benefits; (b) critical precursor conditions, such as awareness of and concern for a problem, receptivity to change, availability of solutions, and adequacy of program resources; (c) mutual adaptation of actors' aspirations so that if the program supported their

Dimensions Subsystems	Passages	Degrees Routines	Niche Saturation
Production			
Maintenance			
Supportive			
Managerial			

FIGURE 88.1 Level of institutionalization matrix.

From Goodman, R. M., McLeroy, K. R., Steckler, A. B., & Hoyle, R. H. (1993). Development of Levels of Institutionalization Scales for Health Promotion Programs. *Health Education Quarterly, 20,* 161–178.

aspirations they became advocates for it; (d) development of a coalition of program advocates whose aspirations are being supported by the program and the presence of a broker positioned at the middle to upper levels of the organization with good intuitive and negotiating skills who brings the coalition together; (e) mutual adaptation of program and organizational norms; and (f) fit with the host organization's mission and core operations (Goodman & Steckler, 1989).

Such a model suggests interventions to facilitate institutionalization as well as what should be measured to determine if institutionalization has occurred.

The Levels of Institutionalization Scales for Health Promotion Programs (LoIn) were developed in a second study of dissemination of health promotion programs in junior high schools in North Carolina. Building on the exploratory model described earlier, LoIn measures the degree to which an innovation is integrated into four subsystems of an organization (production, managerial, maintenance, and supportive) through three stages (passages, routines, and niche saturation). A passage might be the first time an innovation is actually implemented; routines might be included in the annual budget, surviving turnover of staff; niche saturation is defined as the maximum feasible expansion of an innovation within an organization. Figure 88.1 depicts this model. One might say that the more cells that a particular health program occupies, the more embedded into these subsystems and the more institutionalized the program becomes. Scoring guidelines accompany the instrument; no total scores in published sources could be located (Steckler, Goodman, McLeroy, Davis, & Koch, 1992).

PSYCHOMETRIC PROPERTIES

The LoIn was developed from a theoretical base in which relationships between the concepts are specified, important for construct validity. As a result of review by five experts in fields of organizational theory, health care administration, and health education research, the original 32-item instrument was revised to include 15 three-part items. A study of 322 health promotion programs provided data for a confirmatory factor analysis. It supported the hypothesis of an eight-factor model: four factors concern how routinized the program was in each subsystem (more highly correlated with program longevity), and four factors concern the degree of program niche saturation within each subsystem (more highly correlated with managers' perceptions of program permanence). Because the factor analysis did not control for age of programs, further testing is needed to assure that the scale is applicable regardless of the age of a program. Details of the factor analysis may be found in Goodman, McLeroy, Steckler, and Hoyle (1993). Subscale alpha coefficients ranged from .44 to .86. Neither estimates of predictive validity nor of sensitivity to change could be located.

LoIn scales were used by Barab, Redman, and Froman (1998) in a study of institutionalization of diabetes education programs in hospitals and home health agencies. Reliability estimates for routines (alpha = .61) and for niche saturation (alpha = .44) were substandard. Average correlation among the four subsystems for routines was .67 and for niche saturation .38, indicating moderate to large amounts of shared variance among subsystems and challenging claims of discriminant validity. Criterion-related validity was found between length of program existence and the routine factor. Factor analysis lent credence to a two-factor model and raises questions about the efficacy of treating the eight subscales as separate.

CRITIQUE AND SUMMARY

It is first important to affirm that not all programs deserve to be institutionalized. They may not have been successful in reaching their goals, or there may be little demand for them. For those that are serving their clients well, however, it is important to be able to measure the likelihood that they will be sustained and to take action to protect them. LoIn may eventually be helpful in this regard.

The LoIn helps administrators retain the perspective that program institutionalization is largely a political endeavor that entails trade-offs and compromises among key members of the organization in which a program operates. LoIn is based both on organizational theory and empirical research of health promotion programs in organizations. It offers insights both for staff trying to institutionalize a program as well as for funders seeking innovative programs in which their investment will last. The LoIn has recently been used in a study of diabetes education programs (Redman & Barab, 1997).

Penha-Walton and Pichert (1993) compare diabetes foot care educational programs in two Veterans Administration medical centers, using the conceptual framework from the LoIn. Although no formal hypothesis testing was carried out, the primary differences between the program that survived and the one that did not were (a) replacement of the champion who had left, and (b) use of institutional funds for start-up as opposed to use of grant funds (the program ceased when the grant funds ran out). This and others studies suggest that important elements to identify or develop in a patient education program include presence of a well-placed program champion, placing the program in an institution with strong subsystems to provide program support, fitting the program to the host institution's mission, and establishing appropriate periods to sustain the program through institutionalization. The usual three years of funding for a start-up program is insufficient to reach this goal (Steckler & Goodman, 1989).

The relationship between LoIn score and program survival in an institution is still unclear. Perhaps the present usefulness of this tool is more as a checklist for those trying to institutionalize meritorious programs or not institutionalize poor ones. Yet, although LoIn is in the early stages of development, no other tools measuring this construct for health programs could be located.

Scheier (1993) points out that the items in each factor do not always seem to match the factor's conceptual definition raising issues of content validity, questions of whether the eight scales are measuring independent dimensions of institutionalization (discriminant validity), or questions of whether another respondent from the same agency would respond similarly (interrater reliability). She believes that the scales may not yet be ready for widespread use in research projects not focused on measurement development or by practitioners as diagnostic indicators of their organization's progress toward institutionalization of a program. The LoIn authors disagree. Barab, Redman, and Froman's investigation (1998) of psychometric characteristics of the LoIn in studying diabetes education programs showed that there is more work to be done on the scale.

REFERENCES

Barab, S. A., Redman, B. K., & Froman, R. D. (1998). Measurement characteristics of the Levels of Institutionalization Scales: Examining reliability and validity. *Journal of Nursing Measurement, 6,* 19–33.

Goodman, R. M., McLeroy, K. R., Steckler, A. B., & Hoyle, R. H. (1993). Development of level of institutionalization scales for health promotion programs. *Health Education Quarterly, 20,* 161–178.

Goodman, R. M., & Steckler, A. (1989). A model for the institutionalization of health promotion programs. *Family and Community Health, 11*(4), 63–78.

Penha-Walton, M. L. I., & Pichert, J. W. (1993). Institutionalizing patient education programs. *Journal of Nursing Administration, 23*(6), 36–41.

Redman, B. K., & Barab, S. (1997). Diabetes education infrastructure and capacity in hospitals and home health agencies in Maryland and Pennsylvania. *Diabetes Educator, 23*(4), 1–13.

Scheirer, M. A. (1993). Are the Level of Institutionalization Scales ready for "prime time"? A commentary on "Development of Level of Institutionalization (LoIn) Scales for Health Promotion Programs." *Health Education Quarterly, 28,* 179–182.

Steckler, A., & Goodman, R. M. (1989). How to institutionalize health promotion programs. *American Journal of Health Promotion, 3*(4), 34–44.

Steckler, A., Goodman, R. M., McLeroy, K. R., Davis, S., & Koch, G. (1992). Measuring the diffusion of innovative health promotion programs. *American Journal of Health Promotion, 6,* 214–225.

LEVELS OF INSTITUTIONALIZATION (LoIn) SCALES
FOR HEALTH PROMOTION PROGRAMS
PRODUCTION SUBSYSTEM

1a.   Have the program's goals and/or objectives been put into writing?

    (1) ___ Yes   (2) ___ No   (3) ___ Not sure/not applicable
       ↓   ↓

1b.   If yes, for how   Go to Question 2
      many years have
      written goals and
      objectives actual-
      ly been followed?

       ___ Year(s)
        ↓   ↓

1c.   Of all the aspects of this program that could have written goals and objectives, what is your best estimate of the proportion which actually have written goals and objectives?

No aspects of this program have written goals and objectives.	Few aspects of this program have written goals and objectives.	Most aspects of this program have written goals and objectives.	All aspects of this program have written goals and objectives.
1	2	3	4

2a.   Have any of the plans or procedures used for implementing this program been put in writing?

    (1) ___ Yes   (2) ___ No   (3) ___ Not sure/not applicable
       ↓   ↓

2b.   If yes, for how   Go to Question 3
      many years have
      such written plans
      or procedures actu-
      ally been fol-
      lowed?

       ___ Year(s)
        ↓   ↓

2c.   Of all the aspects of this program that could have written plans or procedures, what is your best estimate of the proportion which actually have written plans or procedures?

No aspects of the program have written plans or procedures.	Few aspects of the program have written plans or procedures.	Most aspects of the program have written plans or procedures.	All aspects of the program have written plans or procedures.
1	2	3	4

3a. Has a schedule (e.g., timetable, plan of action) used for implementing program activities been put in writing?

(1) ＿＿ Yes   (2) ＿＿ No   (3) ＿＿ Not sure/not applicable

↓   ↓

3b. If yes, for how many years have such written schedules actually been followed?   Go to Question 4

＿＿＿ Year(s)

↓   ↓

3c. Of all the aspects of this program that could have written schedules, what is your best estimate of the proportion which actually have written schedules?

No aspects of this program have written schedules.	Few aspects of this program have written schedules.	Most aspects of this program have written schedules.	All aspects of this program have written schedules.
1	2	3	4

4a. Have the strategies for implementing this program been adapted to fit local circumstances?

(1) ＿＿ Yes   (2) ＿＿ No   (3) ＿＿ Not sure/not applicable

↓   ↓

4b. If yes, for how many years have locally adapted strategies actually been followed?   Go to Question 5

＿＿＿ Year(s)

↓   ↓

4c. Of all the aspects of this program that could be adapted to fit local circumstances, what is your best estimate of the proportion which have actually been adapted?

No aspects of this program have been adapted.	Few aspects of this program have been adapted.	Most aspects of this program have been adapted.	All aspects of this program have been adapted.
1	2	3	4

5a. Has a formal evaluation of the program been conducted?

(1) ＿＿ Yes   (2) ＿＿ No   (3) ＿＿ Not sure/not applicable

↓   ↓

Go to Question 6

(continued)

5b. If yes, for how
     many times has
     the program been
     formally
     evaluated?

         _____ Year(s)
              ↓   ↓

5c. Of all the aspects of this program that could be formally evaluated, what is your
     best estimate of the proportion which have been formally evaluated?

No aspects of this	Few aspects of	Most aspects of	All aspects of this
program have	this program have	this program have	program have
been evaluated.	been evaluated.	been evaluated.	been evaluated.
1	2	3	4

MANAGERIAL SUBSYSTEM

6a. Has a supervisor (e.g., section chief, department head) been formally assigned to
     oversee this program?

         (1) ___ Yes   (2) ___ No   (3) ___ Not sure/not applicable
              ↓   ↓

6b. If yes, for how   Go to Question 7
     many years has
     such a supervisor
     actually been for-
     mally assigned to
     oversee the pro-
     gram?

         _____ Year(s)
              ↓   ↓

6c. Of all the aspects of this program that could receive supervision, what is your best
     estimate of the proportion which actually receives such supervision?

No aspects of this	Few aspects of	Most aspects of	All aspects of this
program receive	this program re-	this program re-	program receive
supervision.	ceive supervision.	ceive supervision.	supervision.
1	2	3	4

7a. Have formalized job descriptions been written for staff involved with this program?

         (1) ___ Yes   (2) ___ No   (3) ___ Not sure/not applicable
              ↓   ↓
                                                        Go to Question 8

7b. If yes, for how
many years have
formalized job de-
scriptions actually
been followed?

    _____ Year(s)

      ↓   ↓

7c. What is your best estimate of the number of staff involved with this program who
have written job descriptions?

None of the staff involved with this program have written job descriptions.	Few of the staff involved with this program have written job descriptions.	Most of the staff involved with this program have written job descriptions.	All of the staff involved with this program have written job descriptions.
1	2	3	4

8a. Are *evaluation reports* of this program done on a schedule similar to evaluation reports for most other programs in your organization?

    (1) ____ Yes   (2) ____ No   (3) ____ Not sure/not applicable

      ↓   ↓

8b. If yes, for how
many years have
evaluation reports
actually been pro-
duced on a sched-
ule similar to such
reports for most
other programs in
your organization?

                                        Go to Question 9

    _____ Year(s)

      ↓   ↓

8c. What is your best estimate of the extent that evaluation reports for this program are
produced on a schedule similar to evaluation reports for most other programs in
your organization?

No evaluation reports are produced on a similar sched-ule.	Few evaluation reports are produced on a similar sched-ule.	Most evaluation reports are produced on a similar sched-ule.	All evaluation reports are produced on a similar sched-ule.
1	2	3	4

(continued)

MAINTENANCE SUBSYSTEM

9a.   Have any permanent staff been assigned to implement this program?

        (1) ____ Yes   (2)____ No   (3) ____ Not sure/not applicable

           ↓   ↓

9b.   If yes, for how   Go to Question 10
      many years have
      permanent staff
      been assigned to
      implement the pro-
      gram?

        ____ Year(s)

          ↓   ↓

9c.   What is your best estimate of the number of staff who implement the program that
     are in permanent positions?

No staff involved are in permanent positions.	Few staff involved are in permanent positions.	Most staff involved are in permanent positions.	All staff involved are in permanent positions.
1	2	3	4

10a. Has an *administrative-level* individual within your organization been actively in-
     volved in advocating for this program's continuation?

        (1) ____ Yes   (2) ____ No   (3) ____ Not sure/not applicable

           ↓   ↓

10b. If yes, for how   Go to Question 11
      many has this *ad-*
      ministrative-level
      individual active-
      ly advocated for
      this program's con-
      tinuation?

        ____ Year(s)

          ↓   ↓

10c. What is your best estimate of how active this administrative-level individual has
     been in advocating for the program's continuation?

Not active at all	Minimally active	Moderately active	Very active
1	2	3	4

11a. Do staff in your organization, other than those actually implementing the program,
     actively contribute to the program's operations?

        (1) ____ Yes   (2) ____ No   (3) ____ Not sure/not applicable

          ↓   ↓

                                       Go to Question 12

11b. If yes, for how
many years have
such staff in your
organization ac-
tively contributed
to the program's
operation?

_____ Year(s)

↓   ↓

11c. Of all the staff in your organization who could contribute to the operation of this
program, what is your best estimate of the proportion that actually contribute to it?

None of the staff contribute to the program's operation.	Few of the staff contribute to the program's operation.	Most of the staff contribute to the program's operation.	All of the staff contribute to the program's operation.
1	2	3	4

SUPPORTIVE SUBSYSTEM

12a. Has the program made a transition from trial or pilot status to permanent status in
your organization?

(1) ___ Yes   (2) ___ No   (3) ___ Not sure/not applicable

↓   ↓

12b. If yes, for how   Go to Question 13
many years has
this program had
permanent status?

_____ Year(s)

↓   ↓

12c. What is your best estimate of how permanent this program is in your organization?

Not permanent at all	Minimally perma-nent	Moderately perma-nent	Very permanent
1	2	3	4

13a. Has the program been assigned permanent physical space within your organization?

(1) ___ Yes   (2) ___ No   (3) ___ Not sure/not applicable

↓   ↓

Go to Question 14

(continued)

13b. If yes, for how
      many years has it
      maintained such
      permanent space?

            _____ Year(s)
                ↓   ↓

13c. Of all the permanent space that this program needs, what is your best estimate of
      the proportion of permanent space it currently occupies?

This program does *not* occupy any permanent space.	This program occupies only a *small* amount of the permanent space that it needs.	This program occupies *most* of the permanent space that it needs.	This program occupies *all* of the permanent space that it needs.
1	2	3	4

14a. Is this program's source of funding similar to the funding sources for other estab-
      lished programs within your organization?

            (1) _____ Yes   (2) _____ No   (3) _____ Not sure/not applicable
                ↓   ↓

14b. If yes, for how   Go to Question 15
      many years has
      this program's
      funding sources
      been similar to
      those for other es-
      tablished pro-
      grams within your
      organization?

            _____ Year(s)
                ↓   ↓

14c. In your best estimate, how permanent is the program's source of funding?

Not permanent at all	Minimally perma-nent	Moderately perma-nent	Very permanent
1	2	3	4

15a. Is the staff most closely associated with this program's implementation hired from a
      stable funding source?

            (1) _____ Yes   (2) _____ No   (3) _____ Not sure/not applicable
                ↓

15b. If yes, for how
      many years has
      the staff most
      closely associated
      with this pro-
      gram's implemen-
      tation been hired
      from a stable fund-
      ing source?

        _____ Year(s)

          ↓   ↓

15c. What is your best estimate of how permanent the funding is for the staff most close-
      ly associated with this program's implementation?

Not permanent at all	Minimally permanent	Moderately permanent	Very permanent
1	2	3	4

From Goodman, R. M., McLeroy, K. R., Steckler, A., Hoyle, R. H. (1993). Development of Institutionalization (LoIn) Scales for Health Promotion Programs: Health Education Quarterly, RO(2), 161–178. Reprinted by permission of Sage Publications, Inc.

Definitions for Organizational Subsystems
and Degrees of Program Penetration

*Subsystems**

Production:	Concerned with "throughput," or those activities which are product directed.
Managerial:	Concerned with coordinating the operations of the other subsystems.
Maintenance:	Concerned with personnel issues and continuity of production in areas such as recruitment, indoctrination or socialization, rewarding, sanctioning and procurement of resources.
Supportive:	Concerned with hospitable environmental conditions by establishing legitimacy and favorable organizational relationships.

Degrees

Passages:	The first degree of program institutionalization which is signified by one-time sentinel events such as the formalization of program plans, the shift from soft to hard sources of funding, and the program's inclusion on the organizational chart.
Routines:	The second degree of program institutionalization which is signified by the habituation, or routinization of program passages, such as the continued inclusion of the program in the organization's formal plans, annual renewal of stable funding, and continued inclusion of the program in new versions of the organizational chart.
Niche saturation:	The third degree of program institutionalization which is signified by the maximum feasible expansion of the program within the host organization's subsystems, such as the optimum realization of the programs plans, the achievement of optimum levels of funding, and the inclusion of the program in a core (versus peripheral) location on the organizational chart.

---

*The definitions for the subsystems are adapted from Katz and Kahn (1978).

+The definitions for the degrees are adapted from Yin (1979).

Scoring the LoIn Scale

The grid on the next page can be used to score the LoIn Scale in conjunction with the following directions:

Each question has three sub-questions (a, b, and c). Sub-questions "a" and "b" are scored together, resulting in one score for the two sub-items, and sub-question "c" forms is scored separately.

For all "a" and "b" sub-questions, score as follows:

- if you checked "No" or "Not sure/not applicable" for "a," then the score for the sub-item = 0;
- if you checked "Yes" for "a" *and* wrote "0" or "1" for "b," then the score for the sub-item = 1;
- if you checked "Yes" for "a" *and* wrote "2" or "3" for "b," then the score for the sub-item = 2;
- if you checked "Yes" for "a" *and* wrote "4" or "5" for "b," then the score for the sub-item = 3;
- if you checked "Yes" for "a" *and* wrote "6" or more for "b," then the score for the sub-item = 4

For all "c" sub-questions, score them as the number that you circled for that item (e.g., if you circled a "2" then the score for that item = 2).

Each three-part item represents one of the following organizational sub-systems: production (items 1–5), managerial (items 6–8), maintenance (items 9–11), supportive (items 12–15). Using the grid on the next page, add the scores for all sub-items "a" and "b" as indicated and divide by the number listed on the grid. Follow the same procedure for all "c" sub-items.

For sub-items "a" and "b":

- if the mean score is "1" or less then institutionalization is low;
- if the mean score is greater than "1" but less than or equal to "3" then institutionalization is low to moderate;
- if the mean score is greater than "3" but less than or equal to "5" then institutionalization is moderate to high;
- if the mean score is greater than "5" then institutionalization is high.

For sub-items "c":

- if the mean score is less than or equal to "2" then institutionalization is low;
- if the mean score is greater than "2" but less than or equal to "3" then institutionalization is moderate;
- if the mean score is greater than "3" then institutionalization is high.

*In which subsystems did you score **low**? What can you do to increase the institutionalization score for that subsystem?*

SCORE SHEET FOR PROGRAM INSTITUTIONALIZATION ITEMS "A" AND "B"

Subsystem	Item	Item Score	Mean Score		
PRODUCTION	1 "a" and "b"				
	2 "a" and "b"				
	3 "a" and "b"				
	4 "a" and "b"				
	5 "a" and "b"				
		Item sum =	Item sum/5 =		
MANAGERIAL	6 "a" and "b"				
	7 "a" and "b"				
	8 "a" and "b"				
		Item sum =	Item sum/3 =		
MAINTENANCE	9 "a" and "b"				
	10 "a" and "b"				
	11 "a" and "b"				
		Item sum =	Item sum/3 =		
SUPPORT	12 "a" and "b"				
	13 "a" and "b"				
	14 "a" and "b"				
	15 "a" and "b"				
		Item sum =	Item sum/4 =		

SCORE SHEET FOR PROGRAM INSTITUTIONALIZATION
ITEM "C"

Subsystem	Item	Item Score	Mean Score		
PRODUCTION	1c				
	2c				
	3c				
	4c				
	5c				
		Item sum =	Item sum/5 =		
MANAGERIAL	6c				
	7c				
	8c				
		Item sum =	Item sum/3 =		
MAINTENANCE	9c				
	10c				
	11c				
		Item sum =	Item sum/3 =		
SUPPORT	12c				
	13c				
	14c				
	15c				
		Item sum =	Item sum/4 =		

Appendix: Summary of Tools

Author (language)	What is measured	Time to complete	Readability grade	Scoring guide	Validity Content	Construct	Sensitive to intervention	Reliability Int. consist.,	Other[a]
Ailinger	K	5 min	6	Y	Y			.84	
Ali	SE			Y		Y	Y	.87	
Allen	K		5–6	Y	Y	Y	Y	.56–.75	
Anderson	A		10	Y		Y		.63 –.71	
Anderson (Diabetes) Empowerment Scale	SE					Y	Y	.96	.79
Anderson (Karen)	SE			Y	Y	Y		.87–.9	
Ascher-Svanum	K			Y	Y	Y	Y	.85–.89	.83
Austin	A/C			Y	Y	Y		.8	
Austin (Parent, Child)	A				Y	Y		.71–.94	
Barlow	SE			Y	Y	Y		.89–.96	
Barnason	S			Y	Y	Y		.96	
Barry	K			Y	Y	Y	Y	.68	
Bartholomew	SE		6	Y	Y	Y	Y	.88–.94	
Bennett	A			Y	Y	Y		.68 –.91	
Berkenstadt	A			Y	Y	Y	Y		
Bernier	L			Y	Y	Y		.86	

Author (language)	What is measured	Time to complete	Readability grade	Scoring guide	Content	Construct	Sensitive to intervention	Int. consist.,	Other[a]
Brody	SE			Y		Y	Y	.60–.74	.59–.89
Bursch	SE, A				Y	Y		.75–.87	
Callahan	A			Y		Y	Y	.68	.69–.79
Carey	K	7 min	6	Y	Y	Y	Y	.91	.83–.91
Carey (Diabetes)	A	< 5 min		Y	Y	Y		.73	.85
CDC	K			Y	Y	Y	Y	.89	
Dancey	K			Y	Y	Y		.84	.73
DePaola	A		4,7	Y	Y	Y		.72–.85	.8, .87
Eaden	K		4.4	Y	Y	Y		.95	
Evans	K			Y	Y	Y	Y		.78
Ferrell	K			Y	Y	Y	Y	.81	.92
Fife	A			Y	Y	Y		.81	
Fitzgerald	K	15 min	6	Y	Y	Y		mid .70s	
Froman	SE			Y	Y	Y		.98	
Galloway	K	20 min		Y	Y	Y		.93	
Galloway/Bubela	L	20 min		Y	Y	Y		.95–.97	
Gattuso	SE			Y	Y	Y	Y	.90, .92	
Gerard	L	30 min		Y	Y			.91–.95	
Gibson (Sp)	A	10 min		Y	Y	Y		.82	.83, .84
Goel	K	few min	8	Y	Y		Y	.74	.76
Gonzalez-Calvo (Sp)	SE			Y		Y	Y	.70–.80	
Goodman	L			Y		Y	Y	.44–.86	
Gross	SE	5 min		Y	Y	Y	Y	.95	.87

(continued)

Author (language)	What is measured	Time to complete	Readability grade	Scoring guide	Validity Content	Construct	Sensitive to intervention	Reliability Int. consist.,	Other[a]
Gupchup	O			Y	Y	Y		.86	
Hampson	A			Y		Y		.68, .66	.67, .70
Hargreaves	A			Y		Y		.9	
Harris	SM	15–20 min		Y	Y	Y		.76	.67[a]
Hill	K			Y	Y		Y	.72	.81
Hodnett (Da, Fr, He, Sp, Sw)	T	10 min		Y		Y	Y	.91–98	
Holmes-Rovner	S		8			Y	Y	.86	
Kim	A	20 min	6	Y		Y		.71–82	.52–84
	SE			Y		Y		.94	
	K			Y		Y		.69	
Kolbe	K			Y	Y	Y			.8
Kristjanson	O			Y	Y	Y		.83–95	.82–91
Levin	A			Y		Y		.63	
Levin (Jennifer)	SE			Y		Y		.82–92	.68–88
Levinson (Fr, Nw)	SE	10 min		Y	Y	Y	Y	.73	
Lindsay	O					Y		.89–95	
Lineker	K			Y	Y			.76	.91
Lorig (Du, Sp, Sw)	SE			Y	Y	Y	Y	.76–92	.81–91
Lowe	SE		7–8	Y	Y	Y		.86–95	.46–76

462

Author (language)	What is measured	Time to complete	Readability grade	Scoring guide	Validity Content	Validity Construct	Sensitive to intervention	Reliability Int. consist.,	Reliability Other[a]
Lubrano/Veale	K		Easier than standard writing	Y	Y			.85	.77
Maeland	K			Y	Y	Y	Y	.48–.78	
Maly	SE			Y	Y	Y		.91, .83	
Medland	O			Y	Y		Y	.94–.96	
Mesters	K			Y	Y		Y	.81	
	A			Y	Y		Y	.33, .59	
	SE			Y	Y		Y	.93	
	A			Y	Y		Y	.92	
Mobley	K			Y	Y			.51	.88
Moerman	K, O	2 min				Y	Y	.68–.86	.62–.92
Mollem	A			Y		Y		.85	
Nouwen (Fr)	A, SE			Y		Y		.65–.89	
O'Connor	A	5 min	8	Y	Y	Y	Y	.78–.92	.81
Oetker-Black	SE	10–15 min		Y	Y	Y		.84–.98	
Ondrusek	K	5 min	8.2	Y	Y		Y		.76
Pande	K		Easier than standard writing	Y	Y	Y		.84	
Polonsky	L			Y	Y	Y	Y	.95	
Reece	SE	10 min		Y	Y	Y		.86–.91	

(continued)

463

Author (language)	What is measured	Time to complete	Readability grade	Scoring guide	Validity Content	Validity Construct	Sensitive to intervention	Reliability Int. consist.	Reliability Other[a]
Richards	A					Y		.71–.87	
Salmon	A			Y	Y	Y		.47–.87	
Schmaling	A			Y	Y	Y	Y	.77–.86	
Schuster	K			Y	Y			.84	
Shiloh	K	5 min	< 6	Y	Y		Y	.62	
Svarstad	O			Y		Y			
Symonds/Burton	A			Y		Y	Y	.84	
Tinetti	SE			Y	Y	Y	Y	.9	.71
Torabi	A	12 min		Y	Y	Y	Y	.77–.82	.69, .76
Wehby/Brenner	L			Y	Y			.91	
Weinman	A			Y		Y		.57–.82	.49–.84
Weinrich	K			Y			Y	.69–.77	.65
Wigal	SE			Y		Y	Y	.74 –.95	.77
Wysocki	SM		6–7	Y	Y	Y		.91	.78[a]
Zerwic	A				Y	Y			.81–.9
Zimmerman	O			Y	Y	Y			

[a]Represents interobserver reliability; all others in this column are test–retest reliability.

Note: A, attitude/belief/behavior; C, for children; K, knowledge; L, learning assessment/instructional design or delivery; He, Hebrew; S, satisfaction; SE, self-efficacy; SM, self management; O, other; T, theoretical model; Da, Danish; Du, Dutch; Fr, French; Nw, Norwegian; Sp, Spanish; Sw, Swedish; Int. Consist., internal consistency for full scale (unless all that was reported was for subscales).

464

Index

Springer Publishing Company

Assessing and Measuring Caring in Nursing and Health Science

Jean Watson, RN, PhD, HNC, FAAN, with contributors

"A magnificent job... Dr. Jean Watson and her colleagues have focused their careers on the phenomenon of caring, and this book is another one of their great contributions to the scientific community."
—From the Foreword by **Ora L. Strickland**, RN, PhD, FAAN

"This work ... is not an answer to the issue of how to capture caring in nursing practice, rather, the instruments simply serve as indicators along the way. Nevertheless, empirical indicators that move us closer to recognizing and honoring the deeply human nature of nursing's caring work warrant attention and use in clinical inquiry."
—From the Preface by **Jean Watson**

Dr. Jean Watson and colleagues have gathered all the available measurement instruments on caring in nursing in this book, along with discussion of their origins, development, and use. Nurse clinicians, educators, researchers, and managers will find this a valuable resource.

Contents:

Part I: Overview
• Caring and Nursing Science: Contemporary Discourse
• Background for Selection of Caring Instruments, *J. Watson and J. Zuk*

Part II: Summary of Each Instrument for Measuring Caring
• Caring Behavior Assessment
• Professional Caring Behavior
• Nyberg Caring Attributes Scale
• Peer Group Caring Interaction Scale & Organizational Caring Climate Questionnaire
• Methodist Health Care System Nurse Caring Instrument

Part III: Challenges and Future Directions
• The Evolution of Measuring Caring: Moving Toward Construct Validity, *C. Coates*
• Postscript—Free Thoughts on Caring Theories and Instruments for Measuring Caring, *J. Watson*
• Appendix: Master Matrix Blueprint for All Instruments for Measuring Caring

2001   336pp   0-8261-2313-9   hard

536 Broadway, New York, NY 10012-3955 • Tel: (212) 431-4370 • Fax: (212) 941-7842
Order Toll-Free: (877) 687-7476 • **Order On-Line:** *www.springerpub.com*

Springer Publishing Company

Measurement of Nursing Outcomes, 2nd Edition

Volume 1: *Measuring Nursing Performance in Practice, Education, and Research*

Carolyn Feher Waltz, PhD, RN, FAAN
and **Louise Sherman Jenkins,** PhD, RN, Editors

Volume 2: *Client Outcomes and Quality of Care*

Ora Lea Strickland, PhD, RN, FAAN, and
Colleen DiIorio, PhD, RN, FAAN, Editors

Volume 3: *Self Care and Coping*

Ora Lea Strickland, PhD, RN, FAAN, and
Colleen DiIorio, PhD, RN, FAAN, Editors

These thoroughly updated and revised new editions of the award-winning series on measurement presents nearly 80 actual, tested instruments for assessing nursing outcomes in a multitude of settings and situations. Each tool is accompanied by a descriptive essay that includes information on purpose, administration, scoring, and reliability and validity. Whether you are interested in measuring patient outcomes, evaluating patient learning, or assessing the effectiveness of teaching and learning in a nursing school, this compendium can provide the authoritative tools you need.

Volume 1   424pp   0-8261-1417-2   hard
Volume 2   304pp (est.)   0-8261-1427-X   hard
Volume 3   256pp (est.)   0-8261-1795-3   hard
3-Volume Set   0-8261-1606-X   hard

536 Broadway, New York, NY 10012-3955 • (212) 431-4370 • Fax (212) 941-7842
Order Toll-Free: (877) 687-7476 • www.springerpub.com